Home Health Nursing

Assessment and Care Planning

Home Health Nursing

Assessment and Care Planning

† Marie S. Jaffe, RN, MS
Formerly Nursing Faculty,
University of Texas at El Paso
College of Nursing and Allied Health
El Paso, Texas

Linda Skidmore-Roth, RN, MSN, NP
Formerly Nursing Faculty
New Mexico State University
Las Cruces, New Mexico

Formerly Nursing Faculty
El Paso Community College
El Paso, Texas

† Deceased

Third Edition

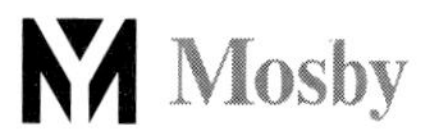

St. Louis Baltimore Boston
Carlsbad Chicago Naples New York Philadelphia Portland
London Madrid Mexico City Singapore Sydney Tokyo Toronto Wiesbaden

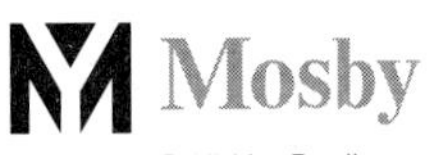

A Times Mirror Company

Publisher: Nancy L. Coon
Executive Editor: N. Darlene Como
Senior Developmental Editor: Laurie Sparks
Project Manager: John Rogers
Production Editor: Cheryl Abbott Bozzay
Designer: Yael Kats
Manufacturing Supervisor: Linda Ierardi

THIRD EDITION

Printed in the United States of America

Mosby–Year Book, Inc.
11830 Westline Industrial Drive
St. Louis, Missouri 63146

Library of Congress Cataloging in Publication Data
Jaffe, Marie S.
Home health nursing: assessment and care planning/Marie S. Jaffe, Linda Skidmore-Roth.—3rd ed.
p. cm.
Rev. ed. of: Home health nursing care plans. 2nd ed. c1993.
Includes bibliographical references and index.
ISBN 0-8151-4877-1
1. Home nursing. 2. Nursing assessment. 3. Nursing cre plans. I. Skidmore-Roth, Linda. II. Jaffee, Marie S. Home health nursing care plans. III. Title.
[DNLM: 1. Home Care Services—handbooks. 2. Nursing Assessment—handbooks. 3. Patient Care Planning—handbooks. WY 49 J23h 1996]
RT120.H65J34 1996
362. 1'4—dc20
DNLM/DLC
for Library of Congress

96-23053
CIP

96 97 98 99 / 9 8 7 6 5 4 3 2 1

Preface

This third edition of *Home Health Nursing: Assessment and Care Planning* has been developed to assist those providing home nursing services with a guide to appropriate interdisciplinary approaches for all aspects of care necessary to achieve an overall goal of optimal health and function of the homebound client. At the same time, it serves to recognize and reflect agency and insurance requirements related to providing nursing care in the home setting.

Nursing care provided in the home generally focuses on treatment of diseases and associated conditions and on client teaching for self-care, since reimbursement is generally available only for those services; however, nurses continue to be forerunners in health promotion and disease prevention. These concepts are integrated throughout the book to assist nurses to promote health while providing treatment-oriented care. Community health nurses, nursing students, and home health ancillary personnel in public and privately owned agencies, as well as clinics and newly emerging home health care divisions in hospitals, will benefit from this small, compact, easily carried reference with its comprehensive home care-specific content and nursing process format.

The most pronounced difference from the second edition is the inclusion of outcomes that are both short term and long term. Outcomes are client specific and include time frames for achievement. An outstanding feature of the revision is a completely updated assessments' section that includes geriatric considerations for all body systems. Terminology has changed to reflect new interpretive guidelines; for example, caretaker is now caregiver. The assessment and teaching functions of the nurse within each nursing diagnosis continue to be highlighted.

The conditions selected for inclusion are identified by medical diagnoses and have been chosen on the basis of their relevance to the population of clients served in the home setting. It is important to note that conditions that may be cared for in the home vary in different regions of the country.

Appropriate care planning and documentation are required by government and third-party payors to justify payment for care given in the home and the future care needs of clients. It is hoped that this third edition will better benefit those giving home care to clients and ultimately will allow them to continue to receive care in a familiar and less threatening environment.

Marie S. Jaffe
Linda Skidmore-Roth

Guidelines For Using This Book

The following outline presents an overview of the book's contents, with an explanation of each section and suggestions for use.

1. *Assessments* are guides to be used as resources for collection of data that will be incorporated into the interventions on the basis of specific problem identification in the nursing diagnosis. Offered are guides that are related to body systems, body functions, psychosocial concerns, family concerns, and environmental considerations. The guides are referred to in most care plans and are to be used as comprehensive tools by which the nurse may view the client by utilizing those items pertinent to a particular problem or condition. The guides may also be used for interventions that are not referred to if the nurse desires to do so, since a complete nursing assessment is usually required for all clients cared for in the home.
2. *Care Plans* are grouped under major body systems in alphabetical order and reflect general practice rather than specialty practice in home nursing care. The organization and content of each plan follow a logical progression and include the following:
   a. An introductory paragraph defining and describing the condition and concluding with the reason and goals for home care.
   b. Nursing diagnoses related to the illness (one to five may be developed), which are taken from the most recent available (1994) approved list of the North American Nursing Diagnosis Association (NANDA). Those that relate to an individual client may be used, and additional diagnoses may be added from the list offered in the Appendixes if needed.
   c. Related or risk factors for each nursing diagnosis follow. One or more may be given that may or may not be used, but the possibility of using other relationships based on specific client problems should not be precluded.
   d. Defining characteristics are signs and symptoms or possible observations that are related to a particular nursing diag-

nostic stem and its related factors. The nursing diagnosis, related factors, and defining characteristics provide a valuable background for each problem in the care plan.

e. Outcomes include a short-term goal and a long-term goal that are expected to be achieved to solve a specific problem area identified by the nursing diagnosis. They are offered as an aid for the nurse to develop goals with the client and include the behaviors and physical evidence that one would expect to suggest goal achievement. As with the nursing diagnosis material, the outcomes may be used as they are or supplemented by client-specific and mutually developed goals and their associated observations. Each short-term or long-term goal includes a time frame for outcomes, which, at best, is an estimate and may be longer or shorter as a client's individual condition would warrant. The time frames serve only as a guide for the nurse to determine what is realistic and workable for a client.
f. Interventions are divided into nurse and client/caregiver actions for each nursing diagnosis. This organization assists in determining who is responsible for what actions to implement the plan of care and is home care user friendly to the extent that it is meant to include any caregiver in the home. The nursing interventions are primarily oriented toward assessments, tasks, and instruction/information to be performed by the nurse; the client/caregiver interventions are listed as the actions to be performed after the nurse performs the instruction/information component of the care plan. Other interventions for the nurse or client may be added as needed. Each nursing intervention includes visit time frames for implementation, which are intended to be suggestions; they are flexible enough to accommodate changes appropriate to individual client needs and agency policy. A special effort has been made to include referral to other disciplines in the interventions, whether these are available within or outside the agency.

3. *Appendixes* contain material that may be used to supplement the care plans. They include a listing of all NANDA-approved nursing diagnoses, procedures for basic life support, universal precautions and medication administration, insurance payment guidelines, tips on documentation, guidelines for client self-

determination, a selection of common laboratory values, and a listing of selected home care resources.

A most important thought and suggestion that the authors would like to leave with the user of the care plans is to modify and/or supplement any material that has been offered to better suit the identified needs of a specific client or family/caregiver.

Contents

Assessments

Assessments

Health History and Review of Systems

IDENTIFYING INFORMATION

Name, residence, telephone, age or date of birth, sex, race, ethnicity, religion, marital status/significant person/contact person, language, education, occupation, financial/insurance, source of information, advance directive (see Appendix)

PAST HISTORY

- Statement about general health
- Other medical conditions and dates of onset or occurrence; health status in past year
- Surgeries and injuries and dates, known or suspected allergies (food, drugs, environmental allergens)
- Hospitalizations for injuries, surgery, or medical problems (condition, date, duration)
- Admittance to long-term care facility (reason, date, duration)
- Immunizations and dates
- Military history, travel and dates
- Childhood diseases and ages of occurrence
- Psychiatric illness and treatment
- Usual health care patterns and kind of practitioner used
- Use of rehabilitative and support personnel, past home care services
- Life-style patterns and personal habits in sleep, nutrition, fluid intake, urinary and bowel elimination, activity, sexual pattern, personal hygiene, others

PRESENT HISTORY

- Chief complaint or health concern (in client's words if possible)
- Onset and development of problem, where it took place, what was done

- Signs and symptoms, location, severity, duration, frequency, changes and effect on client, meaning of illness to client
- Factors that alleviate or aggravate symptoms
- Client's knowledge of disease, procedures, and planned therapy
- Client's adaptation to chronic disorder
- Laboratory and diagnostic tests and procedures performed and results
- Medications and treatments ordered since discharge
- Homebound status

FAMILY HISTORY

- Spouse, children, parents, siblings, including health status, ages, occupations, deaths and causes; pets in the home
- Roles and responsibilities of family members, relationship with family members, activities, response to stress or crisis
- Support systems within family, marital relationship
- History of abuse by family members or relatives
- Adaptation of family members to care of client in the home

PSYCHOSOCIAL HISTORY

- General appearance
- Health goals and practices
- Alcohol, caffeine, and tobacco consumption: type, amount, frequency
- Living arrangement (alone or with others and relations with them)
- Occupation and income, ability to pay for health care, insurance plan (Medicare, Medicaid, CHAMPUS, private insurance, workers' compensation)
- Education, degrees, profession if applicable
- Recreation and interests, social and other activities, hobbies, travel, retirement if applicable
- Friends, community involvement, clubs, organizations, or church activities
- Use of community agencies (Meals on Wheels, hospital or clinic, day care, transportation, home cleaning services, shopping services)
- English as a second language or no English spoken
- Review of a usual day's activities
- Emergency contact and telephone number

MEDICATIONS AND TREATMENTS

- Prescribed and over-the-counter drugs: name, type, dose, frequency, route, length of use, side effects, desired effect, conditions being treated, drug form and how administered, contraindications, and risk for toxicity
- Oxygen and other inhalation medications or treatments
- General compliance with medication regimen
- Street or recreational drug use
- Aids to ensure safe, correct self-administration of medications
- Effect of client's age on absorption and excretion
- Treatment for adverse effects

REVIEW OF SYSTEMS

- Height, weight, vital signs, and temperature

Pulmonary system

- Upper or lower respiratory disease or infections (acute or chronic)
- Dyspnea (at rest or exertional), pain in sinus, nose, throat, or chest; congestion or discharge from nose (rhinorrhea, epistaxis, snoring); hemoptysis; cough (productive or nonproductive, with sputum characteristics); hoarseness; olfactory perception; wheezing; abnormal breath sounds

Cardiovascular system

- Heart disease (chronic, acute, congenital), vascular disease (hypertension, arterial or venous circulatory disorders)
- Chest, arm, throat, or jaw pain; leg pain or claudication; paresthesias; edema; varicosities or ulcer; dyspnea (exertion, nocturnal); palpitations; orthopnea; murmur; abnormal heart sounds

Neurologic system

- Neuromuscular or neurosensory conditions; head or spinal trauma; seizure activity; vertigo or syncope; headache; tremors or spasms; paralysis; paresis; paresthesias; mentation changes (memory, orientation, level of consciousness); motor changes (gait, coordination); sensory perception changes (touch, taste, smell, vision, hearing); presbycusis; presbyopia; tinnitus; eye or ear pain or drainage; pruritus; photophobia; blurring; diplopia; floaters; use of glasses, contact lenses, hearing aid; sleep and rest pattern (rested, fatigue, muscle cramps); speech pattern (aphasia, slurred, alternate speech method)

Gastrointestinal system

- Gastrointestinal, hepatic, biliary disorders; abdominal pain; nausea; vomiting; diarrhea; constipation; indigestion; heartburn; rectal bleeding; hematemesis; flatus; belching or eructation; jaundice; dysphagia (swallowing difficulty); chewing difficulty; anorexia; changes in appetite; presence and fit of dentures; caries; oral pain, bleeding, or lesions; halitosis; changes in gustatory perception; recent weight loss or gain; food intolerances, dislikes, and habits; special diet; 24-hour dietary intake review; bowel pattern review

Endocrine system

- Glandular dysfunction (thyroid, pancreas, adrenal, pituitary), polyuria, polydypsia, changes in metabolic function, skin color and texture, hair, tolerance to heat and cold, Cushing's response to corticosteroid therapy

Hematologic system

- Anemia, type and cause; weakness; pallor; night sweats; lymph node enlargement; skin hemorrhages; bruising; petechiae; bleeding from any site; previous transfusions (blood or blood products)

Musculoskeletal system

- Bone or joint disease; fracture; pain or stiffness in joints and muscles; redness, swelling, or heat at joint sites; deformity; limited range of motion (ROM) and movement; fatigue; weakness; energy and endurance; ability to perform activities of daily living (ADL) (total, assisted), deficits and use of assistive devices; limb prosthesis; exercise or activity pattern review; rehabilitation services; reaction to disability; Katz index of ADL independence

Renal/urinary system

- Upper or lower renal tract disorders, urinary pattern review, difficulty in urination (dysuria, dribbling, urgency, frequency, oliguria, nocturia, retention, incontinence), hematuria, calculi, dialysis, urinary tract infection, presence of catheter, 24-hour fluid intake and output, dialysis

Integumentary system

- Skin color; eruptions; elasticity; turgor; texture; scarring; dryness or moisture; pruritis; alopecia; hair and nails characteristics and changes; corns; calluses; infection; pattern of daily skin, hair, nail care review

Reproductive system

- Breast and male or female genital or organ disorders, sexually transmitted diseases, infection, lesions, discharges, bleeding, pain (testicular, pelvic, dyspareunia), infertility, impotence, pattern of sexual activity and changes, menstrual information (menarche, last period, abnormal bleeding or irregularities, menopause), pregnancies (live births, abortions, complications), penile implant

Psychosocial/psychiatric/mental

- General appearance, depression, sadness, chronic anxiety or worry, dementia, delirium, mood swings, stressors, self-concept and self-esteem, delusions, combativeness, cognitive impairment (memory, attention span, orientation, judgment), intellectual function, disengagement or reclusiveness, thoughts of suicide; Mini-Mental State Exam, Short Portable Mental Status Questionnaire, Beck Depression Inventory, Yesavage Geriatric Depression Scale, OARS Social Resource Scale, Family APGAR

Pulmonary System Assessment

PAST HISTORY

Lung and airway disorders

- Chronic bronchitis (chronic obstructive pulmonary disease) [COPD]
- Asthma

- Emphysema (COPD)
- Tuberculosis (TB)
- Pneumonia
- Pleurisy, pleural effusion
- Lung, larynx malignancy
- Influenza, colds, sinusitis, pharyngitis, and frequency
- Chest surgery (tracheostomy, lobectomy, or pneumonectomy) or trauma (rib fracture, pneumothorax)

Signs and symptoms of respiratory disorders
- Dyspnea with or without exertion, breathlessness
- Coughing and sneezing: amount and frequency
- Sputum: amount, consistency, color
- Chest, throat pain
- Wheezing, prostration

Family history
- Respiratory disorders, acute and chronic
- Allergies, eczema

Allergies
- Plants
- Animals
- Foods
- Drugs
- Environmental, occupational pollutants

Immunizations
- Pneumonia
- Influenza

Activities of daily living (ADL)
- Position during sleep for optimal breathing
- Amount of exercise, tolerance, and effect on breathing
- Abilities for personal ADL self-care

Psychosocial history
- Tobacco, alcohol, and caffeine consumption: type, amount, frequency
- Anxiety and adaptation associated with acute illness or chronic pulmonary disease
- Home environment and exposure to irritants (odors, smoke,

sprays, allergens, air conditioning and heating system, humidity, ventilation)

Past treatments and diagnostic procedures

- Past or recent hospitalizations
- Desensitization therapy
- Pulmonary rehabilitation
- Medications taken for respiratory condition (oral, inhalants, injections)
- Diagnostic procedures and results

PRESENT HISTORY

- Chief complaint, including onset and length of time present

Signs and symptoms

- Respiratory rate, ease, depth, rhythm, use of accessory muscles; factors precipitating increases or other changes
- Dyspnea, orthopnea, tachypnea, bradypnea; cyanosis, pallor
- Chest, throat, sinus pain
- Fatigue, activity intolerance
- Productive or nonproductive cough and characteristics (amount, consistency, color)

Present treatment and diagnostic procedures

- Assisted ventilation
- Use of oxygen
- Medications (bronchodilators, corticosteroids, decongestants, antitussives, expectorants, antihistamines, antimicrobials, antituberculars, oxygen, others)
- Breathing treatments (nebulizer, physiotherapy, breathing exercises)
- Lung biopsy, thoracentesis, bronchoscopy, radiography, nuclear study, pulmonary function, sputum culture, measurement of arterial blood gases (ABG)

Knowledge of disease and planned home therapy

PHYSICAL EXAMINATION

Inspection

- Symmetry of chest (shape, expansion, movement, anterior-posterior diameter ratio)

- Color of lips, ears, nails, nasal and throat mucosa
- Breathing pattern using mouth, diaphragm, chest, abdomen, accessory muscles, chest expansion
- Capillary refill, clubbing of fingers
- Symmetry, discharge, patency of nares; septum for alignment; color, lesions, discharge of pharynx; presence, color, size, exudate of tonsils
- Restlessness, confusion, fatigue, diaphoresis

Palpation

- Chest wall and intercostal muscles for skin smoothness, warmth, firmness, tenderness, bulging or masses, retraction, crepitus, symmetry of movement and chest expansion
- Tracheal midline alignment
- Tactile and vocal fremitus and location of increases or decreases

Percussion

- Posterior, anterior, lateral chest wall resonance for hyperresonance, dullness, flatness, tympany (pitch, intensity, duration with bilateral comparison)

Auscultation

- Posterior, anterior, lateral chest wall for vesicular breath sounds (posterior), bronchovesicular breath sounds (upper right posterior), bronchial breath sounds (over trachea) and whether diminished or absent and location
- Breath sounds heard in areas where not expected
- Voice sounds for intensity at airways and periphery by egophony or bronchophony (clarity, muffled sounds)
- Adventitious sounds, such as crackles, rhonchi, wheezes, friction rub

ANATOMIC AND FUNCTIONAL CHANGES ASSOCIATED WITH THE AGING CLIENT

- Weaker chest muscles, affecting bronchopulmonary movement, and increased use of accessory muscles and diaphragm for breathing
- Increased stiffness of rib cage and anteroposterior chest diameter in relation to lateral diameter, which reduces chest expansion

- Reduced reflex activity, ciliary movement, and drying and atrophy of mucous membranes, affecting ability to cough and efficient bronchoelimination
- Shallow and more rapid respiratory rate, increasing with anxiety or exertion, pattern in rate and depth becoming uncoordinated with exertion or chronic respiratory disease
- Loss of lung elasticity, reduced compliance with air retained in lung bases, causing lower vital capacity, higher residual air, and affecting breathing pattern
- Changes in properties and distribution of elastin and collagen that result in a loss of lung and blood vessel elasticity and change in volume pressure of the lungs and decreased lung recoil, causing collapse of smaller bronchioles
- Progressive hyperventilation as lung elasticity is lost, causing slight hyperresonance on percussion and decreased or slightly quieter breath sounds on auscultation
- Fewer numbers of and increased size of alveoli, the loss of lung capillaries, decrease in respiratory rate, oxygen saturation, and expired carbon dioxide, which results in reduction in gas exchange
- Reduced rate of gas movement across alveolocapillary membrane, increased use of oxygen during stress, which affects perfusion and diffusion, resulting in a greater risk for impaired gas exchange

Cardiovascular System Assessment

PAST HISTORY

Cardiac and vascular disorders

- Hypertension
- Congestive heart failure (CHF)
- Coronary artery disease (CAD)
- Myocardial infarction (MI)
- Stroke
- Arterial insufficiency disorders (atherosclerosis, claudication, Buerger's disease)

- Venous insufficiency disorders (thrombophlebitis, varicose veins, leg ulcer)
- Surgery: heart (bypass, valvular, pacemaker), vascular (endarterectomy, venous ligation)

Signs and symptoms of cardiovascular disorders
- Pain in chest, arms, throat, jaw, or extremities; leg pain at rest or during activity
- Heart palpitations, dizziness, weakness
- Dyspnea, orthopnea
- Neck vein distention
- Dependent edema
- Cold, numbness, tingling of extremities
- Discoloration of extremities

Family history
- Heart or vascular condition, acute or chronic
- Hypertension, stroke
- Diabetes mellitus
- Asthma
- Obesity

Allergies
- Medications
- Foods

Activities of daily living (ADL)
- Sleeping in semi-Fowler's or high Fowler's position
- Abilities for personal self-care and/or ADL
- Exercising and effect on pulse and respirations
- Homebound status

Psychosocial history
- Tobacco, caffeine, and alcohol consumption: type, amount, frequency
- Personality traits
- Occupation and work-related stress
- Adaptation to chronic illness or condition

Past treatments and diagnostic procedures
- Past or recent hospitalizations
- Holter monitor

- Cardiac rehabilitation
- Special diet: low cholesterol and fat, low calorie, low sodium
- Medications taken for cardiac or vascular conditions (oral, sublingual)
- Diagnostic procedures and results

PRESENT HISTORY

- Chief complaint, including onset and length of time present

Signs and symptoms

- Blood pressure, pulse rate (beats/min) and regularity, apical pulse, apical-radial pulse; factors that cause changes in baselines, changes with position or posture (sitting, standing, lying)
- Onset, duration, precipitating factors if any, alleviating factors if relevant to symptoms
- Chest, arm, throat, jaw pain; aching in legs; pain, redness, and swelling in leg calf; slow healing of lesions
- Dyspnea, orthopnea, palpitations, changes in pulse regularity (slow or rapid)
- Edema, weight gain
- Changes in mentation, headache, insomnia, restlessness, fatigue
- Changes in skin color (pallor, redness, cyanosis)

Present treatments and diagnostic procedures

- Use of oxygen
- Medications (antianginals, antiarrhythmics, anticoagulants, antihypertensives, β-adrenergic blockers, calcium channel blockers, diuretics, inotropics, lipid-lowering agents, thrombolytics, vasopressors, others)
- Electrocardiogram, cardiac angiography, echocardiography, cardiac nuclear scan, cardiac enzymes, lipid panel, electrolytes, prothrombin or thromboplastin time

Knowledge of disease and planned home therapy

PHYSICAL EXAMINATION

Inspection

- Symmetry of chest, legs, and arms
- Anterior chest wall for contour or retractions
- Skin of arms, hands, legs, and feet for color and texture (pink, warm, smooth, dry); color change in extremities when dangling or elevated (return to normal in 10 seconds)

- Hair distribution on legs, arms; clubbing fingers
- Rashes, scars, ulcers and exudate, and discoloration of extremities (brownish color, eschar, irregular shape of ulcer, chronic venous stasis)
- Veins flush with skin surface or venous enlargement
- Pulsations in the aortic, pulmonary, right ventricular, apical, or left ventricular areas
- Capillary refill of nail beds of less than 3 seconds

Palpation

- Skin of extremities smooth, dry, warm to touch
- Masses, pain, or tenderness in chest or extremities
- Extremity veins smooth and full or dilated and tortuous
- Edema in legs, dependent or pitting
- Calf for tenderness, tension, redness, warmth, presence or absence of Homans' sign
- Cardiac thrills (pulsations of the heart that feel like the throat of a purring cat) or heaves
- Brachial artery of arms for rate, rhythm, amplitude, symmetry for blood pressure measurement
- Femoral, popliteal, carotid, temporal, and dorsalis pedis pulse for rate, regularity, amplitude, contour, and symmetry (60 to 90 beats/min)
- Radial pulse for rate (tachycardia, bradycardia), regularity (trigeminal, bigeminal, pulsus differens), amplitude (pulsus alternans, pulsus biferiens, bounding pulse, pulsus paradoxus)

Auscultation

- Brachial blood pressure in both arms in lying position (same or no more than 5 to 10 mm Hg variance) and in standing position (decrease of 10 to 15 mm Hg systolic and 5 mm Hg diastolic); pulse pressure calculation
- Apical pulse, point of maximum impulse (PMI) for rate, regularity, intensity
- Apical-radial pulse for rate, regularity, pulse deficit
- Carotid artery for bruits
- Chest for areas of aortic valve (right sternal border at second interspace), tricuspid (midclavicular line at left fifth intercostal), pulmonic valve (left sternal border at second interspace), second pulmonic (left sternal border at third interspace) for heart sounds (S_1 and S_2 heard in all areas) and extra heart sounds (S_3 and S_4, which should be absent)

- Heart murmurs for location, timing, duration, pitch, intensity, quality, sound distribution or pattern
- Pericardial friction rub; clicks, snaps for timing, intensity, and pitch

ANATOMIC AND FUNCTIONAL CHANGES ASSOCIATED WITH THE AGING CLIENT

- Reduced heart size as a result of cardiac chronic illness and immobility; possible heart displacement from abnormal curvature of the spine
- Thickening and sclerosing of endocardium; thickening and rigidity of valves, which causes resistance to blood flow
- Reduced work of left ventricle and blood pumped by the heart at rest that decreases cardiac output and diminishes cardiac reserve; less capable of responding to increased demands when needed
- Loss of muscle fibers in heart from increased collagen and reduced elastin, causing reduced contractility and filling capacity and stiffness and enlargement of intramuscular vessels
- Increased arterial wall changes (atherosclerosis), reducing lumen size; occlusion of coronary arteries, causing decrease in blood flow
- Decrease in ability of heart to utilize oxygen, resulting in oxygen-activity imbalance and ischemia
- Reduced transport of nutrients and oxygen and removal of waste products from tissues, resulting from decreased capillary permeability and circulation
- Loss of elasticity in arterial walls, increased lability of vasopressor control that causes a decrease in the ability of vessels to stretch or expand, affecting blood pressure
- Increases in peripheral resistance from arteriole constriction, causing an increase in blood pressure and work of the heart; systolic increases faster than diastolic, causing a wider pulse pressure; both systolic and diastolic increase up to 70 years of age
- Blood pressure increases with exercise take longer to return to baseline; reduced sensitivity to pressure changes by the baroreceptors in the aorta and carotid arteries, causing slow response to postural changes
- Reduced effectiveness of venous valves and reduced muscle tone, causing decreased return of blood to the heart and distended superficial veins associated with inactivity

- Cellular changes, fibrosis of conduction system, neurogenic effect that impairs vasomotor response of vessels causing changes in electrocardiogram (ECG); prolonged intervals of QRS complex, PR segment, and QT prolongation; possible decreased voltage of all waves

Neurologic System Assessment

PAST HISTORY

Neurologic motor and sensory disorders

- Multiple sclerosis
- Cerebrovascular accident (CVA)
- Transient ischemic attacks (TIA)
- Muscular dystrophy
- Seizure disorder
- Head or spinal cord injury
- Brain or spinal cord tumor
- Motor or sensory aberrations
- Parkinson's disease
- Auditory, visual, speech, tactile impairments
- Surgery: brain (craniotomy), spinal column (laminectomy), eye (cataract, corneal transplant)

Signs and symptoms of neurologic disorders

- Headache, dizziness
- Mentation changes, mental retardation
- Tremors, seizure activity
- Paralysis, gait disturbances
- Speech changes, aphasia
- Behavioral changes (confusion, disorientation, mood, affect)

Family history

- Neurologic disorders, acute or chronic
- Hypertension
- Stroke
- Epilepsy
- Alzheimer's disease, dementia

- Huntington's chorea
- Diabetes mellitus

Allergies

- Medications

Activities of daily living (ADL)

- Abilities for personal self-care and/or ADL
- Amount of independence or dependence
- Use of assistive aids (glasses, contact lenses, hearing aid)
- Rest/sleep/nap patterns (hours/24 hours, frequency, times, length, use and effect of prescribed or over-the-counter sleeping aids, factors that promote or prevent sleep)
- Homebound status

Psychosocial history

- Tobacco, alcohol consumption, daily and over period of years
- Occupational exposure to toxic agents that affect mental function
- Personality traits
- Adaptation to chronic illness or condition

Past treatments and diagnostic procedures

- Past or recent hospitalizations
- Cervical or pelvic traction
- Medications taken for neurologic conditions
- Diagnostic procedures and results

PRESENT HISTORY

- Chief complaint, including onset and length of time present

Signs and symptoms

- Anxiety
- Insomnia
- Headaches, back or neck pain
- Syncope, vertigo
- Fatigue, mood and communication problems
- Memory deficits, changes in level of consciousness and behavior
- Sensory problems (paresthesias, visual, auditory)

- Motor problems (balance, paralysis, rigidity, tic, coordination)
- Quadriplegia, paraplegia

Present treatments and diagnostic procedures

- Medications (sedatives, hypnotics, analgesics, anticonvulsants, antidepressants, antiglaucoma agents, antiparkinson agents, antipsychotics, central nervous system [CNS] stimulants, skeletal muscle relaxants)
- Lumbar puncture, cerebral angiography, electroencephalography, skull or spinal radiography, myography, electromyography, magnetic resonance imaging, nuclear and computerized tomographic scans, visual and auditory tests, cerebrospinal fluid analysis

Knowledge of disease and planned home therapy

PHYSICAL EXAMINATION

Inspection

- Vital signs and temperature
- General appearance (posture, personal hygiene, facial expression)
- Symmetry of muscle size, loss of muscle mass, range of motion in all joints
- Motor function (gait, coordination, balance, tremors during rest or intentional, ataxia, speech difficulty, dysphagia, muscle tone for spasticity or flaccidity, muscle strength in upper and lower extremities, involuntary muscle movements, deep reflexes)
- Sensory function (tactile, pain, proprioception, visual, auditory, discriminatory sensation, temperature)
- Mental function (level of consciousness; orientation to time, place, person and event; memory, attention span, ability to make judgments and solve problems, ability to communicate, anger, agitation, euphoria, lability, depression)

Spinal nerve innervation

- Cervical 4-8 (C4-C8): Motor function from neck downward to include ability to raise arms, flex and extend elbow, dorsiflex wrist, flex finger
- Thoracic 1-12 (T1-T12): Abduct finger, movement of thoracic and abdominal musculature

- Lumbar 1-5 (L1-L5): Flex hip, extend knee and large toe, dorsiflex ankle
- Sacral 1-5 (S1-S5): Plantar flex ankle, movement of perianal muscle

Cranial nerve innervation

1. Olfactory (sensory—smell): Odor identification
2. Optic (sensory—vision): Visual acuity, periphery and confrontation tests
3. Oculomotor (motor—pupil constriction, eyelid and extraocular movements): response to penlight, size and shape of pupil, ptosis, accommodation to finger moving toward nose
4. Trochlear (motor—eye movement inward and downward): convergence of eyes inward when finger moves toward nose
5. Trigeminal (motor—temporal, masseter muscles and lateral jaw movement; sensory-maxillary, mandibular facial and ophthalmic sensitivity): movement of jaw and mastication muscles and ability to open and close jaws; sensitivity to sharp and dull object to area with eyes closed and to cornea with application of cotton wisp
6. Abducens (motor—eye abduction): eye muscle movement for disconjugate gaze, eyes not moving together
7. Facial (motor—facial expressions; sensory—taste): face and scalp muscle movement, grimacing, closing eyes tightly, discriminating salty and sweet tastes
8. Acoustic (sensory—hearing with coclear division and balance with vestibular division): Weber's and Rinne tests for acuity; balance test
9. Glossopharyngeal (motor—pharynx; sensory—taste and pharyngeal sensation): swallowing ability and gag reflex, rise of uvula when saying "ah," taste sensation at posterior tongue, hoarseness
10. Vagus (motor—pharynx, larynx, palate; sensory—pharynx, larynx): ability to speak, phonation, swallowing, and gag reflex with cranial nerve IX
11. Accessory (motor—sternocleidomastoid and trapezius muscle movements): shoulder shrugging and turning head against resistance
12. Hypoglossal (motor—tongue): tongue protrusion, deviation, and strength

Palpation

- Symmetry, shape, masses, depression of head and muscles
- Carotid and temporal pulses, comparing strength and quality bilaterally
- Muscles for tone, shape, size, and atrophy

Skeletal muscle reflexes

- Biceps, brachioradial, triceps, patellar, Achilles tendon (ankle), Babinski's (plantar)

Auscultation

- Bruits over eyes, temples, mastoid processes

ANATOMIC AND FUNCTIONAL CHANGES ASSOCIATED WITH THE AGING CLIENT

- Reduced size and weight of brain, atrophy of convolutions, widening sulci and gyri, increased dilatation of ventricles, appearance of lesions and senile plaques
- Reduced number of neurons, which decreases transmission from brain to body areas, affecting arousal of organ or system
- Reduced dendrites in nerve, synapses, lesions on axons, which decrease peripheral nerve conduction and cause a slowing of reaction time
- Cerebral circulation changes affecting mental acuity, movement, sensory perception and interpretation, and ability to cope with multiple events
- Metabolic changes affecting synapses that cause neurotransmitter effects of brain that influence sleep, temperature control, and mood
- Reflexes slow but deep reflexes unchanged
- Electroencephalography readings are one cycle lower than for younger adults
- Sleep stages I and II last longer, stage III remains the same, and stage IV is reduced or omitted; changes in sleep stages can result in irritability, lethargy, fatigue, anxiety, tension, difficulty in falling asleep, frequently interrupted sleep with easier awakening as intensity of sleep is decreased
- Deterioration of tactile, olfactory, gustatory (reduced number of taste buds) perceptions that affect pain threshold, sensation of pressure and hot or cold, and anorexia or loss of interest in food

Gastrointestinal System Assessment

PAST HISTORY

Gastrointestinal disorders

- Peptic ulcer, gastritis
- Inflammatory bowel disease
- Enteritis, irritable bowel
- Diverticular disease
- Esophageal reflux, varices
- Hepatitis
- Cirrhosis
- Gallbladder disease
- Hernia
- Hemorrhoids, rectal disorders
- Surgery (partial or complete gastrectomy or colectomy, cholecystectomy, liver transplant, herniorrhapy, hemorrhoidectomy, oral surgery)

Signs and symptoms of gastrointestinal disorders

- Nausea, vomiting
- Diarrhea, constipation
- Dysphagia
- Indigestion, heartburn
- Anorexia
- Weight changes
- Malnutrition
- Blood in vomitus, feces
- Abdominal pain, distention
- Rectal pain, itching

Family history

- Gastrointestinal disorders, acute and chronic
- Ulcers
- Hemorrhoids
- Colorectal malignancy
- Hepatitis
- Obesity

Allergies
- Foods
- Medications

Patterns of bowel elimination and nutritional intake
- Food likes and dislikes, appetite, cultural influences, eating pattern (meal frequency and time)
- Ability to chew and swallow, dentures and fit
- Caloric intake for 24 hours, special diet of high or low calories, high fiber, bland or low residue
- Bowel elimination pattern, characteristics, amount, color, frequency, flatus
- Laxative or enema use, type and frequency

Activities of daily living (ADL)
- Abilities for self-care (feeding and toileting)
- Use of assistive aids for meals and elimination
- Homebound status

Psychosocial history
- Tobacco, alcohol, and caffeine consumption: daily and over period of years
- Personality traits
- Stress, anxiety, chronic illness and effect on elimination and nutrition
- Adaptation to chronic illness or condition

Past treatments and diagnostic procedures
- Past or recent hospitalizations
- Presence of bowel diversion (type, care, response)
- Medications taken for gastrointestinal conditions (oral, rectal)
- Diagnostic procedures and results

PRESENT HISTORY

- Chief complaint, including onset and length of time present

Signs and symptoms
- Pain and characteristics
- Anorexia, nausea, vomiting
- Heartburn, flatulence, eructation
- Constipation, diarrhea, impaction

- Weight changes
- Jaundice, pruritis
- Blood in vomitus (coffee-ground), feces (black, tarry)

Present treatments and diagnostic procedures

- Medications (antacids, antiemetics, antidiarrheals, H_2 receptor antagonists, laxatives, stool softeners, suppositories, vitamins, anticholinergics, antidiabetics, antimicrobials, lipid-lowering agents)
- Proctoscopy; gastroscopy; colonoscopy; esophagoscopy; gastric and bowel radiography; gallbladder radiography; gastrointestinal and hepatobiliary nuclear and computerized tomography scans; paracentesis; tissue biopsy; ultrasonography; gastric acid tests; motility tests; feces for culture, occult blood, ova, parasites, toxins; liver function tests; enzymes; complete blood count; electrolytes
- Enemas, bowel irrigation
- Nasogastric, gastrostomy feedings; total parenteral nutrition
- Gastric decompression, suctioning

Knowledge of disease and planned home therapy

PHYSICAL EXAMINATION

Inspection

- Weight: actual and ideal for age, size, sex, and frame; height in relation to weight
- Contour of abdomen; shape, size, and protrusion of umbilicus
- Abdominal skin smoothness, rash, scars, ascites
- Oral cavity for pain, color, texture, caries, mucositis, lesions, bleeding, odor, irritation by dentures
- Teeth number, color, surface
- Tongue color, texture, coating, lesions; hard and soft palate color, shape, movement
- Anus for pain, itching, inflammation, bleeding, drainage
- Jaundice of skin, sclera, mucous membranes
- Feces and vomitus for abnormal constituents or consistency
- Drainage from nasogastric tube or ostomy, condition of stoma

Auscultation

- Presence of bowel sounds in four quadrants, including frequency, pitch, loudness, rushing, swishing, gurgling

- Absence of bowel sounds for 5 minutes in any quadrant

Percussion

- Four quadrants for dull (bladder distention), tympanic (stomach and intestinal distention or gas), or wavelike sounds
- Liver and spleen for dullness

Palpation

- Abdominal tone, masses, pain, distention, tautness, warmth or coldness in four quadrants
- Smooth, firm palpable liver and kidneys or nonpalpable organs
- Contour, mobility, and tenderness of palpable inguinal nodes or nonpalpable
- Rectal sphincter for tightness, smooth rectal walls

ANATOMIC AND FUNCTIONAL CHANGES ASSOCIATED WITH THE AGING CLIENT

- Thinning of teeth and wearing down of grinding surfaces with erosion of roots and crowns, which affects biting and chewing; saliva pH becomes alkaline, causing tendency for tooth decay; denture fit affected as oral structures change and bone loss occurs
- Thinning and drying of oral epithelium as volume of saliva decreases; reduced salivary enzyme that affects the beginning digestion of starches; taste buds reduced in number, affecting taste and appetite
- Decreased metabolic rate with gradual weight reduction; change in fat distribution with increased body fat and decreased lean body mass and subcutaneous tissue
- Weaker abdominal and pelvic musculature, affecting defecation
- Reduced size of liver; pancreatic atrophy occurs
- Reduced stomach, hepatic, pancreatic enzymes and thinning and atrophy of tract mucosa, slowing digestion and absorption, drug metabolism and detoxification
- Decreased gag reflex, affecting swallowing, which can result in aspiration
- Reduced peristalsis and motility, affecting delayed emptying and esophageal reflux, gastrocolic reflex, and contraction of sphincter muscles, which contribute to constipation

Endocrine System Assessment

PAST HISTORY

Endocrine gland disorders

- Diabetes mellitus
- Diabetes insipidus
- Addison's disease
- Hyperthyroidism or hypothyroidism
- Hyperparathyroidism or hypoparathyroidism
- Thyroid malignancy
- Pituitary tumor
- Surgery (thyroidectomy)

Signs and symptoms of endocrine disorders

- Weight, appetite, hydration changes
- Vital sign changes, presence of dyspnea, palpitations
- Mentation, visual disturbances
- Weakness, fatigue, changes in muscle activity
- Elimination pattern changes (bowel and urinary)
- Frequent infections

Family history

- Endocrine disorders, acute or chronic
- Diabetes mellitus
- Thyroid disease
- Hypertension
- Obesity

Allergies

- Foods
- Medications
- Iodine

Activities of daily living (ADL)

- Abilities for self-care and/or ADL
- Ability to follow regimen for diabetes mellitus
- Exercise requirements
- Homebound status

Psychosocial history

- Tobacco and alcohol consumption: daily and over periods of years
- Personality traits
- Stress from occupation or chronic condition
- Cultural preferences in diet, special diet of diabetic, low calorie, low fat
- Adaptation to chronic illness

Past treatments and diagnostic procedures

- Past or recent hospitalizations
- Exposure to or treatment with radiation
- Medications taken for endocrine conditions (oral, subcutaneous)
- Diagnostic procedures and results

PRESENT HISTORY

- Chief complaint, including onset and length of time present

Signs and symptoms

- Weakness, fatigue, muscle weakness, twitching, spasms, numbness, tingling, cramping, tremors, wasting, reduced strength
- Bone pain, aching
- Polyuria, polydipsia, polyphagia
- Anorexia, nausea, vomiting
- Headache, malaise
- Nervousness, irritability, drowsiness, confusion, insomnia
- Anxiety, depression, apathy, syncope
- Pruritis, thick leathery skin, brittle nails, coarse hair
- Libido, impotence, amenorrhea

Present treatments and diagnostic procedures

- Medications (hormones, antidiabetics, antithyroid agents, β-adrenergic blocking agents, glucocorticoids)
- Radiography, nuclear scans, biopsy, complete blood count, electrolytes, glucose studies, ketones, thyroid function studies, growth hormone studies, cortisol, aldosterone, urinalysis

Knowledge of disease and planned home therapy

PHYSICAL EXAMINATION

Inspection

- Vital signs, height, and weight
- Symmetry of extremities, edema (location, type, grade)

- Skin color, turgor, dryness, oiliness, texture, edema, distribution of fat
- Nail texture; hair amount, texture, and distribution
- Moon face, protruding eyeballs, thickening of tongue, hoarseness, odor of breath
- Symmetry of neck; masses visible on swallowing

Palpation

- Decreased or absence of deep reflexes
- Thyroid size, shape, hardness, nodules; nodes for size, fixation

ANATOMIC AND FUNCTIONAL CHANGES ASSOCIATED WITH THE AGING CLIENT

- Reduced weight of pituitary gland with increased connective tissue and decrease in vascularity, some atrophy of the parathyroid gland, and follicular distention and fibrosis of thyroid gland
- Decreased triiodothyronine hormone by the thyroid, follicle-stimulating hormone by the pituitary, parathyroid hormone by parathyroid, cortisol hormone by the adrenals, anabolic steroids by gonads, progesterone by ovaries, testes and adrenals, testosterone in males; cessation of estrogen in females
- Changes in metabolic rate; atrophy of uterus, vagina, and ovaries; menopause; muscle loss; decreased sexual drive resulting from reduced production and secretion of the hormones
- Pancreatic alveolar degeneration and duct obstruction, reduced number of insulin receptors on cells, decreased insulin release with carbohydrate intake, reduced glucose tolerance and amount of insulin secreted, placing one at risk for diabetes type II

Hematologic System Assessment

PAST HISTORY

Blood and blood-forming organ disorders

- Anemias
- Leukemias, lymphomas
- Hemophilia

- Immune disorders
- Other blood dyscrasias
- Surgery (splenectomy)

Signs and symptoms of hematologic diseases
- Weight loss
- Fatigue, weakness, pallor, shortness of breath
- Pain in bones or joints
- Bleeding from any site, bruising on body parts
- Enlarged nodes

Family history
- Hematologic disorders, acute and chronic
- Anemias
- Hemophilia
- Sickle cell trait
- Malignancies

Allergies
- Foods
- Medications
- Chemicals

Activities of daily living (ADL)
- Abilities for self-care and/or ADL
- Amount of dependence on independence
- Homebound status

Psychosocial history
- Tobacco, caffeine, and alcohol consumption: amount, type, frequency
- Personality traits and life-style
- Occupation and exposure to chemicals, heavy metals, other toxic agents, or environmental pollutants
- Adaptation to chronic illness or condition

Past treatments and diagnostic procedures
- Past or recent hospitalizations
- Bone marrow transplant
- Transfusions of blood or blood products and response
- Medications taken for hematologic conditions (oral, parenteral)
- Special diet of high iron, folate
- Diagnostic procedures and results

PRESENT HISTORY

- Chief complaint, including onset and length of time present

Signs and symptoms

- Change in behavior, level of consciousness, orientation
- Fatigue, weakness, dizziness, headache, pallor, dyspnea
- Pain in bones or joints, mouth or tongue
- Anorexia, nausea, emaciation
- Night sweats
- Infections
- Skin hemorrhages, bleeding from any site (prolonged or excessive)

Present treatments and diagnostic procedures

- Medications (antimicrobials, antianemics, antineoplastics, glucocorticoids, immunosuppressants, analgesics, antianxiety agents)
- Bone marrow analysis, node biopsy, nuclear scan, complete blood count, platelet and reticulocyte counts, prothrombin and thromboplastin time, iron studies

Knowledge of disease and planned home therapy

PHYSICAL EXAMINATION

Inspection

- Vital signs, height, and weight
- General appearance for dehydration, cachexia
- Ecchymoses or petechiae
- Skin color, texture, pruritis
- Oral cavity for redness, edema, bleeding, ulceration

Palpation

- Liver and spleen size
- Joint swelling
- Lymph node enlargement: tenderness, mobility, consistency in neck, axilla, and inguinal areas

ANATOMIC AND FUNCTIONAL CHANGES ASSOCIATED WITH THE AGING CLIENT

- Lymphoid tissue changes affecting immunity, decreased immunocompetence reducing chances for survival from illness

- Degeneration of thymus gland, affecting secretion of thymic hormone and production and efficiency of T-lymphocytes, which reduces ability to respond to antigen stimuli and prevent tumor formation
- Reduced ability to produce leukocytes and erythrocytes by bone marrow, which affects response to infection and anemia
- Decreased antibodies, which affects response to antigens, and increased autoantibodies, affecting susceptibility to autoimmune disease

Musculoskeletal System Assessment

PAST HISTORY

Muscle, bone, and joint disorders

- Arthritis and type
- Bursitis
- Fractures
- Low back syndrome
- Osteoporosis
- Paget's disease
- Ruptured disk
- Bone malignancy
- Bone infections
- Deformities
- Neuromuscular disease
- Musculoskeletal surgery or trauma (amputation, laminectomy, hip or knee replacement)

Signs and symptoms of musculoskeletal disorders

- Pain, swelling in joints
- Muscle weakness, twitching, or deterioration
- Coordination or balance in walking and other movements
- Range of motion (ROM) and activity and mobility
- Paralysis
- Burning, numbness, tingling in extremities
- Contractures, abnormal body alignment
- Pathologic fractures

Family history
- Joint or bone disorders, acute and chronic
- Neurologic motor deficits
- Neuromuscular disease
- Musculoskeletal disease

Allergies
- Foods
- Medications
- Chemicals

Activities of daily living (ADL)
- Ability for self-care and/or ADL
- Ability to use hands and fingers to grasp, hold objects
- Ability to walk, energy and endurance and effect on joints
- Use of aids for eating, toileting, dressing, personal hygiene, and grooming
- Homebound status

Psychosocial history
- Tobacco, alcohol, caffeine, and chemical consumption: daily and over period of years
- Personality traits
- Occupation and need for mobility and dexterity, proneness to accidents
- Adaptation to disability or chronic illness

Past treatments and diagnostic procedures
- Past or recent hospitalizations
- Cast, splint, or traction for bone or joint disorder or surgery
- Physical and occupational therapy and rehabilitation
- Transcutaneous electrical nerve stimulation (TENS), cold or heat applications
- Medications taken for musculoskeletal conditions (oral, injections)
- Diagnostic procedures and results

PRESENT HISTORY

- Chief complaint, including onset and length of time present

Signs and symptoms
- Pain in affected area

- Redness, swelling, warmth in affected area
- Weakness, fatigue
- Loss of mobility, coordination or balance, or weight-bearing ability
- Limited ROM
- Loss of sensation in extremity
- Muscle spasms, reduced muscle strength and mass
- Diminished peripheral pulse in extremities, delayed capillary refill

Present treatments and diagnostic procedures

- Medications (anticholinergics, antimicrobials, antigout agents, antiparkinson agents, analgesics, nonsteroidal analgesics, glucocorticoids, immunosuppressants, skeletal muscle relaxants, antianxiety agents, minerals)
- Radiography, nuclear and computerized tomography scans, myelography, electromyography, biopsy, electrolytes, uric acid, rheumatoid factor, complete blood count, sedimentation rate, alkaline phosphatase
- Special diet, high calcium, low calorie
- Use of trapeze, cast, brace, traction, aids for ADL
- Bed rest, chair, amount of activity allowed
- Limb prosthesis

Knowledge of disease and planned home therapy

PHYSICAL EXAMINATION

Inspection

- Symmetry of legs and arms, shoulders, clavicles, scapulas, musculature (hypertrophy or atrophy)
- Full ROM of all joints, degree of motion and symmetry
- Ability to sit, lie, get up, stand, walk, and posture in all positions
- Deformities or contractures, deviations, changes in contour
- Presence of scoliosis, kyphosis, lordosis, hammer toe
- Gait, coordination, balance, and endurance
- Body alignment in supine, prone, side-lying positions
- Amputation (arm or leg and site of amputation)
- Enforced immobilization
- Circulatory and neurologic function of casted extremity or body part

Palpation

- Warmth, swelling, tenderness at joint(s) or injury
- Crepitus from joint motion
- Muscles for strength, mass, tone, spasticity, flaccidity, rigidity
- Presence of reflexes
- Tenderness on pressure or movement
- Thickening, bony enlargement around joints

ANATOMIC AND FUNCTIONAL CHANGES ASSOCIATED WITH THE AGING CLIENT

- Loss of muscle fiber, muscle mass, bone minerals, and bone mass, causing muscle wasting and reduction in weight, strength, endurance, and agility; and brittle bones as bone resorption is faster than new bone formation, resulting in an increased risk for fractures
- Shortened vertebral column, hip and knee flexion, and curvature of spine, reducing height and effecting postural change that causes change in body balance and risk for falls
- Reduced motor coordination and manual skills, affecting reaction time, and change in extrapyramidal system, causing muscle stiffness, slowness, and tremors at rest
- Decreased storage of muscle glycogen and change in enzyme function, causing loss of energy and muscle fatigue
- Joint changes from increased synovial membrane and synovial fluid thickness
- Muscle cramping and paresthesias of legs, resulting in pain and loss of sleep
- Mechanical and dermatologic changes in feet caused by long-term stress of weight bearing on feet

Renal/Urinary System Assessment

PAST HISTORY

Kidney and bladder disorders

- Renal failure
- Urinary tract infection (cystitis, pyelonephritis)
- Glomerulonephritis

- Calculi
- Neurogenic bladder
- Prostatic hypertrophy
- Hypertension
- Malignancy
- Surgery: kidney (nephrectomy, nephrostomy, transplant), bladder (urinary diversion, cystectomy, prostatectomy)

Signs and symptoms of renal/urinary disorders
- Pain in kidney or bladder area
- Urinary incontinence, bladder distention
- Retention, hesitancy, dribbling, urgency, frequency, burning, nocturia, dysuria
- Polyuria, oliguria, anuria
- Urine amount, color, odor, sedimentation, hematuria, pus, mucus, clarity
- Type of fluid intake and output (I&O) for 24 hours
- Weight gain
- Edema, fever, bruising, restlessness, insomnia
- Skin dryness, itching, poor turgor, lip and mucous membrane dryness
- Mentation changes

Family history
- Renal or bladder disorders, acute or chronic
- Congenital or familial renal or urinary conditions
- Hypertension
- Connective tissue disorder
- Diabetes mellitus

Allergies
- Foods
- Medications

Activities of daily living (ADL)
- Abilities for personal self-care (toileting)
- Use of assistive aids for elimination
- Homebound status

Psychosocial history
- Tobacco, alcohol and caffeine consumption: type, amount, frequency

- Personality traits
- Sexually transmitted diseases
- Exposure to environmental or occupational nephrotoxic substances (heavy metals, carbon tetrachloride, phenols, pesticides)
- Adaptation to chronic illness or condition

Past treatments and diagnostic procedures

- Past or recent hospitalizations
- Presence of urinary diversion (type, care, response)
- Medications taken for renal or urinary conditions (oral, injections)
- Diagnostics and results

PRESENT HISTORY

- Chief complaint, including onset and length of time present

Signs and symptoms

- Pain
- Weight gain, edema
- Changes in urinary pattern
- Changes in urinary characteristics
- Anorexia, nausea, vomiting
- Thirst, dry skin, poor skin turgor
- Weakness, muscle cramping
- Pruritis, visual changes
- Fluid imbalance
- Electrolyte imbalance

Present treatments and diagnostic procedures

- Medications (analgesics, diuretic, antimicrobials, anticoagulants, cholinergics, electrolytes, immunosuppressants, glucocorticoids)
- Intravenous pyelography, cystography, radiography, nuclear scan, ultrasonography, kidney biopsy, blood urea nitrogen, creatinine and creatinine clearance, urinalysis, urine culture
- Use of urinary drainage devices or catheterization
- Fluid inclusions or restrictions
- Hemodialysis or peritoneal dialysis
- Special diet, low salt, potassium, calcium, or protein

Knowledge of disease and planned home therapy

PHYSICAL EXAMINATION

Inspection

- Blood pressure for elevation
- Skin color, pruritis, petechiae, ecchymoses, dryness, urate crystals
- Edema of hands, feet, sacral region, legs; abdominal distention, neck vein distention
- Urinary output and characteristics with or without an indwelling catheter
- Behavior changes (alertness, confusion, cognitive ability, level of consciousness)
- Fruity or urine odor to breath, foul odor to urine
- Condition of urinary diversion site, dialysis shunt or abdominal site, urinary catheter site

Palpation

- Size and movement of kidneys
- Pain in kidney, bladder area
- Bladder or abdominal distention

Percussion

- Dullness over bladder if distended

ANATOMIC AND FUNCTIONAL CHANGES ASSOCIATED WITH THE AGING CLIENT

- Reduced renal tissue growth and number of nephrons, decreasing kidney size and affecting renal function efficiency
- Sclerosis of glomeruli and atrophy of afferent arterioles, which results in degeneration of glomeruli and glomerular filtration rate (GFR)
- Reduced cell mass and water content of adipose tissue, causing decreased intracellular body water and total body water with extracellular body water remaining unchanged
- Reduced blood flow, GFR, and tubular function, affecting ability to concentrate urine and drug clearance
- Reduced resorption of gucose and sodium, creatinine production and clearance; increased blood urea nitrogen (BUN), causing prolonged time for acid-base abnormalities to return to normal and age adjustments in evaluating lab values

- Bladder becomes funnel shaped and capacity and smooth muscle tone are decreased, causing urinary frequency and nocturia
- Enlarged prostate in men, resulting in urgency, frequency, and dribbling
- Increased weakness of bladder and perineal muscles in women, causing retention and stress incontinence
- Bladder emptying incomplete, resulting in urinary stasis and risk for urinary tract infection
- Reduced inhibitory neural impulses to the bladder, affecting bladder contractions and voluntary control over bladder function, which causes incontinence

Integumentary System Assessment

PAST HISTORY

Integumentary disorders

- Dermatitis
- Eczema
- Infestations, scabies, pediculosis
- Infections of skin, nails, scalp
- Skin malignancy
- Surgery (graft, cosmetic)

Signs and symptoms of integumentary disorders

- Alopecia
- Dandruff
- Itching, breaks in skin
- Brittleness, ridging, redness, edema of nails and cuticles
- Tendency to skin infections, herpes simplex
- Sensitivity to sun, soaps, deodorants, perfumes, others
- Dryness, oiliness, excessive moisture, body odor
- Skin color changes
- Lumps or growth on the skin
- Bruising, delayed healing
- Ulcer on extremity

Family history

- Integumentary disorders, acute and chronic
- Allergies, eczema

Allergies

- Foods
- Medications
- Cosmetics
- Environmental contacts

Activities of daily living (ADL)

- Abilities for personal self-care (bathing, grooming, dressing)
- Pattern of bathing, frequency and time, soap, toothpaste, shaving cream, powder, lotions used, razor or electric shaver, use of assistive aids for personal hygiene
- Pattern of hair and nail care, shampoo, rinse, nail polish, hair tint used, trimming of toenails and fingernails, use of assistive aids or professionally done
- Homebound status

Psychosocial history

- Home environment exposure to allergens or irritants
- Personality traits, anxiety
- Occupational exposure to irritants such as dyes, sprays, perfumes, allergens
- Effect on body image if dermatitis or scarring present
- Adaptation to chronic skin condition

Past treatments and diagnostic procedures

- Past or recent hospitalizations
- Medications used for integumentary conditions (topical, oral)
- Diagnostic procedures and results

PRESENT HISTORY

Chief complaint, including onset and length of time present

Signs and symptoms

- Changes in skin color, eruptions, breaks, and precipitating factors
- Hair loss and precipitating factors
- Nail changes and precipitating factors

- Injury from burns, with extent and degree of damage to skin and pain

Present treatments and diagnostic procedures
- Medications (antipruritics, antianxiety agents, antimicrobials, glucocorticoids, antihistamines, sedatives, analgesics)
- Skin biopsy, skin culture, complete blood count
- Desensitization therapy
- Braden scale for decubitus prediction

Knowledge of disease and planned home therapy

PHYSICAL EXAMINATION

Inspection
- Skin for cyanosis, redness, jaundice, pallor, pigmentation, bleeding, bruising
- Skin for striae, rashes, urticaria, bites, wrinkling
- Skin dryness, moisture, oiliness, sweating, peeling, scaling, crusting
- Pruritis, odor, exudate, cleanliness
- Edema, pain, breaks, incisions and scars, sagging parts
- Blisters, cellulitis, calluses, corns, superficial infection
- Lesions, lipomas, keloids, warts, nevi, with location and distribution
- Senile lentigines, senile ectasias, seborrheic keratosis, sebaceous hyperplasia in the aging client
- Nail cleanliness, texture, thickness, angle, infection, ingrown nails or hangnails
- Hair cleanliness, quantity, texture, distribution, color, odors, brittleness, oiliness or dryness, baldness
- Scalp infestation, lesions, dandruff

Palpation
- Skin temperature (warm, hot, cold), texture (rough, bumpy, smooth, thin, thick)
- Skin turgor, elasticity, moisture, mobility, elevated lesions with measurement
- Tumors, cysts, or any lumps on skin or scalp
- Bony prominences and response to pressure
- Capillary return in nails and movement of nail plate when pressure applied

ANATOMIC AND FUNCTIONAL CHANGES ASSOCIATED WITH THE AGING CLIENT

- Change in distribution of body fat with loss of subcutaneous fat, especially over the arms and legs, which causes loss of body insulation and support for vessels
- Reduced formation of collagen with loss of elasticity of skin, causing sagging, wrinkles, lines in face and neck, ptosis of eyelids, and elongation of ear lobes
- Reduced cell replacement in dermis and epidermis, affecting wound healing and risk for decubitus ulcers
- Atrophy of skin layers and reduced vascularity and elasticity, which causes loss of water content and storage in skin layers, reduced skin turgor, stiffness, and loss of pliability
- Reduced water content of skin and function of eccrine and sebaceous glands, causing rough, scaly texture and pruritis from dryness, risk for pressure ulcers, trauma, and reduced ability of body to cool itself
- Decreased circulation to skin and appendages, affecting blood supply of oxygen and nutrients to skin
- Neurosensory changes in skin, affecting tactile perception of pain associated with lesions or tumors
- Excessive skin pigmentation on exposed areas, causing aging spots, and overgrowth epidermal tissue, causing senile telangiectasia and hyperkeratotic warts
- Nail ridges; thickness, brittleness, and splitting of nails increased, causing reduced growth and strength, increased risk for fungal infections with lifting of nail plate
- Density of hair follicles reduced; loss of axillary, pubic, head hair, and melanin production, causing graying, increased hair growth in ears, nares, eyebrows

Reproductive System Assessment: Female

PAST HISTORY

Reproductive disorders

- Sexually transmitted diseases

- Pelvic inflammatory disease (PID)
- Endometriosis
- Tubal pregnancy
- Abortions
- Infertility
- Menstrual disorders
- Breast, uterine, ovarian, vaginal malignancy
- Surgery: breast (simple or radical mastectomy), uterus (hysterectomy), pelvic reproductive organs (salpingectomy, oophorectomy, tubal sterilization), vaginal (cystocele or rectocele repair)

Signs and symptoms of reproductive organ disorders
- Breast tenderness, discharge, lump or mass; change in nipple
- Dyspareunia
- Dysmenorrhea, amenorrhea, other menstrual irregularities
- Rashes or irritations of genitalia with pruritis
- Discharge from meatus, vagina
- Dysuria, urinary frequency, retention, incontinence

Family history
- Breast or reproductive organ malignancy
- Reproductive organ disorders, acute or chronic

Allergies
- Scented feminine powders, pads, tampons

Activities of daily living (ADL)
- Ability for personal self-care and/or ADL (toileting, menstrual hygiene)
- Amount of independence or dependence
- Presence of indwelling catheter and ability for care
- Breast self-examination and frequency
- Birth control use and effectiveness
- Homebound status

Psychosocial history
- Age at menarche; menstrual frequency, amount, duration, regularity, and pain; last menstrual period
- Number of pregnancies, children
- Date or age of menopause, hot flashes, discharge, pain
- Intercourse frequency if active, satisfaction level

- Sexual orientation, multiple partners if appropriate
- Ability to carry out role function to satisfaction
- Adaptation to infertility or other chronic condition

Past treatments and diagnostic procedures

- Past or recent hospitalizations
- Intrauterine device, birth control implant
- Medications taken for gynecologic conditions (oral, vaginal)
- Diagnostic procedures and results

PRESENT HISTORY

- Chief complaint, including onset and length of time present

Signs and symptoms

- Abdominal pain, menstrual dysfunction
- Vaginal discharge and characteristics
- Genital irritation, pruritis
- Dyspareunia, dysuria

Present treatments and diagnostic procedures

- Medications (hormones, antimicrobial, analgesics, fertility agents, antineoplastic agents, birth control agents)
- Ultrasonography, mammography, laparoscopy, amniocentesis; breast, endometrial or cervical biopsy; complete blood count, typing and Rh factor; pregnancy test, pap smear
- Presence of urinary catheter, birth control device

Knowledge of disease and planned home therapy

PHYSICAL EXAMINATION

Inspection

- Size, symmetry, contour, dimpling, texture, rash, moles, venous pattern, color of breast(s)
- Size, shape, color, discharge, induration of nipple(s); size, shape, and surface of areolae
- External genitalia (urethra, clitoris, introitus, perineum) color, inflammation, swelling, ulcerations or lesions, discharge, episiotomy
- Pediculosis pubis
- Vaginal wall bulging, mucous membrane color, inflammation, masses, and lesions
- Cervical color, position, ulceration, bleeding, discharge

Palpation

- Breast elasticity, fullness, tenderness, nodes, nipple elasticity and discharge with pressure
- Size, shape, location, consistency, tenderness, mobility of breast mass
- Axillary nodes present or absent
- Bulging of perineum, smoothness, discharge from glands or duct openings
- Vaginal wall smoothness, muscle tone, tenderness, nodules
- Cervical size, shape, position, mobility, patency
- Uterine size, position, shape, consistency, mobility, tenderness, mass

ANATOMIC AND FUNCTIONAL CHANGES ASSOCIATED WITH THE AGING CLIENT

- Sparser pubic hair
- Reduced size of uterus, cervix, and ovaries; size and firmness of breast tissue
- Reduced subcutaneous tissue, which causes sagging breasts and flattening and folding of labia
- Shorter and narrower vaginal canal with increased thinning and loss of elasticity of the lining, which causes atrophic vaginitis and dyspareunia
- Vaginal secretions alkaline and reduced in amount, causing a need for more lubricant prior to intercourse
- Pelvic muscle tone weakness, which increases risk for uterine prolapse and stress incontinence
- Decreased estrogen secretion, which results in hot flashes, and follicular maturation, which affects the stimulation to the uterine lining, and Bartholin's gland secretion, which results in reduced lubrication of the vagina

Reproductive System Assessment: Male

PAST HISTORY

Reproductive disorders

- Sexually transmitted diseases

- Prostatitis, prostatic hypertrophy
- Epididymitis
- Hydrocele
- Hernia
- Malignancy (prostate, testis)
- Surgery (prostatectomy, orchiectomy, penile implant, vasectomy, herniorrhaphy)

Signs and symptoms of reproductive organ disorders

- Pain in scrotum, testes
- Discharge from penis
- Lesions on penis
- Impotency, libido or sexual dysfunction
- Urinary difficulty with urgency, frequency, weak stream, difficulty in starting or stopping, incontinence, inability to empty bladder

Family history

- Reproductive disorders, acute or chronic

Activities of daily living (ADL)

- Ability for self-care and/or ADL (toileting, genital hygiene)
- Presence of indwelling catheter and ability for care
- Use of incontinence pads or undergarments
- Homebound status

Psychosocial history

- Personality traits
- Intercourse frequency if active, satisfaction level
- Sexual orientation, multiple partners if appropriate
- Ability to carry out role functions to satisfaction
- Effect of sexual dysfunction on self-concept
- Adaptation to illness, impotence, or other chronic condition

Past treatments and diagnostic procedures

- Past or recent hospitalizations
- Penile implant or device
- Scrotal self-examination and frequency
- Medications taken for reproductive conditions (oral)
- Diagnostic procedures and results

PRESENT HISTORY

- Chief complaint, including onset and length of time present

Signs and symptoms

- Pain
- Urinary dysfunction
- Bleeding or discharge from penis
- Genital irritation, pruritis
- Penile lesions, ulcers, soreness

Present treatments and diagnostic procedures

- Medications (hormones, analgesics, antimicrobials, antispasmodics, antineoplastics)
- Cystoscopy, nuclear scan, prostate biopsy, complete blood count, urinalysis, urine culture, anal and meatal smear
- Use of aids or device for impotence
- Presence of urinary catheter

Knowledge of disease and planned home therapy

PHYSICAL EXAMINATION

Inspection

- Breast and nipple symmetry, lesions, drainage, induration
- Pediculosis pubis, pubic hair distribution
- Penis, urethral meatus, scrotum for ulceration, scars, rashes, discharge, swelling, tenderness
- Circumcision and cleanliness
- Size and shape of penis for age, contour of scrotal sac with testes in place, position of urethral meatus

Palpation

- Breasts and nipples for masses, tenderness, discharge on pressure
- Penile shaft for masses, tenderness, induration
- Testes for size, shape, consistency, tenderness, symmetry, irregularities
- Hernia via inguinal ring and canal
- Prostate via rectal examination for softness, contour, enlargement, tenderness

ANATOMIC AND FUNCTIONAL CHANGES ASSOCIATED WITH THE AGING CLIENT

- Increased size of prostate with urinary problems, and decreased size and firmness of testes, which causes reduced sperm production; scrotum sac hangs lower and more loosely

- Reduced volume and viscosity of seminal fluid, which decreases force of ejaculation
- Erection time increased with need for more stimulation, affecting orgasm and enhanced satisfaction
- Decreased testosterone secretion, causing reduced sexual energy

Eye, Ear, Nose, and Throat Assessment

PAST HISTORY

Eye, ear, nose, and throat disorders

- Infections (tonsillitis, conjunctivitis, otitis, pharyngitis)
- Glaucoma
- Cataracts
- Retinal detachment
- Deviated septum, nasal polyps
- Allergic rhinitis
- Macular degeneration
- Dry eye
- Presbyopia, presbycusis
- Surgery: eye (cataract, keratoplasty, corneal transplant, enucleation), ear (tympanoplasty, stapedectomy), nose (polypectomy, submucous resection), throat (tonsillectomy)

Signs and symptoms of eye, ear, nose, or throat disorders

- Pain, headaches
- Discharge from eye, ear, nose
- Multiple colds
- Halitosis
- Buzzing or roaring in ears
- Vertigo, loss of equilibrium
- Nystagmus
- Hoarseness
- Runny or stuffy nose, epistaxis
- Changes in visual, auditory acuity

Family history

- Eye, ear, nose, and throat (EENT) disorders, acute and chronic
- Allergies

Allergies

- Foods
- Medications
- Animals
- Chemicals
- Environmental pollutants

Activities of daily living (ADL)

- Ability for self-care and/or ADL
- Effects of visual or auditory impairment on independence or dependence
- Use of glasses, contact lenses, eye prosthesis, hearing aid, lip reading, signing
- Ability to care for assistive visual and auditory aids and instill eyedrops, eardrops, or nose drops
- Response to noise levels, mouthwash or rinses, hair sprays, ear cleansing with cotton swabs
- Homebound status

Psychosocial history

- Effect of impairment on self-concept and occupation
- Effects of age and emotions on impairments or disease
- Personality traits, anxiety, or depression
- Home environment exposure to allergens and irritants
- Adaptation to impairment or illness

Past treatments and diagnostic procedures

- Past or recent hospitalizations
- Last hearing or vision test
- Desensitization therapy
- Medications taken for EENT conditions (oral, inhalant, topical)
- Diagnostic procedures and results

PRESENT HISTORY

- Chief complaint, including onset and length of time present

Signs and symptoms

- Pain or soreness in affected area
- Onset, duration, precipitating factors

- Dysphagia, hoarseness, loss of voice
- Discharge from eye, ear, nose, throat
- Redness, swelling of eye, throat, nasal mucosa
- Epistaxis
- Temperature elevation
- Changes in visual or auditory perception and acuity

Present treatments and diagnostic procedures

- Medications (antimicrobials, glucocorticoids, antihistamines, analgesics, antiglaucoma agents, antipyretics)
- Radiography, computerized tomography, complete blood count, culture of throat, nasal, ear, eye secretions
- Eye, ear, throat irrigations
- Nasal packing, eye covering and dressing

Knowledge of disease and planned home therapy

PHYSICAL EXAMINATION

Inspection

- Ophthalmoscopic and otoscopic examination
- Visual acuity, visual fields, extraocular muscle intactness and movement tests
- Eyelids for symmetry, position, blinking, color, edema, lesions; eyebrows for movement, quantity and distribution, symmetry
- Conjunctiva and sclera color, edema, lesions, opacities; iris marking, color, and shape
- Cornea surface, transparency, sensitivity
- Pupil size, shape, equality, reaction to light and accommodation
- Round, intact lacrimal glands, moisture or dryness of eyes
- External ears and auricles for lesions, deformities, color, size, and symmetry of position
- Ear canals for redness, edema, swelling
- Nose deformities, shape, symmetry, color, edema, drainage, bleeding, and septal alignment
- Lips for color, dryness, cracking, edema, ulcers
- Throat color, swelling, bleeding, inflammation, lesions
- Tonsils (if present) for redness, swelling, pus, or other exudate

Palpation

- Pinnae for firmness, masses, elasticity, pain
- Structure of nose
- Tenderness of frontal or maxillary sinuses and lacrimal glands

ANATOMIC AND FUNCTIONAL CHANGES ASSOCIATED WITH THE AGING CLIENT

- Reduced size of pupils, affecting night vision or a slow adaptation to the dark
- Reduced sensitivity of cones in retina, which causes decreased discrimination and blending of colors
- Sclera that becomes yellow with pigmented deposits and cornea with white-yellow deposits around iris (arcus senilis), which becomes more translucent; inner canthus develops yellow plaques (xanthelasma)
- Loss of elasticity and increased opacity of lens, affecting focus and accommodation, night vision, color vision, reduced peripheral vision and tolerance to glare, and high risk for development of cataracts
- Reduced secretion by lacrimal glands, which causes dry conjunctiva and eye irritation; resorption of intraocular fluid; and a shallower anterior chamber which can all increase risk for glaucoma
- Thinner and more wrinkled lids, loss of supporting tissue, which causes a sunken appearance of the eye into the socket
- Atrophy or sclerosis of tympanic membrane and increased rigidity of middle ear bones, which affect the transmission of nerve impulses from the ear to the brain, causes difficulty in hearing high-frequency sounds that later progresses to include low-frequency sounds, hearing if noise if present, sound distortion, and phonetic regression; keratin in cerumen is increased, hardens, and accumulates, affecting hearing

Psychosocial Assessment

MENTAL/COGNITIVE/LEARNING

Past history

- Educational level and achievements
- Attitude toward learning, motivation
- Difficulty in achieving educational or vocational goals
- Learning disabilities
- Interest in and willingness to learn about care and procedures
- Ability to listen to and comprehend information given

- Ability to read and follow written instructions
- Vocabulary level and attention span
- Memory and ability to recall events, past and present
- Hearing, visual impairments
- English spoken or English as a second language

Present history

- Knowledge and understanding of illness and prognosis
- Cerebral function, including orientation, memory, recall, attention and concentration, comprehension, judgment, dementia, level of consciousness, communication pattern (articulation)
- Thought processes with ability to think rationally and logically and to solve problems
- Sensory function, including vision, hearing
- Physical ability, strength for self-care
- Ability to express needs and maintain record of care and procedures
- Administration of Short Portable Mental Status Questionnaire or Mini-Mental State Examination

PSYCHIATRIC

Past history

- Psychiatric conditions, treatments, therapist
- Institution, including length of stay and discharge date
- Attitude toward treatments
- Medications taken (prescribed, over the counter, recreational, street)
- Alcohol intake, amounts and length of time
- Hypochondriasis
- Suicide potential and precipitating factors
- Family history of mental disorders
- Relationships with family members and feelings about family

Present history

- Personal appearance, including hygiene, clothing, physical characteristics, posture, mannerisms, facial expression, gestures
- Communications, including tone, quality, flow, speed, use of associative looseness, flight of ideas, blocking, mutism, circumstantiality, word salad, echolalia, eye contact
- Mood, effect, stressors present
- Orientation to time, place, person, and event

- Delusions, hallucinations, illusions, paranoia
- Coping ability and skills, use of defense mechanisms
- Presence of chronic anxiety, worry, depression, insomnia
- Lives alone or with others, isolates self, support of significant others
- Participation in social interactions and activities
- Administration of Beck Depression Inventory, Yesavage Geriatric Depression Scale

ADVANCE DIRECTIVES

- Patient Self-Determination Act and its requirements and need for written information about advance directives (see Appendix)
- Presence of an advance directive or form for health care and location of the document(s) or a copy available
  - Living will
  - Durable power of attorney for health care
- Family understanding of and conflicts about client's directives
- Knowledge of rights of autonomy and consent to or refusal of care in the home, initiation of 911 call for client in home

SPIRITUAL

- Religious beliefs and practices, identified spiritual leader
- Feelings about a supreme being and how this view affects illness
- Feelings about what will happen during illness
- Specific people helpful in religious life
- Religious symbols of importance (Bible, prayer, rosary, literature)
- Rituals of importance (communion, Sacrament of the Sick, lighting Sabbath candles, quiet time)
- Religious restrictions (dietary laws, fasting, blood transfusion, medical treatment, birth control, abortion, autopsy)
- Need for church attendance, priest, minister, or rabbi visits

OCCUPATIONAL/RECREATIONAL

Past history

- Type of and feelings about past employment
- Effects on health
- Reasons for leaving or changing vocation, profession
- Presence of occupational hazards
- Hobbies and avocational activities

PRESENT HISTORY

- Type of present employment or retirement, loss of employment
- Feelings about work or retirement
- Activity involved in work
- Effect of work environment on health (stress, chemicals, allergens)
- Plans for returning to work
- Housekeeping tasks (amount, kind, and participation)
- Need for more education or wish for vocational retraining
- Type, frequency, and degree of participation in play, recreational activities
- Effect of illness on recreational interests or hobbies
- Alternative interests and activity options during illness
- Need to change recreational activities permanently
- Adaptation to retirement and role changes

FUNCTIONAL CHANGES ASSOCIATED WITH THE AGING CLIENT

- Intelligence remains basically the same but can be affected by sensory deficits
- Learning capacity can be slowed initially but can keep pace with other learners, and there is a tendency to continue with familiar solutions for problems rather than develop new attitudes and methods
- Retention ability more limited and easily affected by external distractions
- More difficult to perform more than one task at a time
- Slowing of memory if information not continued to be used
- Personality traits remain the same but can become more psychologically diverse

Functional Assessment

GENERAL

- Homebound status, complete bed rest, activity restrictions
- Independence or dependence in self-care and activities of daily living (ADL) and desire and willingness to perform and adapt to limitations

- Degree of disability or handicap or deficit
- Presence of artificial limb, eye, dentures
- Rehabilitation therapy by physical and/or occupational therapist
- General review of activities of a typical day to include personal care, social, and leisure routines
- Katz index of ADL for actual functional status

BATHING/GROOMING

- Ability to wash body (shower, tub bath, sponge bath)
- Use of aids to bathe (long handles for sponge, mitt on hand, bars, skidproof mat, and stool in bath or shower stall, soap on rope hanging around neck)
- Ability to brush teeth, cleanse dentures, comb or brush hair
- Use of aids to brush teeth (long and built-up handles, extension handles, cup for soaking teeth, mounted dryer or brush with suction cup, squeeze bottles for shampoo and toothpaste)
- Ability to shave or apply makeup (electric or safety razor, makeup kit)
- Use of aids to shave and apply makeup (shaving cream, built-up handles, mirror mounted with suction cups or hanging around neck)

DRESSING/UNDRESSING

- Type of clothing that is easy to put on and remove (loose fitting, elastic at waist, closures with zipper or velcro, wide openings to slip over head or slip on with front opening, shoes that slip on or have velcro closures)
- Ability to dress and undress (buttons, zipper, tie laces, putting on shoes and hose)
- Use of aids for dressing (hooks, zippers, long handles for shoes)

TOILETING

- Ability to use bathroom, commode, bedpan, urinal
- Use of aids for toileting (grab bars, mounted toilet seat with side arms, tongs or mounts for toilet tissue)

FEEDING

- Ability to feed self, partial or total assistance, ability to prepare meal
- Use of aids for eating (china and flatware with suction cups, flatware with swivel, extension handles on flatware, bumper guard on plate, bib for droppings, cuff to hold utensils)

- Use of aids for drinking (grippers on cup or glass, large handles, long and bending straws, suction cups for cup or glass)

MOBILITY

- Ability to walk, sit, stand, or lie down, amount of assistance needed
- Use of aids for mobility and movement (wheelchair, walker, crutches, cane, brace, elevated chair, adjustable seat or ejector chair, footstool, trapeze, holding rails, mechanical lift, electric or semielectric hospital bed)

GENERAL ACTIVITIES

- Book holder, tilted table, clipboard, holder for pencil, card or pad holder, mounts on chair for radio and books, and remote control for electric appliances
- Cars with special modifications, use of vans or buses with wheelchair lift
- Magnifiers, large-print reading materials and telephone amplifier, special wiring for turning lights on or to alert deaf client
- Automatic dialer and speaker phone attachment
- Pets for visual and auditory assistance

Environmental Assessment

HOME EXTERIOR

- Primary entrance
- Steps or ramp available if needed
- Homebound or able to leave home safely

HOME INTERIOR

- Condition and cleanliness, noise, waste disposal
- Space storage for extra equipment and supplies
- Counter space for preparation of supplies, cleaning of equipment
- Refrigeration for foods, medications, supplies
- Location of fuse or circuit breaker box
- Proper lighting, frayed or loose wiring or electrical connections, grounding of equipment
- Heating and air conditioning adequacy

- Woodstove or kerosene heater use and ability to fuel fire
- Ventilation, temperature control, drafts
- Laundry facilities for clothing, linens, supplies
- Doorways and if adequate to move through easily, to accommodate wheelchair, commode, and to allow for delivery of equipment
- Floors and pathways clear, dry, and not slippery; arrangement of furniture out of pathways but close enough to use for support when ambulating; small rugs and carpet edges out of pathways
- Stairway, number of stairs and height of stairs; room on first floor or need for client to be transported upstairs
- Safety bars and holding aids for movement within environment
- Hot and cold running water or means to heat water, indoor plumbing versus drawn water
- Bathroom, commode within easy access
- Presence of allergens, dust, animals, plants, sprays, odors

SAFETY FACTORS

- Client's feeling of safety in home
- Hospital bed, trapeze connection
- Side rails up or bed in low position if using hospital bed
- Call bell, water, tissues, wastebasket, telephone within reach
- Chair to assist to standing position
- Scales for weight in bathroom or near bed
- Proper body alignment and positioning if on bed rest
- Use of restraints, smoking and precautions taken
- Isolation or protective isolation procedures needed
- Nonslip mats in bath or shower
- Night-lights if out of bed at night to use bathroom or commode
- Safety aids for ADL to prevent falls, promote self-care; amount of assistance needed, proper fitting nonskid foot covering
- Proper hand-washing technique when required
- Proper administration of medications and use of aids to ensure accuracy
- Proper cleansing and disinfection of reusable supplies, removal and disposal of hazardous wastes
- Available emergency numbers to call

Family Assessment

PHYSICAL HISTORY

- Chronic illness of family members
- Functional abilities or disabilities
- Energy levels of family members and how physical needs of its members are met
- Physical strength and ability to perform procedures
- Rigidity in functioning within family system
- Health practices
- Types of practitioners used
- Medications taken by family members

PSYCHOSOCIAL HISTORY

Emotional status/mental status

- Changes in family life and roles caused by client needs
- Family unable to meet emotional needs of its members
- Ability of family members to express feelings
- Ability of family to accomplish developmental tasks
- Ability to communicate clear message, solve problems, and make decisions
- Family attitude, overconcern toward illness or disability, relationship of client and family members
- Family patterns in use of coping mechanisms (denial, rationalization, projections, defensiveness) and ability to adapt
- Family organization (arguments, separations, divorces)
- Willingness to perform procedures and care for client
- Support of client by member most likely to become caregiver
- Family APGAR for family function

PSYCHIATRIC DISORDERS

- General mental health of family
- Psychosomatic tendency
- Chronic anxiety in family members
- Depression in family members
- Behavior disorder of family member
- Presence of alcoholism, family violence, suicides, drug abuse

CULTURAL INFLUENCES

- General values and ethnic identity of family
- Spiritual beliefs, religious affiliation
- Language barriers, English as a second language
- Beliefs regarding health care and health professionals

Economic Assessment

FINANCIAL RESOURCES

- Ability to perform financial responsibilities and handle money, power of attorney to manage finances
- Ability to access preventive health care and screening
- Ability to purchase food, pay for rent and utilities
- Ability to purchase or rent equipment, supplies, and services used in the home
- Retirement income and/or effect of illness on limited or fixed income
  - Social security
  - Retirement program
  - Private pensions
  - Public assistance
- Occupation, effect of illness on work and ability to continue with the same occupation
- Programs available to assist
  - Social Security Supplement (SSS)
  - Foundations
  - Churches
  - National associations
  - Voluntary agencies and support groups
  - Government grants
- Insurance for health, home, or hospital care
  - Medicare, Medicare gap or supplemental health insurance
  - Medicaid
  - Health maintenance organization (HMO)
  - Private health insurance
  - Private home care insurance
  - Private long-term care insurance
  - Workers' compensation

Veterans Administration
CHAMPUS
Catastrophic health insurance

RESOURCES FOR EQUIPMENT AND SUPPLIES

- Pharmacy and supply companies
- Home health agencies
- Home infusion and supply companies
- Durable equipment companies (purchase or rental)
- Medical supplies companies (disposable and reusable)
- Community organizations that offer medical supplies, financial assistance

Care Plans

Pulmonary system

Asthma

Asthma is an airway-reacting, obstructive pulmonary disease characterized by an irritation and constriction of the bronchi and bronchioles, resulting in bronchospasms, excessive mucus production, dyspnea, and frequently wheezing, especially in acute episodes. The causes may be extrinsic (associated with allergic responses) or intrinsic (associated with stress, activity or exercise, or respiratory infection) or a combination of these.

Home care is primarily concerned with the teaching of medication regimens to prevent or control attacks, prevention of upper and lower pulmonary and sinus infections, and assistance in reducing stressors.

Nursing diagnosis

Anxiety

Related factors: Threat of death; threat to or change in health status

Defining characteristics: Dyspnea, fear of suffocation, apprehension regarding recurrence of attacks, feelings of helplessness and tension, change in life-style needed to control breathing

OUTCOMES

Short-term

Reduction in anxiety, as evidenced by verbalization of anxiety and concern, relaxed posture, respirations slower and more quiet, statements that client feels better, is less anxious, able to sleep better (expected within 2 to 7 days)

Long-term

Anxiety reduced to optimal coping capabilities, as evidenced by avoidance of physical and emotional stressors, compliance with treatment regimen with positive responses, control of anxiety during dyspneic episodes (expected within 2 weeks and ongoing)

NURSING INTERVENTIONS/INSTRUCTIONS

1. Assess mental and emotional status and effect of stressors on breathing (see Psychosocial Assessment, p. 7, for guidelines) (first visit).
2. Establish rapport and exhibit a caring, accepting attitude while client expresses anxiety and concerns about the condition, its symptomatology, chronicity, and any perceived disability (each visit).
3. Assess client's inner personal resources and coping abilities; note reactions and responses to instructions and various treatment modalities (first visit).
4. Assist client in identification of stressors and realistic adaptation in avoiding them (first and second visits).
5. Instruct client in guided imagery and relaxation techniques and in music therapy (first and second visits).
6. Instruct client in the importance of a measured, paced routine for all activities of daily living (ADL) and to avoid those that cause fear and uncertainty (first visit).
7. Provide continuing information about client's condition, tests, treatments, and progress; answer all questions honestly. Set up a telephone appointment to respond to these questions if information is not immediately available (each visit).
8. Initiate referral to self-help or support groups or to counseling if indicated (any visit).

CLIENT AND FAMILY/CAREGIVER INTERVENTIONS

1. Client attempts to prevent or discourage stressful situations and noxious stimuli.
2. Client practices guided imagery and visualization techniques during stressful and nonstressful episodes.
3. Client identifies present coping skills and refines or develops more effective ones to decrease anxiety.
4. Client has someone present during attack so that he or she is not alone; has telephone numbers for emergency assistance nearby and available.
5. Client asks questions about condition and reason for treatments if needed.

6. Client consults physician if unable to control anxiety and respirations are affected.
7. Client consults psychological counselor to control breathing pattern and reduce anxiety if necessary.

Nursing diagnosis

Ineffective airway clearance

Related factors: Tracheobronchial secretions, obstruction

Defining characteristics: Altered breath sounds (wheezing), changes in rate or depth of respirations, cough with or without sputum, excessive mucus, dyspnea

OUTCOMES

Short-term

Adequate oxygenation, as evidenced by respiratory rate, depth, and ease within baseline determinations; usual speech pattern; absence of dyspnea, cough, or wheezing; absence of complaints of chest tightness, pressure, or feelings of suffocation; pulse and blood pressure within preestablished baselines; airway clear of mucus, with chest clear and with normal breath sounds and air movement; skin pink, warm, and dry (expected within 1 to 2 days)

Long-term

Adequate respiratory functioning, as evidenced by breathing with optimal level of ease necessary to maintain desired or limited lifestyle (expected within 1 to 2 weeks)

NURSING INTERVENTIONS/INSTRUCTIONS

1. Assess respiratory status, rate, depth, and ease; wheezing that is more pronounced on expiration; dyspnea; difficulty in speaking; use of accessory muscles; hyperinflated appearance of chest; cough; tachycardia; diaphoresis; and factors that precipitate these signs and symptoms (see Pulmonary System Assessment, p. 6) (each visit).
2. Instruct client to take own respirations and pulse and record in log; allow for return demonstration (first visit).

3. Instruct client to avoid known allergens, noxious stimuli, emotional stressors, and environmental temperature changes (first visit).
4. Assess effect of activity on respiratory status and energy level; reinforce need to exercise moderately and regularly and to maintain activity tolerance. Instruct client to pace activities and rest if breathing is affected (first visit).
5. Instruct client in positioning during rest or sleep, generally semi-Fowler's (first visit).
6. Instruct client in breathing exercises (first and second visits).
7. Instruct client to drink 2 to 3 liters (2 to 3 quarts or 10 to 12 glasses) of fluid daily unless restricted (first visit).
8. Administer oxygen by nasal cannula at 2 L/min as ordered, using compressed cylinder, concentrator, or liquid system; instruct in self-administration, safety precautions, and care of equipment (each visit).
9. Instruct client in use of humidifier, incentive spirometer, nebulizer, and handheld inhaler (first visit).
10. Instruct client in use of prophylactic cromolyn bronchodilators (oral and inhalation), steroids, mucolytics, and expectorants; include dose, time, frequency, food and drug interactions, method of administration, and side effects. Instruct client to stop drug and call physician if side effects occur (first visit; reinstruct on second visit).
11. Initiate referral to respiratory therapist and durable equipment company as indicated (first visit).

CLIENT AND FAMILY/CAREGIVER INTERVENTIONS

1. Client and caregiver take and record rate and depth of respirations twice daily and log any changes in breathing pattern.
2. Client performs deep breathing and physical exercise regimen daily.
3. Client uses humidifier and breathing apparatus as ordered.
4. Client and caregiver safely administer oxygen by cannula when needed.
5. Client maintains predetermined fluid intake over 24 hours.
6. Administer medications correctly by proper route. Client avoids taking any other drugs unless approved by physician;

reports any adverse effects of medication to physician; carries bronchodilator inhaler at all times.

7. Client has laboratory tests for theophylline level when ordered.
8. Client avoids exposure to allergens and irritants, including house dust, dirty heating or air conditioning filters, pet hair, molds, pollens, and environmental pollutants; eliminates offending foods, odors, passive smoking, and other known irritants.
9. Client wears identification bracelet or carries card with information about condition, medications, and allergies.
10. Client is referred to American Lung Association and self-help groups for information and support.

Nursing diagnosis

Risk for infection

Related factors: Inadequate primary defenses (decrease in ciliary action, stasis of body fluids); chronic disease; increased environmental exposure to infectious agents

Defining characteristics: Inability to mobilize and remove secretions, change in sputum color and breathing pattern, temperature elevation, chest pain

OUTCOMES

Short-term

Prevention of respiratory infection, as evidenced by normal range of temperature; sputum clear, thin, and easily coughed up and removed (expected with daily assessment)

Long-term

Maintenance of a pulmonary system free of acute infection (acute bronchitis, pneumonia, influenza) (expected to be ongoing).

NURSING INTERVENTIONS/INSTRUCTIONS

1. Assess temperature for elevation; note amount and characteristics of sputum and compare with tenacious, yellowish or green or brown sputum of infectious process (each visit).

2. Instruct client to avoid exposure to infection potential (first visit).
3. Instruct client in administration of antiinfectives, including dose, frequency, method, route, food and drug interactions, and side effects (first visit).

CLIENT AND FAMILY/CAREGIVER INTERVENTIONS

1. Client takes temperature if feeling chilled or experiencing malaise or if sputum changes color, and reports to physician.
2. Client avoids exposure to persons with upper respiratory or pulmonary infections.
3. Client and caregiver maintain an environment that is free of irritants, well ventilated, and of optimal temperature and humidity.
4. Client covers mouth and nose when sneezing and coughing. Client disposes of tissues and contaminated articles in a waterproof bag; seals and disposes of properly.
5. Client washes hands frequently and when necessary to prevent transmission of infectious agents.
6. Client disinfects reusable equipment and supplies; air dries and stores in clean plastic bag.
7. Client administers prescribed antiinfectives correctly; takes full course of medication, and reports responses.

Nursing diagnosis

Ineffective management of therapeutic regimen (individual)

Related factors: Excessive demands made on individual; decisional conflicts

Defining characteristics: Inappropriate choices of daily living for meeting the goals of a treatment or prevention program; verbalization that client did not take actions to include treatment regimens in daily routines or take actions to reduce risk factors for exacerbation of illness

OUTCOMES

Short-term

Performance of health behaviors consistent with therapeutic regimen, as evidenced by verbalization of specific behaviors needed for optimal health and prevention of complications or exacerbation of symptoms (expected within 1 week)

Long-term

Compliance with management of therapeutic regimen, as evidenced by active participation in therapy, demonstration of health behaviors consistent with goals of therapy, and dealing with social situations that oppose or present a conflict with regimen (expected within 1 month and ongoing)

NURSING INTERVENTIONS/INSTRUCTIONS

1. Provide client with detailed written instructions and a plan for specific behavior, such as medications via oral and inhalation routes, control of activity and environment, respiratory exercises, foods and other allergens to avoid, and other measures specific to client (first visit).
2. Advise client to use reminders or clues to perform or change a behavior (first visit).
3. Instruct client in monitoring behavior(s) regularly and recording for analysis and in need for alternative behavior(s) or strengthening behavior(s) (first and second visits).
4. Instruct client in use of a structured method of performing aspects of therapeutic regimen, such as a checklist, calendar, or pill dispenser (first visit and reinforce second visit).
5. Encourage client to seek ongoing support groups for long-term opportunities to reinforce behavior(s) and comply with regimen (any visit).

CLIENT AND FAMILY/CAREGIVER INTERVENTIONS

1. Client demonstrates accurate performance of specific health behavior(s) consistent with goals of therapeutic regimen.
2. Client engages in activities that assist in compliance with therapeutic regimen and strengthen coping ability.
3. Client uses alternative resources and support groups.
4. Client verbalizes plan to deal with situations that oppose therapeutic goals and exacerbate condition.
5. Client verbalizes, plans, and performs specific health-related activity, with recording and analysis of behavior(s) to modify.

Chronic Obstructive Pulmonary Disease (COPD)

Chronic obstructive pulmonary disease is a progressive disorder of the lungs and airways. It includes diseases such as emphysema and chronic bronchitis. The disorder is characterized by long-term destruction of the walls of the alveoli, which affects oxygen and carbon dioxide gas exchange, and chronic inflammation and narrowing of the bronchioles, affecting air outflow. COPD is caused by smoking, air and chemical pollutants, α_1-antitrypsin deficiency, and the aging process. Changes in the respiratory system associated with the aging process, such as loss of elasticity, decreased vital capacity, and increased residual air, contribute to the prevalence and severity of the disorder.

Home care is primarily concerned with the teaching of medication regimens, which involve various routes, depending on the progression and severity of the disease; the maintenance of daily well-being as the disease progresses to the end stage; and the use of assistive mechanical ventilation. Emphasis is also placed on infection protection and control.

Nursing diagnosis

Anxiety

Related factors: Threat of death; change in health status

Defining characteristics: Apprehension, uncertainty about outcome, fear of suffocation, increased helplessness and tension

OUTCOMES

Short-term

Reduction in anxiety level, as evidenced by verbalization of anxiety and concerns and their causes; anxiety reduced and within manageable level during dyspneic episodes (expected within 2 days)

Long-term

Anxiety reduced and controlled, as evidenced by avoidance of anxiety-producing situations and by positive responses to therapy (expected within 1 month)

NURSING INTERVENTIONS/INSTRUCTIONS

1. Assess mental and emotional status and effect of stressors on breathing and life-style; inner personal resources and ability to cope and respond to treatment; environment for excessive stimuli (first visit).
2. Provide an accepting environment for expression of anxiety and concerns (each visit).
3. Identify coping mechanisms used by client and encourage client to use those that are effective (each visit).
4. Instruct client in relaxation techniques, music, guided imagery, and the use of autogenic technique during periods of dyspnea (first and second visits).
5. Instruct client to avoid stressful situations, excessive activity, and medications that are taken for anxiety that affect respiration (first visit).
6. Provide client with continuing information about status or condition, improvements, and treatments, and answer all questions (each visit).
7. Initiate referral to counseling or psychotherapy as indicated (any visit).

CLIENT AND FAMILY/CAREGIVER INTERVENTIONS

1. Caregiver maintains calm, caring attitude during episodes of dyspnea; stays with client.
2. Client attempts to prevent or discourage stressful situations.
3. Client develops and uses effective coping skills that decrease anxiety.
4. Client asks questions about medications, equipment, or the disease when information is needed.
5. Client adapts to chronic illness and long-term treatments.
6. Client seeks out assistance from psychotherapist to manage anxiety.

7. Client consults physician if unable to control anxiety and respiration is affected.

Nursing diagnosis

Ineffective breathing pattern

Related factors: Anxiety; decreased energy and fatigue; decreased lung expansion; tracheobronchial obstruction

Defining characteristics: Dyspnea; tachypnea; cough with or without sputum; changes in rate and depth of respiration; use of accessory muscles; altered chest excursion; crackles, rhonchi; assumption of three-point position; prolonged expiratory phase; increased anteroposterior diameter of chest; abnormal arterial blood gas levels

OUTCOMES

Short-term

Return to adequate breathing pattern and airway clearance, as evidenced by satisfactory respiratory rate, ease, and depth at baseline and by reduction in dyspneic episodes, hypoxia, stasis of secretions, and abnormal breath sounds (expected within 1 to 2 days)

Long-term

Maintenance of respiratory baselines, evidenced by breathing at optimal level within disease parameters (expected within 1 month)

NURSING INTERVENTIONS/INSTRUCTIONS

1. Assess respiratory status, including rate, depth, and ease; presence of dyspnea; use of accessory muscles, with lengthened expiratory phase; energy and fatigue level; ability to mobilize and remove secretions by coughing; breath sounds on auscultation for crackles or wheezes; hyperresonance on percussion; tactile fremitus (see Pulmonary System Assessment, p. 6, for guidelines) (each visit).
2. Provide postural drainage using gravity and percussion, avoiding any positions that may compromise the elderly client (first visit and as needed).

3. Instruct client to drink 2 to 3 liters (10 to 12 glasses) of fluids per day, unless restricted, and to follow an activity regimen within tolerance level (first visit).
4. Demonstrate for and instruct client in deep breathing and coughing exercises, with pursed-lip breathing and abdominal breathing (first visit).
5. Inform client of positions for sleeping that will allow for ease in breathing and chest expansion (first visit).
6. Instruct client in administration of oral bronchodilators; use of small-volume nebulizer and handheld measured-dose inhaler (carry at all times); and administration of corticosteroids orally and by handheld measured-dose inhaler (first visit).
7. Instruct client in oxygen administration via nasal cannula from compressed cylinder, concentrator, or liquid oxygen system (first and second visits).
8. Encourage continued participation in pulmonary rehabilitation program at home (first visit).
9. Initiate referral to respiratory therapist and durable medical equipment agency (first visit).
10. Instruct client to cease smoking and to enter program for support if necessary.
11. Draw blood sample, or advise client to visit laboratory, for theophylline level check when ordered by physician.
12. Report to physician dyspnea not controlled by medication, inability to clear secretions from airway, confusion, or change in mentation.
13. Instruct client to wear identification bracelet or carry card in purse or wallet stating condition and medications.
14. Instruct client to utilize American Lung Association for information and support services.

CLIENT AND FAMILY/CAREGIVER INTERVENTIONS

1. Assess respiration for rate and ease twice daily.
2. Perform deep breathing exercises, four breaths 4 times per day.
3. Perform isometric exercises to strengthen diaphragm and intercostal muscles and lift 3-pound weights for upper-body strengthening daily as part of a pulmonary rehabilitation regimen, which should also include swimming, walking, or bicycling.
4. Maintain fluid intake of 8 to 10 glasses per day unless restricted.

5. Use positioning and foam-rubber wedge or pillows for sleeping.
6. Administer medications correctly; avoid over-the-counter drugs unless advised by physician; report adverse effects to physician.
7. Administer oxygen correctly at 2 to 3 L/min (portable and stationary), and take safety precautions in presence of oxygen.
8. Avoid exposure to outside and home pollutants, such as sprays, fumes, smog or particulates in air, pet hair, or other allergens.
9. Use humidification in home and change air conditioner and furnace filters monthly. Humidification unit and filter should be cleaned weekly.

Nursing diagnosis

Activity intolerance

Related factors: Generalized weakness; sedentary life-style; imbalance between oxygen supply and demand

Defining characteristics: Tired, weak feeling; fatigue, exertional discomfort and dyspnea; awakening caused by dyspnea; hypoxia; increased pulse rate and blood pressure during activity

OUTCOMES

Short-term

Increased endurance and ability to perform ADL, as evidenced by maintenance of respiration, pulse, and blood pressure while independently caring for self and performing routine tasks (expected within 1 week)

Long-term

Optimal activity level achieved and maintained within baseline respiratory and energy parameters (expected to be ongoing)

NURSING INTERVENTIONS/INSTRUCTIONS

1. Assess activity tolerance, pulse, and respirations before and after activity; assess for presence of dyspnea and increased work of breathing during activity; assess amount of sleep and rest (first visit).

2. Instruct client to rest after each activity and to pace activities around rest periods and use of bronchodilator (first visit).
3. Instruct client to use oxygen during activities if appropriate (first visit).
4. Instruct client in use of energy-saving devices and aids (first and second visits).
5. Instruct client to build endurance by increasing activities every 2 to 3 days (each visit).
6. Arrange for home health aide (HHA) visits to assist with ADL.

CLIENT AND FAMILY/CAREGIVER INTERVENTIONS

1. Client exercises moderately and for short periods of time, as tolerated, and increases as energy and endurance increase.
2. Client takes pulse before and after activity; checks for increases of 10 or more beats/min.
3. Client rests every 3 hours and following activity such as bathing, walking, or using stairs.
4. Client uses stool to sit in shower, arm rests, aids for dressing, hand bars for support, aids for reaching and walking, wheelchair if necessary.
5. Client uses inhaler before activity; performs activity when systemic bronchodilator is at optimal effect.
6. Client asks for assistance in ADL.
7. Client uses proper inspiration and expiration pattern when participating in an activity, such as lifting during expiration.
8. Client avoids continuing activity if dyspneic or fatigued.

Nursing diagnosis

Risk for infection

Related factors: Inadequate primary defenses; chronic disease

Defining characteristics: Stasis of secretions, inability to mobilize and remove secretions, loss of ciliary action, reduced pulmonary macrophages

OUTCOMES

Short-term

Prevention of pulmonary infection, as evidenced by normal temperature and sputum that is clear and thin for easy removal (expected with daily assessment)

Long-term

Maintenance of pulmonary system free from acute infection (expected to be ongoing)

NURSING INTERVENTIONS/INSTRUCTIONS

1. Assess for temperature elevation, chest pain, change in color of sputum to yellow or green, and increased viscosity (each visit).
2. Instruct client in antibiotic administration (first visit).
3. Inform client of precautions to take to avoid exposure to potential infection (first visit).

CLIENT AND FAMILY/CAREGIVER INTERVENTIONS

1. Client takes temperature if feeling chilled and sputum changes color.
2. Client avoids smoking and exposure to groups or to persons with upper respiratory infections.
3. Client washes hands frequently, especially before treatments or eating and after using tissues for coughing and expectorating.
4. Client covers nose and mouth when coughing; disposes of tissues in bag that is waterproof; seals and discards daily.
5. Client and caregiver maintain environment that is humidified and well ventilated.
6. Client secures pneumonia and flu immunizations.
7. Client washes, rinses, and disinfects reusable equipment and supplies; air dries on clean toweling or hangs over shower rail.
8. Client discards disposable supplies in sealed waterproof bag.
9. Client reports temperature elevation, chills, yellow or green sputum, or chest pain to physician.
10. Client takes prescribed antibiotics at proper intervals around the clock until all is used.

Pneumonia

Pneumonia is an inflammation of the lungs caused by bacteria, viruses, fungi, or protozoa. It may also be caused by aspiration of food, water, or gastric contents into the alveolar system. It is usually the result of an upper respiratory infection and may involve segments, a lobe, or an entire lung. The disease progresses from an initial filling of the alveoli and bronchioles with exudate to consolidation of the lung area as leukocytes attempt to destroy the organisms. The disease is especially life threatening in the elderly or chronically ill.

Home care is primarily concerned with teaching of medication regimen (antiinfectives based on identified causative pathogen) and prevention of complications.

Nursing diagnosis

Ineffective breathing pattern

Related factors: Chest pain; decreased energy and fatigue; inflammatory process; tracheobronchial obstruction

Defining characteristics: Dyspnea; tachypnea; respiratory depth changes; altered chest excursion; diminished breath sounds; cough with tenacious, purulent sputum; abnormal arterial blood gas values

OUTCOMES

Short-term

Adequate oxygenation, as evidenced by respiratory rate, depth, and ease within normal baseline determinations, absence of dyspnea, cough less frequent, chest clear with normal breath sounds and air movement (expected within 7 to 10 days)

Long-term

Adequate respiratory functioning, as evidenced by breathing with optimal level of ease to maintain usual life-style (expected within 1 month)

NURSING INTERVENTIONS/INSTRUCTIONS

1. Assess physical status of respiratory system (see Pulmonary System Assessment, p. 6, for guidelines); note life-style, history, and trends (e.g., frequent upper respiratory infections, chronic respiratory disease, chronic illness, smoking, alcoholism, immunosuppressive therapy) to identify predisposing factors and to determine their implications for care and future teaching (first visit).

2. Monitor respirations for ease, rate, and depth; auscultate and percuss chest for diminished breath sounds and dullness (each visit). Instruct client to take respirations and record in log (first visit).
3. Assess skin color, constitutional symptoms, chills and fever, and pleuritic chest pain, and note sputum and its viscosity, amount, and change in color (each visit).
4. Assess fluid maintenance needs on the basis of age, weight and height, sex, general health, and insensible fluid losses. Instruct client to double maintenance needs, unless his or her status would be compromised (as with an elderly client or a client who has a cardiac or renal disorder) (first visit).
5. Note allergies to medications and instruct client in antiinfective therapy (penicillins, cephalosporins, oxacillin, nafcillin, tetracycline, erythromycin, lincomycin or clindamycin), including dose, frequency, food or drug interactions, and side effects (first visit).
6. Instruct client in splinting, deep breathing and coughing exercises, and how to expectorate; allow for return demonstration (each visit).
7. Monitor sputum culture results and x-ray results as available.
8. Refer client to respiratory therapy as indicated.
9. Instruct client to avoid indiscriminant or trivial use of antibiotics (last visit).
10. Suggest visit to physician for influenza and pneumonia immunizations, especially if client is elderly (last visit).

CLIENT AND FAMILY/CAREGIVER INTERVENTIONS

1. Client takes respirations and records in log.
2. Client monitors sputum (not saliva) and reports changes in color, amount, or consistency to physician.
3. Client administers antiinfective, antitussive, and expectorant as ordered and takes complete course of antiinfective prescription.
4. Client drinks predetermined amount of liquid at specified intervals over 24 hours.
5. Client and caretaker humidify environment; maintain optimal temperature and ventilation of environment.
6. Client performs deep breathing and coughing exercises 3 to 4 times per day as tolerated.
7. Client disposes of used tissues properly and washes hands when appropriate.

Nursing diagnosis

Hyperthermia

Related factors: Illness

Defining characteristics: Increase in body temperature above normal range; increased respiratory rate

OUTCOMES

Short-term

Absence of temperature elevation, as evidenced by normal temperature and absence of chills, shaking, or diaphoresis (expected within 3 to 4 days)

Long-term

Afebrile; comfort at optimal level without recurrence of temperature elevation (expected within 1 week to 1 month)

NURSING INTERVENTIONS/INSTRUCTIONS

1. Monitor temperature for deviations from normal and instruct client to take own temperature and record in log and to return demonstration (first visit).
2. Assess for presence of chills and diaphoresis with temperature elevation (each visit).
3. Supervise administration of antiinfectives (first visit; reinstruct on second visit).
4. Instruct client in administration of antipyretics on the basis of temperature elevation (first visit).
5. Instruct client in use of sponge bath and appropriate clothing and room temperature for comfort (first visit).
6. As temperature decreases, monitor white blood cell (WBC) count and sputum culture results if available.

CLIENT AND FAMILY/CAREGIVER INTERVENTIONS

1. Client takes temperature twice daily, when feeling chilled or as needed, and records in log.
2. Client takes antipyretics correctly.
3. Client maintains increased fluid intake unless restricted.
4. Client bathes by sponging or tub bath; maintains dry linens and room free of drafts at comfortable temperature and ventilation.

Nursing diagnosis

Pain

Related factors: Injuring agent of inflammatory process

Defining characteristics: Verbal expression of pain descriptors; holding chest to guard or protect it; changes in respiratory pattern

OUTCOMES

Short-term

Control of pain, as evidenced by relaxed expression and posture, effortless respiration, and statements that pain has been relieved (expected within 2 to 7 days)

Long-term

Optimal comfort level, as evidenced by continued freedom from pain during respiration or ADL (expected within 1 week to 1 month)

NURSING INTERVENTIONS/INSTRUCTIONS

1. Assess pain location, frequency, severity, and characteristics and its relationship to condition and activity (each visit).
2. Instruct client in proper splinting (position, comfort, aids) before coughing and deep breathing exercises (first visit).
3. Instruct client in administration of mild analgesic 1 hour before pulmonary exercises and before pain becomes severe (first visit).
4. Encourage rest periods and pacing of activities (first visit).

CLIENT AND FAMILY/CAREGIVER INTERVENTIONS

1. Caregiver provides rest; assists with ADL.
2. Client administers analgesic correctly; avoids use if it affects respiration.
3. Client schedules activities around medication administration.
4. Client notifies physician if pain persists or symptoms escalate.
5. Client takes time to participate in activities; rests when needed, and resumes activity if possible.

Nursing diagnosis

Risk for activity intolerance

Related factors: Presence of respiratory disease; deconditioned status; work of breathing (weakness, fatigue)

Defining characteristics: Weakness, fatigue, inability to perform ADL

OUTCOMES

Short-term

Minimal fatigue expressed and increased activity tolerance as measured by increasing periods of wakefulness and progressive ability to perform ADL without fatigue (expected within 1 week)

Long-term

Independence in return to self-care, as evidenced by optimal level of care achieved and return to wellness (expected in 1 month)

NURSING INTERVENTIONS/INSTRUCTIONS

1. Obtain history, including ADL, levels of independence and endurance, family assistance and support (first visit).
2. Instruct client in performing personal hygiene and comfort measures; stress accessibility to personal items needed for care and to ask for assistance when needed (first visit).
3. Provide privacy, encourage rest, and instruct client to progressively increase activity at own pace (first and second visits).
4. Instruct client to exercise moderately for short periods of time as tolerated (first visit).

CLIENT AND FAMILY/CAREGIVER INTERVENTIONS

1. Client performs daily personal care with assistance or independently as able, without rushing and at tolerable pace.
2. Client schedules periods of activity and rest on the basis of endurance and individual need.

Nursing diagnosis

Knowledge deficit

Related factors: Lack of information about disease, preventive measures, relapse, or complications

Defining characteristics: Expression of need for information about disease process, causes, risk for reinfection or other complications

OUTCOMES

Short-term

Adequate knowledge, as evidenced by statements of signs and symptoms of disease, transmission and causes of disease, complications of disease, and actions to take (expected within 3 to 7 days)

Long-term

Adequate knowledge, as evidenced by client's meeting requirements to achieve optimal level of health and functioning during progress to wellness (expected within 1 month)

NURSING INTERVENTIONS/INSTRUCTIONS

1. Assess life-style and ability to adapt, learning abilities and interests, family participation and support (first visit).
2. Instruct client to avoid exposure to upper respiratory infections, smoking, and changes in environmental temperature (first visit).
3. Instruct client in signs and symptoms and complications that may occur (e.g., chest pain, dyspnea, persistent temperature) and to report to physician (first visit).
4. Initiate referral to social services and support groups for educational materials and to stop smoking (first visit).
5. Suggest influenza and pneumonia immunization if appropriate (last visit).

CLIENT AND FAMILY/CAREGIVER INTERVENTIONS

1. Client avoids respiratory irritants, persons with infections, cigarette or cigar smoke.
2. Client complies with suggested physician visits for follow-up evaluation and to report any complaints.

3. Client contacts and participates in community support groups focusing on respiratory health.
4. If elderly, client secures influenza and pneumonia immunizations.

Mechanical Ventilation/ Tracheostomy

Mechanical ventilation, also known as artificial or assisted ventilation, is a method of applying positive or negative pressure to support inflation of the lungs. It can provide temporary or permanent assistance to take over the action of the diaphragm and chest wall muscles. Clients with neuromuscular, skeletal, or hypoventilation conditions are candidates for part-time or continuous 24-hour assisted ventilation, depending on the status or severity of the disease. Negative pressure devices are applied to the outside of the chest wall to pull it out and initiate inspiration to allow respiratory muscles to rest. Positive pressure ventilators increase airway pressure above atmospheric pressure to inflate the lungs by pushing a volume of air into the lungs during inspiration and improve gas exchange by better distribution of gases within the lung. They can be invasive (artificial airway such as a tracheostomy tube) or noninvasive (facial or nasal mask). These are the most common type of ventilators used in the home and are small, portable, and easily moved within the environment. The type of ventilator selected depends on the medical diagnosis and is based on regulating the cycle (pressure, volume, and time cycled) prior to discharge from the hospital, daily requirements, needed oxygen concentration, and resources to acquire, maintain, and repair the equipment.

A tracheostomy is a surgically created opening in the skin of the neck and into the trachea (between the second and fourth tracheal cartilage rings) to allow for passage of air in and out of the airways. It is performed when upper airway obstruction is present (infections, edema, tumor, foreign body); in cases of underlying pulmonary disease; following lung, larynx, neck, or cardiac surgery; or in conditions that require long-term assisted ventilation. It can be temporary or permanent with a healed stoma (laryngectomy) related to the reason for the procedure. Tracheostomy tubes are made of plastic or metal (nondisposable) and consist of an inner and outer cannula. The tube can be cuffed or without a cuff and have a fenestration for those able to speak when off the ventilator.

Home care is concerned primarily with total management of the ventilator-dependent client and the various levels of interventions needed to preserve respiratory status and to support the psychophysiologic adaptive capacities of the client and family. Essential is the assessment and instruction in the management of tracheostomy care with prevention of skin, tube, or infection complications (patent inner cannula, change of tube, stoma care, inflation of cuff), ventilator monitoring (settings, alarms, patency and cleanliness of circuitry, troubleshooting), and activities of daily living and special needs (alternate feeding pattern, urinary catheter, ambulation, and other activities). Of additional importance is the ability and capacities of the family to become trained and participate in the total care of the technology-dependent client.

Nursing diagnosis

Anxiety/fear (client and family)

Related factors: Change in health status; presence of ventilator and tracheostomy; threat of death; threatening situations (tube obstruction or accidental dislodgment, ventilator dysfunction)

Defining characteristics: Difficult breathing, feeling of fear of suffocation, apprehension, restlessness, facial tension, inability to speak, fear of responsibility of providing tracheostomy care

OUTCOMES

Short-term

Progressive reduction in anxiety and fear associated with care of tracheostomy, as evidenced by verbalizing increased ability to remain calm and by acquaintance with and competence in care measures as needed (expected within 2 to 4 weeks)

Long-term

Fear and anxiety at a manageable level, as evidenced by effective and ongoing support and performance of adequate care required for ventilator and tracheostomy (expected within 1 month and ongoing)

NURSING INTERVENTIONS/INSTRUCTIONS

1. Assess emotional and mental status of client and family members and their ability to adapt to the presence of assisted ventilation/tracheostomy, anxiety, fear, and concerns about care (see Psychosocial Assessment, p. 7, for guidelines) (first and any visit as needed).
2. Provide information about reasons for assisted ventilation, inform of treatments and procedures involved in home management and how the client's safety and comfort will be facilitated; use easily understandable language (first and second visits).
3. Maintain a calm, quiet environment and comfort client who is fearful when unable to produce sounds and inform that voice will return when the tube is removed, if temporary and if speech rehabilitation is provided, or when off ventilator as appropriate (first visit).
4. Provide opportunity for family and/or caregiver to verbalize fears and concerns, encourage modes of communication to replace lack of vocal sounds (each visit).
5. Suggest that caregiver stay with client during anxious times (first visit).
6. Assist caregiver to reduce feelings of apprehension, anxiety, fear about the client's condition (each visit).
7. Provide link of communication between family and health professional referrals for information and problem solving (any visit as needed).
8. Initiate referral to a support group or community agency or to counseling as appropriate (any visit).

CLIENT AND FAMILY/CAREGIVER INTERVENTIONS

1. Client and family recognize anxiety associated with care of ventilator/tracheostomy, possibility of tube obstruction or other complications.
2. Client and family verbalize anxiety, frustration, fatigue, and stress related to management of total care.

3. Client and family maintain calm, supportive environment, controls stimuli.
4. Client and family use relaxation techniques such as music, TV, reading, imaging.
5. Client and family use appropriate coping mechanisms and support resources if needed.

Nursing diagnosis

Ineffective breathing pattern/airway clearance/gas exchange/ risk for aspiration

Related factors: Decreased energy and fatigue; tracheobronchial obstruction (thick mucus); altered oxygen supply; loss of lung function; inflammatory/infectious process; decreased lung expansion; presence of tracheostomy tube; impaired swallowing

Defining characteristics: Dyspnea, tachypnea, use of accessory muscles (retractions), nasal flaring, grunting, cyanosis ("dusky" skin color), tachycardia, irritability, diaphoresis, elevated temperature, restlessness, abnormal breath sounds (crackles or ronchi), inability to clear increased thick secretions, hypoxia, hypercapnia, elevated peak inspiratory pressure on ventilator or ventilator asynchrony, inability or refusal to remove and clean tube

OUTCOMES

Short-term

Optimal ventilator function and airway patency with adequate ventilation (caregiver response to alarms), and oxygenation (determined by pulse oximetry) via tracheostomy, as established and evidenced by clearance or removal of loosened secretions by cough or suction, prevention of tube dislodgment, maintenance of skin and mucous membrane color based on racial baseline parameters with absence of hypoxia, breath sounds clear and equal bilaterally, adequate rest, sleep, relaxation, and comfort (expected within 2 days and ongoing)

Long-term

Management of home respiratory care, as evidenced by respiratory baselines and gas exchange maintained with ventilator, absence of signs of respiratory distress with clear breath sounds, absence of injury associated with tracheostomy, complete and effective tracheostint care demonstrated, progressive withdrawal of oxygen and/or ventilation support when and if appropriate (expected within 1 month and ongoing)

NURSING INTERVENTIONS/INSTRUCTIONS

1. Explain importance of and ensure that caregiver has been trained in cardiopulmonary resuscitation (CPR) prior to hospital discharge; collaborate with caregiver to develop a protocol to activate emergency medical service (EMS) (first visit and reinforce on subsequent visits).
2. Assess caregiver knowledge and understanding of disease etiology, status and need for assisted ventilation, ability to adapt and manage ventilator and care of tracheostomy (first visit, continue on second visit).
3. Provide information and instruction in pulmonary assessment and signs and symptoms to note and collaborate with caregiver to plan daily care based on respiratory status; use language that is easily understood or provide written instructions (first visit, reinstruct in plan changes as needed).
4. Assess and instruct caregiver to assess and monitor respiratory status for distress, chest expansion for symmetry, counting respiratory rate with ventilator cycle and child's respiratory efforts that include absence or presence of effort, depth, and normal rate and rhythm to determine effectiveness of assisted ventilation and if settings need changing; include color of skin, oral mucous membranes, and nail beds for hypoxia; abnormal breath sounds on auscultation; presence and characteristics of secretions in assessment (see Pulmonary System Assessment, p. 6, for guidelines), (first and every visit).
5. Assess client comfort on ventilatory and follow orders for settings of rate, control or assist/control mode, tidal and sigh volume, fraction of inspired oxygen, peak flow, pressure limits; note stability of these parameters (each visit).
6. Assess and instruct caregiver to assess all ventilator connections, settings, alarms, and function daily and monitor for possible need in changes in ventilatory settings if infection or other stressors are present (first and every visit).
7. Instruct client in how to become synchronous with the ventilator; inform caregiver to stay with client and provide

emotional support when anxious (first and repeat on second visit).

8. Instruct caregiver in the daily cleaning and changing of the circuits, the machine, the suctioning equipment and supplies, and the resuscitation bag (first visit and reinstruct second visit and as needed).
9. Administer and assist and instruct caregiver to provide supplemental humidified oxygen with ventilator via tracheostomy, based on ordered pressure input and flow rate requirements of the ventilator, and portability and availability of the oxygen system; advise caregiver to have a portable oxygen unit and resuscitation bag available (first and second visits).
10. Instruct client and caregiver in safety measures in use of oxygen (first visit).
11. Instruct caregiver to humidify inspired air by cascade, jet nebulizer, or humidifier to prevent drying of secretions and loss of body fluids and heat (first visit).
12. Instruct client and caregiver in medications administration ordered in conjunction with ventilation therapy (first and each visit as needed).
13. Instruct caregiver in tracheostomy tube care, including changing and cleaning inner tracheostomy tube and ties; perform the procedure for tube removal, cleansing and disinfecting, and reinsertion to remove mucus accumulation and to maintain airway patency (first visit and subsequent visits based on need).
14. Instruct caregiver in suction of secretions using clean technique if unable to remove by coughing via tube at the correct amount of pressure, correct number of thrusts for appropriate amount of time, and using resuscitation bag to preoxygenate and between each suctioning event (first visit and subsequent visits based on auscultation or sounds of gurgling).
15. Instruct client and caregiver to assess for possible tube dislodgement or decannulation and measures to take to secure tube, adjust ties; assist in devising an emergency kit containing an extra tube, clean ties, suction tube, and scissors to keep on hand and nearby (first and second visits).
16. Instruct client and caregiver in deflation when off the ventilator and during food ingestion, regardless of the method, and reinflation of cuff when on the ventilator (first and second visit).

17. Instruct caregiver to offer small amounts of easy-to-swallow food and to place client in upright position during meals to prevent aspiration or to perform nasogastric feedings as appropriate (first visit).
18. Demonstrate elevation of the head of the bed, positions of optimal comfort for sleeping and resting that will allow for diaphragmatic movement and chest expansion (first visit).
19. Provide information and instruction using language that is easily understood and provide written instructions and care plan (first visit, reinforce regularly).
20. Assess response to ventilatory assistance and tracheostomy status and report untoward responses or any deviations from the established norm to the physician (each visit).
21. Suggest loose, nonrestrictive clothing near neck (first visit).
22. Inform caregiver and family of availability of American Lung Association and local support groups for information and services (first visit).

CLIENT AND FAMILY/CAREGIVER INTERVENTIONS

1. Caregiver becomes CPR certified prior to client's discharge from hospital, obtains training in emergency procedures associated with ventilator, places list of emergency activities and telephone numbers in strategic place for easy access.
2. Caregiver completes training or classes in all aspects of care prior to independent care of client receiving assisted ventilation.
3. Caregiver locates a resource and acquires special equipment and supplies (oxygen source and back-up tank with gauge, ventilator and accessories, suctioning equipment and supplies, extra tracheostomy tubes, ties, dressings); collaborates with social services to secure financial assistance if needed
4. Caregiver develops trust in home care providers (nurse, respiratory therapist, nursing assistant) and confidence in own competence in managing total care.
5. Caregiver verbalizes understanding and rationale for physical care, airway management, treatments and procedures, and need for constant monitoring.
6. Caregiver assesses respirations for rate and effort compared to ventilator effectiveness, client's color during suctioning, and signs of respiratory distress or deterioration to report.

7. Caregiver demonstrates maintenance of ventilator function using ventilator checklist; complies with treatments, monitoring schedules, equipment care and cleaning.
8. Caregiver correctly administers humidified oxygen (continuous or intermittent) and use of resuscitation bag when needed, provides adequate humidification to airway by increasing humidity to environment.
9. Caregiver follows safety precautions in oxygen use, including posting a sign stating oxygen in use, no sparks, no open flames, no oil or grease, no smoking.
10. Caregiver reviews potential nonmedical problem solving or troubleshooting of equipment malfunction, management of ventilator settings, and alarms outlined in the manufacturer's guidelines and corrective actions to take.
11. Caregiver provides tracheostomy tube care, removes ties and tube, cleanses with soapy water and pipe cleaners and rinses with water, reinserts, secures in place with clean ties; inflates or deflates cuff as appropriate.
12. Caregiver suctions tracheostomy at correct pressure and length of time as frequently as needed using clean technique to remove thick mucus or mucus that is difficult to cough up or if respiratory status changes as a result of airway obstruction caused by mucus accumulation.
13. Caregiver cleanses reusable suction catheter and tracheostomy tube with soap and water and stores in clean plastic bags.
14. Caregiver ensures availability of portable suction apparatus with back-up batteries, portable oxygen tank, and resuscitation bag on hand.
15. Caregiver positions client with foam-rubber wedge or pillows to elevate head for sleep and rest, reports change in mentation or orientation following naps or changes in sleep patterns caused by hypercapnia.
16. Caregiver provides rest prior to frequent small high-caloric meals.
17. Client complies with ordered medication regimen.
18. Caregiver provides oral care for mouth dryness and comfort.
19. Caregiver and client make list of questions to ask for each home care visit.
20. Caregiver identifies any deterioration in respiratory status and reports to physician in a timely manner.

21. Caregiver notifies local electric company and emergency services of client on ventilator.
22. Caregiver utilizes emergency services when life-threatening changes occur and cannot be resolved.

Nursing diagnosis

Risk for infection

Related factors: Inadequate primary defenses (stasis of secretions); invasive procedure (tracheostomy); insufficient knowledge of caregiver to avoid exposure of client to pathogens

Defining characteristics: Ineffective cough to remove secretions, change in odor and color of secretions from tracheostomy to yellow or green, increased secretions, temperature elevation

OUTCOMES

Short-term

Early detection of signs and symptoms of respiratory infection and use of clean technique to perform procedures, as evidenced by airway patency with colorless and odorless secretions removed, afebrile status (expected with daily assessment)

Long-term

Adaptation to a life-style that promotes a clean, safe environment and preventive measures performed to minimize risk for pulmonary infections, as evidenced by patent, infection-free respiratory system (expected to be ongoing)

NURSING INTERVENTIONS/INSTRUCTIONS

1. Assess home and living hygienic conditions (see Environmental Assessment, p. 53 for guidelines) (first visit and follow up for additional modifications on second visit).
2. Assess for changes in respiratory status and for diminished breath sounds on auscultation, changes in oxygen saturation (each visit).
3. Assess temperature for increases or decreases from baseline norm, increased viscosity, change in color or odor of secretions from trachesotomy that indicate pulmonary infection (each visit).

4. Instruct caregiver in taking axillary temperature (first visit).
5. Instruct caregiver in washing hands and importance of washing hands before and after care of a child.
6. Instruct caregiver in use of clean technique during tracheostomy suctioning procedure, cleansing tube, and changing dressing (first visit and review on subsequent visits).
7. Instruct caregiver in administration of ordered prophylactic or therapy and responses to expect with oral antibiotic and antipyretic in proper form based on ability to swallow (first visit and reinforce on subsequent visits).
8. Instruct client and caregiver in precautions to prevent infection, such as washing hands, and avoiding contact with those having an upper respiratory infection, and in importance of adequate nutritional intake and rest (first visit and ongoing).
9. Obtain sputum specimen if possible for culture if ordered (any visit).

CLIENT AND FAMILY/CAREGIVER INTERVENTIONS

1. Caregiver observes for yellow or green color, foul odor, or increased amount of sputum from tube, any blood from the tube and reports changes to the physician.
2. Caregiver suctions the tracheostomy using clean technique at correct suction pressure and length of time if mucus is copious or thick to prevent stasis.
3. Client or caregiver takes axillary temperature if sputum color or respirations change and reports elevations specified by physician.
4. Caregiver administers oral antibiotic therapy correctly until all medication is taken; notes and reports side effects.
5. Caregiver maintains personal hygiene and avoids use of contaminated articles when performing care and possible exposure of client to family members or others with suspected upper respiratory infections; wears face mask if appropriate.
6. Caregiver washes hands properly, especially before caring for client, uses clean technique during care and procedures and washes and stores supplies appropriately.
7. Caregiver properly disposes of all articles and supplies according to universal precautions.

Nursing diagnosis

Risk for impaired skin integrity

Related factors: External factor of irritants (secretions); mechanical pressure of tracheostomy tube

Defining characteristics: Moisture caused by secretions; irritation, excoriation, or damage of peristomal skin or tissue around tube insertion site; redness and accumulation of crusting at site

OUTCOMES

Short-term

Skin at tracheostomy site dry and intact, as evidenced by absence of redness, irritation, or bleeding, and pressure resulting from tube movement during care (expected within 1 to 2 days)

Long-term

Optimal skin integrity maintained, as evidenced by absence of any abnormal color, irritants, bleeding and breakdown at tracheostomy tube site, stenosis or strictures at the stoma site (expected within 1 week and ongoing)

NURSING INTERVENTIONS/INSTRUCTIONS

1. Assess skin at tube site for signs indicating risk for breakdown, such as excessive moisture, irritation and redness, rash, or excoriation, lack of cleanliness and crusting, tube not secured in proper position (see Integumentary System Assessment, p. 36 for guidelines) (first and every visit).
2. Demonstrate and instruct caregiver in assessing skin at least twice daily, cleansing procedure around tube and softening and removal of dried secretions twice/daily with careful attention to avoid manipulation of the tube; allow to return demonstration (first visit and reinstruct second visit if needed).
3. Instruct caregiver in application of antiseptic or antibiotic ointment at site if ordered (first visit).
4. Instruct and inform caregiver to change tracheostomy ties and pad when needed and rotate position of knots on ties to avoid pressure areas; allow to practice procedure under supervision (first and second visits).
5. Inform caregiver to increase environmental humidity to prevent dry skin and mucous membranes (first visit).

6. Instruct client to report any bleeding, rash, or excoriation at the tube site to the physician (first visit).

CLIENT AND FAMILY/CAREGIVER INTERVENTIONS

1. Caregiver assesses skin at tracheostomy site daily and reports changes or breakdown.
2. Caregiver maintains clean, dry, tracheostomy site with tube in secure position.
3. Caregiver avoids allowing secretions to accumulate or dry at tube site by cleansing, and redressing, changing ties and pad if wet, soiled, or loose.
4. Caregiver applies ointment or protective skin barrier at site as ordered.
5. Caregiver notes fit of tube and, if manipulation irritates site, consults with physician to replace tube if fit is not proper (too tight or loose).
6. Caregiver provides optimal humidity by cool room vaporizer to prevent drying or excess moisture of skin.

Nursing diagnosis

Impaired verbal communication

Related factors: Tracheostomy

Defining characteristics: Inability to speak with tube in place, unwilling to attempt other methods of communication

OUTCOMES

Short-term

Alternate modes of communication attempted, as evidenced by satisfactory nonverbal interactions among client, caregiver, family members (expected within 3 to 4 days)

Long-term

Effective method of communication adopted (expected within 1 week and ongoing)

NURSING INTERVENTIONS/INSTRUCTIONS

1. Assess client's, caregiver's and family's willingness to attempt different methods of communication, fenestrated tube in place,

adaptation to possible alternative methods of communications, coping skills and presence of frustration, anger, depression (first and subsequent visits as needed).

2. Assist or suggest various modes of communications, such as slate, paper and pencil, flash cards, and letters of the alphabet, to aid in communication compatible with preference or lifestyle (first and second visits).
3. Initiate order for speech pathologist consultant (any visit).

CLIENT AND FAMILY/CAREGIVER INTERVENTIONS

1. Client maintains effective use of alternate modes of communication, such as computer, magic slate, paper and pencil, hand grasps, signs and signals, eye blinking or movements, mouth sounds, picture cards.
2. Caregiver displays patience and anticipates client's needs.
3. Client speaks using valve device available for use on tracheostomy tube or in-line while on ventilator, with fenestrated tube in place in those able to be off the ventilator for a time and speak.

Nursing diagnosis

Impaired physical mobility

Related factors: Decreased strength and endurance; intolerance to activity and limited movement with ventilator use; anxiety

Defining characteristics: Inability to purposefully move within physical environment, imposed restriction of movement including mechanical apparatus, difficulty in performing ADL

OUTCOMES

Short-term

Progressive mobility independently or with assistance and with or without ventilator, evidenced by position changes, use of assistive aids (expected within 1 week)

Long-term

Optimal independent movement and use of extremities within level of endurance while attached to ventilator, evidenced by participation in self-care as able (expected within 3 weeks and ongoing)

NURSING INTERVENTIONS/INSTRUCTIONS

1. Assess energy level, physical restrictions while attached to ventilator, neuromuscular or musculoskeletal impairments, ability to participate in movement and activities (first visit).
2. Assess availability of portable ventilator and wheelchair to support ventilator to enhance movement within environment; instruct client in use of devices to operate on chair (first and second visit).
3. Assess for response to activity such as respiratory changes or distress (first and each visit).
4. Perform range-of-motion (ROM) exercises and instruct caregiver to perform these daily (first and reinforce on subsequent visits).
5. Instruct client in different position changes as needed for use of extremities in performing self-care (first visit).
6. Obtain an order for physical therapy referral or reinforce teaching by therapist for exercises and mobility while receiving assisted ventilation, occupational and speech therapy if appropriate.

CLIENT AND FAMILY/CAREGIVER INTERVENTIONS

1. Client schedules and assists or participates in daily activities for periods of time as tolerated.
2. Client avoids extremes in activity while allowing for as much independence as possible.
3. Client discontinues activity if fatigue or respiratory distress results.
4. Client follows recommendations of physical therapist to maintain mobility, muscle tone, and range of motion.
5. Client utilizes resource to acquire wheelchair with a mount for ventilator if appropriate.

Nursing diagnosis

Caregiver role strain

Related factors: Amount of caregiving tasks; duration of caregiving required; unpredictable illness course or instability in the care receiver's health; discharge of client with significant home care needs

Defining characteristics: Worry about client's health, having enough time and energy to provide care needed, conflict in family about issues of providing 24-hour care and supervision of client, family disorganization and role changes, significant person's expression of inability to cope and feelings of fear, anxiety, guilt, and anger related to providing care, stress causing impatience with client's needs and physical changes (ventilator/tracheostomy)

OUTCOMES

Short-term

Identification of role strain, as evidenced by verbalization of stress or nervousness, worry, interference with other important roles in life, loss of independence, and need for assistance and support, ability of family to plan and care for client (expected within 1 week)

Long-term

Resolution of role strain, as evidenced by provision of normal environment and continued, progressive, and safe care without compromise to caregiver's or family's physical and emotional needs (expected within 1 month and ongoing)

NURSING INTERVENTIONS/INSTRUCTIONS

1. Assess extent of care needs of client and ability and feeling of adequacy of caregiver to perform role and care, feelings of caregiver about the demands and complexity (exhaustion and resentment) of care, feeling of being alone and no pride in caregiving activities (first visit).
2. Assess relationship between caregiver and family and stressors placed on the relationship caused by the receiver of care, breakdown in family relationships, and role confusion or competing demands from family and care responsibilities (first visit and ongoing).
3. Assist caregiver to monitor continued ability to perform care and treatments, day-to-day needs that need to be changed or learned, changes in strains or stressors, maintenance of routines, and need for additional resources or assistance (each visit).
4. Provide time for caregiver and family to discuss frustrations, anxiety, fear, and fatigue; praise attempts and accomplishments in coping and providing care (each visit).
5. Assist caregiver to locate respite care for client to give relief from constant attendance and care by the caregiver (any visit).

6. Encourage sharing of caregiver roles and responsibilities among family members, friends, and extended family to provide relief to immediate family (any visit).
7. Listen to family feelings, concerns, expectations, and preferences for caregiving; answer all questions (each visit).
8. Instruct caregiver in methods to develop appropriate coping skills and to meet family's medical and other needs (emotional, financial, food, respite, supplies, and equipment) by referral to social or counseling services (initiate on first visit and each visit as needed).

CLIENT AND FAMILY/CAREGIVER INTERVENTIONS

1. Caregiver prepares for emotional changes associated with caregiving during the discharge planning and teaching, develops trust in home care personnel, and collaborates in developing and modifying daily care.
2. Caregiver develops ability to cope with caregiver role; incorporates flexibility into day-to-day functioning.
3. Caregiver explores and utilizes community resources (United Way or others) to provide physical and psychological assistance and relief from role strain (respite care).
4. Caregiver maintains own health and well-being in caregiver role, and as much independence and privacy as possible; becomes involved in outside activities.
5. Caregiver develops new coping skills and strategies for role changes by family members needed to support and/or participate in the care of the client.
6. Caregiver and family members preserve family relationships and minimize stressors by sharing feelings, fears, and concerns with one another.
7. Progressive adaptation and acceptance of ventilatory care by caregiver and family members.
8. Caregiver participates in outside support groups, refers to clergy or counseling as needed.

Tuberculosis

Tuberculosis is an infectious disorder of the lungs but may affect other organs or systems, such as bones and joints, the central nervous system, the genitourinary tract, or the adrenal glands. It is caused by *Mycobacterium tuberculosis* and usually is contracted and transmitted by inhalation of air contaminated by droplets containing the organisms. This inflammatory pulmonary disorder forms tubercles that lead to formation of necrosis, caseation, fibrosis, and calcification in the affected areas of the lungs. The most susceptible groups include persons who are malnourished, persons who exhibit a low host resistance to the causative agent, and immunosuppressed individuals as in AIDS.

Home care concentrates on the teaching of daily personal hygiene, nutrition, rest, and a medication regimen.

Nursing diagnosis

Ineffective breathing pattern

Related factors: Decreased energy and fatigue; inflammatory process

Defining characteristics: Shortness of breath, fremitus, respiratory depth changes, diminished breath sounds, altered chest expansion, productive or nonproductive cough, blood-tinged sputum

OUTCOMES

Short-term

Adequate oxygenation, as evidenced by respiratory rate, depth, and ease within preestablished baselines and by reduced frequency of productive coughing (expected within 1 to 2 weeks)

Long-term

Adequate respiratory functioning, as evidenced by client breathing with optimal level of ease to maintain desired or limited life-style, by x-ray study showing arrested or inactive stage of the disease, and by sputum culture conversion from positive to negative (expected within 2 to 5 months)

NURSING INTERVENTIONS/INSTRUCTIONS

1. Assess physical status of respiratory system (see Pulmonary System Assessment, p. 6, for guidelines) (first visit).
2. Monitor respirations for ease, rate, and depth; temperature for elevation; cough and mucus production for frequency, type, and characteristics; check for hemoptysis and dyspnea; also note dullness on percussion and crepitant crackles and

rhonchi on auscultation. Instruct client in procedure for taking respirations and temperature and recording in a log (each visit).

3. Evaluate level of endurance when client is performing ADL; note onset of fatigue, cough, or pain. Instruct client in measures to minimize or reduce energy expended and in establishing a rest schedule (first visit; reinstruct monthly).
4. Instruct client in effective cough procedure that does not cause stress to the chest wall and in how to collect an early-morning sputum specimen for laboratory analysis (first visit).
5. Suggest oral hygiene for frequent coughing and expectoration (first visit).
6. Monitor results of x-ray studies and sputum analysis as available, and incorporate information into clinical profile.
7. Refer client to self-help or support groups and local branches of organizations such as the American Lung Association and Smokenders (first visit).

CLIENT AND FAMILY/CAREGIVER INTERVENTIONS

1. Client takes and records temperature and respiratory rate and depth as needed.
2. Client adapts ADL to physical tolerance.
3. Client performs oral hygiene 2 to 3 times daily or as needed.
4. Client has laboratory tests done on sputum (collect and transport sputum specimen to laboratory as ordered).
5. Client reports acute dyspnea or hemoptysis to physician.

Nursing diagnosis

Altered nutrition: less than body requirements

Related factors: Inability to ingest nutrients because of biologic factors

Defining characteristics: Anorexia, lack of interest in food; weakness; fatigue; weight loss; inadequate nutritional intake

OUTCOMES

Short-term

Adequate nutrition, as evidenced by stable weight, stable arm circumference, and energy level adequate to perform ADL (expected within 2 to 4 weeks)

Long-term
Optimal nutritional status maintained, as evidenced by normal weight for height and frame and compliance with prescribed diet, rest, and activity regimens (expected within 1 to 3 months)

NURSING INTERVENTIONS/INSTRUCTIONS

1. Assess nutritional status, food likes and dislikes, cultural and religious restrictions, caloric requirements and economic resources (first visit).
2. Take height and weight and compare with standardized charts; instruct client in taking weight (first visit).
3. Take arm measurements for baseline and later comparisons (first visit).
4. Instruct client to maintain a food diary for 1 week, including type and amount of food consumed with times and method of preparation (first and second visits).
5. Instruct client in food selections for a high-protein, high-carbohydrate diet. Incorporate assessment data and food diary into menu planning (first and second visits).
6. Provide information for vitamin supplements (first visit).
7. Suggest oral hygiene before each meal (first visit).
8. Suggest eating more frequent meals in smaller amounts if appetite is poor (first visit).
9. Refer HHA to assist with ADL and meal preparation.

CLIENT AND FAMILY/CAREGIVER INTERVENTIONS

1. Client weighs self weekly using same scale, at same time of day, and wearing same amount of clothing, and records in a log.
2. Client maintains a 7-day food diary listing types, times, and amounts of all foods eaten.
3. Client performs oral hygiene with mouthwash before meals, and brushes teeth after meals.
4. Client eats a high-protein, high-carbohydrate, high-calorie diet.
5. Client uses high-calorie supplements as needed.
6. Client takes daily vitamins.
7. Caregiver prepares foods that are preferred and related to cultural needs and that provide calorie requirements and social interaction.

Nursing diagnosis

Knowledge deficit

Related factors: Lack of information about measures to comply with medical regimen and about prevention of transmission of disease

Defining characteristics: Expression of need for information about the disease, how it is transmitted, long-term medication regimen, rest and activity requirements and limitations

OUTCOMES

Short-term

Adequate knowledge, as evidenced by client describing the causes, transmission, susceptibility, and progression of the disease; signs and symptoms of complications; and medication side effects; skin testing of contacts; compliance with medication regimen (expected within 1 to 2 weeks)

Long-term

Adequate knowledge, as evidenced by continued compliance with medication regimen and life-style adaptations and by x-ray films showing that the disease is in a dormant state; disease prophylaxis of contacts (expected within 2 to 5 months)

NURSING INTERVENTIONS/INSTRUCTIONS

1. Assess client's ability to perform ADL, life-style, ability and willingness to adapt and learn, and family support system. Integrate information with disease staging and progression (see Functional Assessment, p. 51, and Psychosocial Assessment, p. 48, for guidelines) (first visit).
2. Assess respiratory, renal, hepatic, hematopoietic, neurologic, visual, and auditory changes; note known allergies and ascertain pregnancy status (first visit and then monthly) (see respective assessments for guidelines).
3. Instruct client in causes, dormancy, and progression of disease, and relate them to plan for care (first visit).
4. Instruct client contacts (within last 3 months) to obtain skin testing and possible follow-up x-ray films at local health department (first visit and reinstruct each visit).

5. Inform client contacts that medication is provided by the health department for both treatment and prophylaxis (first visit).
6. Instruct client to schedule rest and activity to avoid fatigue while maintaining endurance (first visit).
7. Instruct client in respiratory isolation procedures if necessary; suggest provision of a well-ventilated room supplied with disposable supplies and utensils and a waterproof bag for disposal (first visit).
8. Instruct client to cover nose and mouth when coughing or sneezing and in proper disposal of tissues and other used supplies (first visit).
9. Instruct client in proper hand-washing technique and in when to perform procedure (first visit).
10. Instruct client in administration (including names, times, side effects, dose, and food/drug/alcohol interactions) of isoniazid, ethambutol, rifabutin, rifampin, and streptomycin (and possibly capreomycin, pyrazinamide, ethionamide, clyceoserine, kanamycin, and amikacin); instruct client to avoid over-the-counter or nonprescribed drugs (first visit and reinstruct on second visit).
11. Instruct client contacts in administration and side effects of isoniazid (first visit).
12. Instruct client and family contacts to comply with scheduled appointments with private physician or public health department for follow-up testing and medication (each visit).
13. Inform client to report hypersensitivities (rash, urticaria), pruritis, difficulty in breathing, jaundice, urinary changes, peripheral neuritis, or changes in visual or hearing acuity (first visit).
14. Encourage client to be tested for human immunodeficiency virus (HIV), since the incidence of tuberculosis is high among persons with HIV infection.
15. Initiate referral to public health agencies and social services and to self-help and support groups (first visit).
16. Refer HHA to assist when necessary.

CLIENT AND FAMILY/CAREGIVER INTERVENTIONS

1. Client administers prescribed medications correctly using checkoff sheet, labeled tablet compartments, or another method as a reminder.

2. Client secures medication in advance from public health services or home nurse to facilitate compliance.
3. Caregiver and family comply with diagnostic procedures (skin testing and x-ray films, with return for test reading) and with prophylactic medication regimen as prescribed for family contacts.
4. Client notifies health care provider of pregnancy.
5. Client performs ADL according to needs, resting before and after to avoid fatigue; secures physician permission to return to usual activities and work patterns.
6. Client avoids alcohol, smoking, and any nonprescribed drugs.
7. Caregiver washes hands after each contact with client and used supplies and disposes of used supplies and utensils in a sealed, waterproof bag.
8. Client notifies physician of untoward or toxic reactions to medications.
9. Client and caregiver utilize community resources.

Cardiovascular system

Angina Pectoris/Coronary Artery Disease (CAD)

Coronary artery disease, also known as arteriosclerotic heart disease, is the narrowing or obstruction of the arteries of the heart by atherosclerotic plaque, causing a decrease in blood flow. It leads to a decrease in oxygen supply to the heart (ischemia), resulting in retrosternal or substernal chest pain or pressure that may extend to the left arm or jaw with varying degrees of severity and frequency. Typically, the pain is precipitated by exertion and relieved by a smooth-muscle relaxant or a vasodilator. Predisposing or risk factors include hypertension, elevated lipid panel, obesity, cigarette smoking, and diabetes mellitus.

Home care is primarily concerned with the teaching of medication regimens to prevent or control attacks and the control of risk factors by compliance with exercise and dietary regimens.

Nursing diagnosis

Pain

Related factors: Biologic injuring agents

Defining characteristics: Verbalization of pain descriptors (dull, crushing, tightness, choking, pressing feeling in chest); grimace; holding or guarding chest or arm; clenched fist over sternum; pain with activity and awakening from sleep; elevated pulse and blood pressure

OUTCOMES

Short-term

Absence of pain, as evidenced by client's statement that pain is relieved or controlled by measures to prevent discomfort; relaxed posture and expressions (expected within 1 to 7 days)

Long-term

Optimal comfort level and freedom from anginal pain, as evidenced by continued absence of pain and compliance with medication regimen related to anticipatory need and activity restrictions (expected within 1 month)

NURSING INTERVENTIONS/INSTRUCTIONS

1. Assess, and instruct client to assess, pain and characteristics, and precipitating and alleviating factors, with emphasis on early recognition of onset; have client maintain a diary with a record of each pain episode and characteristics (first visit).
2. Monitor pain for type, location, intensity, and duration to establish individual anginal pattern, and instruct client to report any aberration in established pattern to physician (each visit).
3. Instruct client in administration of sublingual nitroglycerin for use at onset of pain (first visit):
   - Use at first sign of an attack (relate to pain diary).
   - Administer prescribed dose in tablet form under the tongue or in the buccal pouch and allow to dissolve; avoid swallowing the tablet.
   - Repeat dosage up to 3 times at 5-minute intervals if pain is not relieved.
   - Notify physician and call ambulance and go to emergency room if total of 3 tablets taken over 15 minutes does not relieve pain.
4. Instruct client in alternative form and route (inhalation amyl nitrite) if prescribed (first visit).
5. Instruct client to rest during acute episode and to maintain supine or semi-Fowler's position to reduce oxygen requirement (first visit).

CLIENT AND FAMILY/CAREGIVER INTERVENTIONS

1. Client maintains pain diary; identifies trends and reports to physician when necessary.
2. Client administers and records medication to prevent or treat angina.
3. Client uses positions of comfort and takes rest periods as needed.
4. Client schedules medication regimen around activities.
5. Client calls physician and/or ambulance if 3 doses of nitroglycerin are ineffective.

Nursing diagnosis

Activity intolerance

Related factors: Imbalance between oxygen supply and demand

Defining characteristics: Abnormal response to activity (pulse, blood pressure, difficulty breathing, pain); electrocardiogram (ECG) changes reflecting arrhythmias or ischemia; known presence of CAD

OUTCOMES

Short-term

Increase in activity tolerance and endurance, as evidenced by client's statement that stressors have been avoided and pain episodes associated with activity have decreased (expected within 1 to 7 days)

Long-term

Optimal activity and self-care achieved with adaptation to established limitations in functioning (expected within 2 weeks)

NURSING INTERVENTIONS/INSTRUCTIONS

1. Assess life-style, participation in activities of daily living (ADL), and effects of activity on angina (first visit).
2. Identify activities that increase oxygen consumption and cause pain (first visit).
3. Assist client to plan a progressive daily self-care schedule, and instruct him or her to refrain from any activity that precipitates symptoms, including exposure to cold, exertion after a meal, exertion from sexual intercourse (first visit).
4. Advise client that activity may be continued by modifying it in order that no symptoms of angina are elicited; that nitroglycerin may be prescribed prophylactically before activity is to be performed (first visit).
5. Initiate referral to physical and/or sex therapist as indicated (any visit).

CLIENT AND FAMILY/CAREGIVER INTERVENTIONS

1. Client maintains activity and rest schedule as planned.
2. Client progresses in ADL and endurance level without angina response.

3. Client ceases activity and rests when angina occurs.
4. Client seeks assistance to increase activity tolerance and sexual activity if needed.

Nursing diagnosis

Anxiety

Related factors: Threat of death; threat to or change in health status

Defining characteristics: Verbalization of fear of death from heart attack; increased tension and apprehension; feeling of uncertainty with life-style changes; fear of unspecific consequences

OUTCOMES

Short-term

Decrease in anxiety, as evidenced by client's statement expressing reduction in and control of anxiety to manageable level (expected within 1 week)

Long-term

Continuing manageable level of anxiety with optimal psychic and emotional functioning, as evidenced by resumption of daily living pattern with modifications to prevent angina episodes (expected within 2 weeks)

NURSING INTERVENTIONS/INSTRUCTIONS

1. Establish rapport and allow time and supportive environment for client to communicate concerns and fears (each visit).
2. Provide information about all tests and treatments to monitor and control condition (first visit).
3. Allow time for questions, and answer in understandable terms and with honesty (each visit).
4. Reaffirm positive life-style changes (each visit).
5. Refer client to counseling if anxiety becomes chronic (last visit).
6. Teach relaxation techniques if client is agreeable (first visit or when needed).

CLIENT AND FAMILY/CAREGIVER INTERVENTIONS

1. Client inquires about condition and methods to control anxiety.
2. Client initiates necessary life-style changes.
3. Client contacts self-help groups or counseling.
4. Client uses relaxation techniques to control anxiety.

Nursing diagnosis

Knowledge deficit

Related factors: Lack of information about medical regimen

Defining characteristics: Request for information about medications, disease process, nutritional and activity restrictions, and health measures to prevent complications and decrease risks

OUTCOMES

Short-term

Adequate knowledge, as evidenced by client's ability to describe signs and symptoms and progression of the condition; compliance with exercise and dietary controls; and reduction in known stressors and smoking (expected within 1 week)

Long-term

Adequate knowledge of and compliance with medical regimen, as evidenced by client's meeting the requirements of a changed life-style to achieve optimal level of wellness and functioning (expected within 1 month and ongoing)

NURSING INTERVENTIONS/INSTRUCTIONS

1. Assess life-style and ability to adapt, dietary patterns, learning and coping abilities and interest, and family participation and support in the medical regimen (first visit).
2. Assess cardiovascular status (see Cardiovascular System Assessment, p. 10, for guidelines) and note blood pressure, pulse changes, angina pain patterns, history of chronic illness, use of caffeine, alcohol, and tobacco; assess for more distant heart sounds, fourth heart sound, more diffuse apical pulse, presence of nausea, diaphoresis, cool extremities, and vertigo during acute episodes of angina (each visit).

3. Instruct client to maintain an activity diary and relate activities to angina episodes; teach from the known to the unknown, allow client to verbalize signs and symptoms, precipitating factors, and first indication of onset (first visit and reinforce on second visit).
4. Instruct client to identify stressors, including heavy meals, exertion, exposure to cold, emotional upsets, or any combination of these (first visit).
5. Instruct client to closely follow prescribed health regimen for any chronic condition such as hypertension or diabetes mellitus (first visit).
6. Advise client to stop smoking, and refer client to support group if needed (first visit).
7. Instruct client to maintain a food diary; instruct client in lowering caloric intake for reducing weight if indicated, avoiding foods high in saturated fats and cholesterol, and limiting low-fat foods that contain monounsaturated and polyunsaturated fats; include low sodium–intake instructions if recommended, and supply client with food lists and sample menus during teaching sessions (first visit and reinforce when needed).
8. Advise client to follow a paced, incremental walking program (first week).
9. Instruct client in administration of long-acting nitrites, β-adrenergic blocking agents, calcium channel blockers, antilipidemics, and prophylactic antiplatelet agents, including dose, route, frequency, side effects, and food/drug/alcohol interactions; instruct client to avoid skipping doses or abrupt discontinuation of medications and to avoid over-the-counter (OTC) drugs unless advised by physician (first visit).
10. Instruct client in administration of nitroglycerin before or during angina attack and to note vertigo, syncope, or headache with initial dose and tolerance to drug (first visit).
11. Advise client to carry medication at all times (away from body heat), to store it in a dark container, and to replace tablets every 3 months (first visit).
12. Instruct client to report any aberration in anginal pattern and pain that is not relieved by medication (first visit).
13. Instruct client to carry or wear identification information indicating condition and medications being taken (first visit and check for compliance on second visit).

14. Inform client of available social services, community agencies, resources, and groups for information and support (first visit).

CLIENT AND FAMILY/CAREGIVER INTERVENTIONS

1. Client administers medication appropriately and accurately.
2. Client avoids identified stressors, and manages anginal episodes quickly and effectively.
3. Client complies with dietary and exercise programs as instructed.
4. Client limits alcohol intake and reduces or ceases cigarette smoking.
5. Client notifies physician of medication side effects, unrelieved pain, or changes in vital signs.
6. Client utilizes social services, nutritionist, or physical therapist as needed.

Congestive Heart Failure (CHF)

Congestive heart failure (CHF) is a chronic, progressive syndrome characterized by the inability of the heart to act as a pump. The result is a cardiac output that is inadequate to meet the body's metabolic requirements. CHF results from myocardial infarction, coronary artery disease, inflammatory diseases of the heart, hypertension, valvular disorders, or any other condition that strains the heart over a long period of time. The compensatory mechanisms of increased heart rate and cardiac dilatation and hypertrophy are adaptive responses to diminished cardiac output. The cause determines whether hypertrophy occurs on the left or right side or involves both sides. Treatment is directed at management of specific etiologic and pathophysiologic factors, reversal of compensatory mechanisms, and elimination of contributing factors.

Home care is primarily concerned with assessment and with teaching the client about the disorder, the medical regimen designed to prevent the occurrence of heart failure, and measures to treat this chronic condition.

Nursing diagnosis

Decreased cardiac output

Related factors: Mechanical factors causing alteration in preload and afterload; inotropic changes in the heart; structural factors

Defining characteristics: Alterations in hemodynamic readings (pulse, blood pressure); fatigue; dyspnea; rales; cyanosis; pallor; oliguria; left-sided heart failure with overlapping of symptoms of fluid excess as condition progresses

OUTCOMES

Short-term

Adequate cardiac output, as evidenced by reduction in signs and symptoms of lowered cardiac output; compliance with medical regimen, resulting in return of vital signs to baseline ranges (expected within 2 to 7 days)

Long-term

Optimal cardiac status within disease limitations, as evidenced by ability to resume and maintain adapted life-style without distress or complications (expected within 2 to 4 weeks)

NURSING INTERVENTIONS/INSTRUCTIONS

1. Assess circulatory status, noting rate and rhythm of apical and peripheral pulses, blood pressure, presence of cough or dyspnea, activity intolerance levels, presence of S_3 or S_4 heart sounds, accentuated S_2, summative gallop (S_3 with S_1) (see Cardiovascular System Assessment, p. 10, for guidelines) (each visit).
2. Perform complete physical assessment, including renal, hepatic, and neurologic systems, and note any stressors that increase cardiac output, such as chronic inflammatory or infectious diseases, increased blood pressure, pulmonary emboli, arrythmias, anemia, or thyrotoxicosis (first visit).
3. Assess life-style and relate it to contributing factors as a basis for teaching, noting tobacco use, excessive alcohol use, sodium and caffeine intake, stress, or overweight problems (first visit).
4. Instruct client to monitor and record apical and radial pulses; stress alterations that should be reported to physician rather than absolute values (first visit).

5. Instruct client to avoid fatigue by pacing activities and rest periods; instruct client to rest and sleep in semi-Fowler's position (first visit).
6. Instruct client in administration of vasodilators and advise client to note side effects, implication of decreased blood pressure on position, resultant headaches, and altered renal function; instruct client to avoid OTC drugs unless approved by physician (first visit).
7. Instruct client in administration of cardiotonics; advise client to take pulse before administration and to withhold drug if pulse is lower than 60 beats/min; inform client of signs and symptoms of toxicity, including nausea, vomiting, anorexia, diarrhea, confusion, visual changes, and new or worsening pulse irregularities (first visit).
8. Instruct client to report deteriorating condition, including increasing fatigue with activity, dyspnea, pallor, diaphoresis, thready pulse or alteration in pulse baseline, persistent cough, feelings of suffocation, cyanosis, restlessness, anxiety, or panic (first visit).

CLIENT AND FAMILY/CAREGIVER INTERVENTIONS

1. Client monitors and records daily pulses, blood pressure, capillary refill, skin for any change in color.
2. Client administers medications correctly and states implications and expected results.
3. Client avoids fatigue, stressors, and excessive activity.
4. Client lists signs and symptoms of digitalis toxicity and reports if present.
5. Client reports changes in vital signs that indicate change in cardiac output.

Nursing diagnosis

Fluid volume excess

Related factors: Compromised regulatory mechanisms

Defining characteristics: Edema, unexplained weight gain, shortness of breath, orthopnea, change in respiratory pattern, oliguria, jugular vein distention, pulmonary effusion, congestion on x-ray films, abnormal breath sounds (crackles), right-sided failure with overlapping symptoms of decreased cardiac output as condition progresses

OUTCOMES

Short-term

Fluids in balance, as evidenced by intake and output returned to baselines, weight maintained, and edema reduced or absent (expected within 3 to 4 days)

Long-term

Fluid and electrolytes in balance, as evidenced by optimal weight and by achievement of optimal renal and pulmonary function for life-style requirements (expected within 1 month)

NURSING INTERVENTIONS/INSTRUCTIONS

1. Assess fluid requirements; calculate for age and weight (usually about 2 L/day unless restricted) (first visit).
2. Measure height and abdominal girth, and instruct client to take daily weight at same time, on same scale, wearing same clothing, and to record and report weight gains (first visit).
3. Monitor for discrepancies between estimated intake and output and for pedal and ankle swelling, increasing fatigue, abdominal fullness, ascites, oliguria, and weight gain (each visit).
4. Assess chest sounds for crackles and changes in respiration (each visit).
5. Monitor and instruct client in diuretic therapy and potassium levels when they are available; encourage foods high in potassium, including citrus fruits, bananas, poultry, potatoes, and raisins, and/or administer potassium replacement if prescribed (first visit).
6. Monitor and instruct client in dietary sodium intake and for compliance with restrictions (first visit).
7. Instruct client to inform physician of edema, breathing changes or difficulties, or weight gain (first visit).

CLIENT AND FAMILY/CAREGIVER INTERVENTIONS

1. Client monitors weight and fluid intake and urinary output estimations.
2. Client administers diuretics and electrolyte replacement properly.
3. Client complies with sodium restriction.

4. Client reports weight gains, edema, or any other symptoms of fluid retention.

Nursing diagnosis

Fatigue

Related factors: Increased energy requirements, overwhelming physical and psychological demands

Defining characteristics: Verbalization of lack of energy, fatigue, inability to maintain usual routine; poor oxygenation of tissues; bed rest causing deconditioning

OUTCOMES

Short-term

Decreasing fatigue, as evidenced by client's statement of increased energy and endurance and by participation in paced activities (expected within 1 week)

Long-term

Energy and endurance returned to baseline levels, as evidenced by achievement of self-care and mobility for optimal functioning within condition limitations (expected within 1 to 2 months)

NURSING INTERVENTIONS/INSTRUCTIONS

1. Assess life-style, ADL abilities, and limitations imposed by illness (first visit).
2. Identify activities that elicit symptoms and deplete energy reserves (first visit).
3. Assist client in progressive plan for daily care; instruct client to avoid any activity that precipitates symptoms, to pace activities, and to provide rest periods (first visit).
4. Employ energy-saving devices and techniques for ADL (each visit).
5. Inform client to avoid strenuous activity or exercise (first visit).
6. Refer home health aide (HHA) to assist with ADL.

CLIENT AND FAMILY/CAREGIVER INTERVENTIONS

1. Client identifies physical and mental stressors and avoids them when possible.

2. Client progresses in ADL within established limits.
3. Client satisfies rest and sleep needs.

Nursing diagnosis

Ineffective individual coping

Related factors: Multiple life changes, inadequate coping methods

Defining characteristics: Verbalization of inability to cope or ask for help, inability to solve problems, chronic worry and anxiety; inappropriate use of defense mechanisms

OUTCOMES

Short-term

Improved coping, as evidenced by client's statement of understanding of need for adaptations in life-style and positive coping strategies (expected within 1 week)

Long-term

Optimal coping, as evidenced by adaptations in life-style and by compliance with medical regimen to achieve health and optimal functioning (expected within 1 to 2 months)

NURSING INTERVENTIONS/INSTRUCTIONS

1. Assess mental and emotional status, coping abilities, use of defense mechanisms, and problem-solving skills (first visit).
2. Provide an accepting environment for expression of concerns (each visit).
3. Assist client to identify goals and positive coping mechanisms (each visit).
4. Allow client to participate in and plan care and to practice effective problem-solving skills (each visit).
5. Initiate referral to counseling or psychotherapist if indicated (any visit).

CLIENT AND FAMILY/CAREGIVER INTERVENTIONS

1. Client develops and uses effective coping mechanisms.
2. Client shares concerns with family members and requests assistance and support when needed.

3. Client plans care and solves problems that arise from inadequate care.
4. Client manages care effectively and maintains a positive attitude.

Nursing diagnosis

Knowledge deficit

Related factors: Lack of information about condition

Defining characteristics: Request for information about disease and its effect; compliance with daily medical regimen

OUTCOMES

Short-term

Adequate knowledge, as evidenced by client's description of disease process, signs and symptoms, complications, and effect of disease on body systems and general health (expected within 3 days)

Long-term

Adequate knowledge, as evidenced by compliance with the medical regimen to meet requirements of a changed life-style for achievement of an optimal level of health and functioning (expected within 1 month)

NURSING INTERVENTIONS/INSTRUCTIONS

1. Assess life-style and ability to adapt, learning abilities and interest, and family participation and support (first visit).
2. Outline a program to teach disease process and preventive measures (first visit):
   - Medication administration, with complete information for accuracy and desired effects
   - Signs and symptoms of disease and of complications
   - Activity and rest program
   - Bowel hygiene and prevention of change in normal pattern
   - Diet for weight reduction, low in sodium, fats, and cholesterol
   - Cessation of smoking; limitations on caffeine and alcohol
   - Review of laboratory tests and changes needed
   - Foods to avoid and include in dietary regimen

3. Instruct client to comply with physician and laboratory appointments and to check with physician for results and possible changes in therapy (first visit).
4. Instruct client to carry or wear medical identification information (first visit).
5. Refer client to agencies and support groups to assist in compliance with medical regimen if needed (any visit).

CLIENT AND FAMILY/CAREGIVER INTERVENTIONS

1. Client follows medical regimen as taught.
2. Client reports known signs and symptoms of complications if present.
3. Client administers medications safely, with awareness of side effects or untoward effects to report.
4. Client manages care with assistance of agency or group if needed.
5. Client verbalizes understanding that measures to maintain cardiac status are lifelong.

Coronary Bypass Surgery

Coronary bypass is a surgical procedure that circumvents obstructed coronary arterial vessels through a process of myocardial revascularization. The resulting unobstructed blood flow oxygenates previously ischemic heart muscle. Autogenous blood vessels frequently used to bridge the occluded areas are the internal mammary arteries or the saphenous veins. The clinical profile would include a history of arteriosclerotic heart disease and CAD, notably unstable angina pectoris and localized rather than diffuse disease. Some controversy exists about the surgical procedure because, although it offers dramatic relief from pain and other symptoms, it may not necessarily positively affect the prognosis of the disease.

Home care is primarily concerned with postoperative teaching of the medical regimen to prevent complications and with life-style changes that will promote wellness within limitations imposed by the procedure and the underlying heart condition.

Nursing diagnosis

Ineffective individual coping

Related factors: Multiple life changes, personal vulnerability

Defining characteristics: Verbalization of inability to cope, meet role expectations, solve problems; inappropriate use of defense mechanisms; alterations in societal participation; chronic worry and anxiety about outcome of surgery

OUTCOMES

Short-term

Improved coping behaviors, as evidenced by statement of feeling more able to handle stressors and by use of appropriate and effective coping and defense mechanisms (expected within 1 to 2 weeks)

Long-term

Adequate and positive coping, as evidenced by progression from sick-role behaviors to relaxation and adaptive behaviors and by resumption of ADL and other activities within limitations imposed by convalescence (expected within 1 to 2 months)

NURSING INTERVENTIONS/INSTRUCTIONS

1. Establish rapport and provide an accepting environment for expression of concerns and questions (each visit).
2. Assess mental status, ability to adapt, use of coping mechanisms, and internal resources, and explore with client the most effective coping mechanisms and selection of positive options (first visit).
3. Assess client's interest in and participation in activities and resumption of role and place in family (first visit).
4. Allow client to actively participate in plan of health care regimen (first visit).
5. Arrange for contact with support group.

CLIENT AND FAMILY/CAREGIVER INTERVENTIONS

1. Client expresses feelings and concerns.
2. Client identifies and uses coping mechanisms that are the most effective and develops coping skills as needed.

3. Client participates in own health care planning.
4. Client utilizes support group for information and help.

Nursing diagnosis

Knowledge deficit

Related factors: Lack of information about postoperative care

Defining characteristics: Request for information regarding medications, cardiac rehabilitation, dietary restrictions, life-style changes, sexual function, and signs and symptoms to report to physician

OUTCOMES

Short-term

Adequate knowledge of follow-up care, as evidenced by client's ability to describe the condition, risk factors, and required life-style adaptations and by compliance with medication, diet, and rehabilitation program (expected within 1 week)

Long-term

Adequate knowledge, as evidenced by client's complying with postoperative recommendations to achieve optimal level of health and functioning without complications (expected within 1 month and ongoing).

NURSING INTERVENTIONS/INSTRUCTIONS

1. Review physician's postoperative health regimen, amount and type of teaching done, and reinforcement needed in order that home care becomes a continuum of previous teaching (first visit).
2. Facilitate establishment of an environment that is conducive to learning and free of outside distractions, in which the client is free of pain and excessive anxiety, and teach care based on identified needs for information and demonstration (each visit).
3. Assess cardiovascular and respiratory status (see Cardiovascular System Assessment, p. 10, and Pulmonary System Assessment, p. 6, for guidelines); note vital signs (compare to

baselines), point of maximal impulse (PMI), and presence of irregularities or pain (each visit).

4. Instruct client to monitor and record pulse daily for 1 full minute after a 5-minute quiet period and to notify physician of changes or deviation from usual pulse rate and regularity (first visit).
5. Instruct client to take weekly weights at same time, with same clothing, and on same scale and to report unexplained gains or losses to physician (first visit).
6. Instruct client in need for rest, and plan to schedule activities around rest periods; suggest 8 hours of sleep per night or more; inform client of importance of following cardiac rehabilitation program without exception (first visit).
7. Inform client that activity progression will be determined by results of rehabilitation participation, and advise that sexual activity may begin 6 to 8 weeks after surgery, based on physician recommendation and feelings of client and spouse (first visit).
8. Assess for incisional healing, discomfort at operative area, or change in wound, including redness, swelling, or drainage (each visit).
9. Assess for presence of chest pain, and differentiate between preoperative and postoperative pain (anginal or cardiac); instruct client in administration of analgesics (each visit).
10. Evaluate exercise tolerance, and advise against driving or sitting for long periods, abruptly changing positions from lying to sitting or sitting to standing, or lifting heavy objects (first visit).
11. Instruct client in administration and implications of antihypertensives, antiarrhythmics, cardiotonics, diuretics, anticoagulants, and analgesics (first visit and reinforce on second visit).
12. Instruct client to continue prescribed regimen for control of chronic conditions such as hypertension or diabetes mellitus (first visit).
13. Instruct client in low-calorie, low-cholesterol, low-fat, low-sodium diet; instruct client to avoid caffeine and alcohol except in small amounts (first visit and reinforce on second visit).
14. Instruct client to avoid Valsalva maneuver during bowel elimination and to administer stool softeners to prevent constipation (first visit).

15. Remind client that smoking should be reduced and preferably eliminated, and suggest group support to assist in stopping (first visit).
16. Instruct client to report signs and symptoms of complications or regression to preoperative profile, including erratic pulse, chest pain, activity intolerance, fatigue, or unexplained anxiety and restlessness (first visit).
17. Instruct client to carry or wear identifying information about condition and medications (first visit).
18. Inform client of importance of compliance with medical regimen that includes cardiac rehabilitation and of follow-up appointments with physician and laboratory (first visit).
19. Monitor changes in medical orders and laboratory results when applicable (each visit).
20. Initiate referral to social worker, home health aide, and other support personnel and groups as appropriate (any visit).

CLIENT AND FAMILY/CAREGIVER INTERVENTIONS

1. Client monitors and records pulse daily and notifies physician of changes.
2. Client monitors weight weekly and reports significant gains or losses.
3. Client integrates rest periods with increasing activities; tries to get 8 hours of sleep per night.
4. Client participates in cardiac rehabilitation program, with a monitored walking program between sessions.
5. Client resumes sexual activity.
6. Client manages incisional discomfort with medication; provides care for incisional site (hand washing, bathing, dressing).
7. Client avoids sitting for extended periods, lifting heavy objects, or participating in strenuous exercises or sports.
8. Client administers prescribed medications as instructed.
9. Client continues medical regimens for treating chronic conditions.
10. Client maintains diet that promotes ideal weight.
11. Client prepares and eats diet with restrictions in sodium, cholesterol, and fat; limits caffeine and alcohol intake.
12. Client maintains bowel elimination based on individual pattern.

13. Client identifies signs and symptoms of incisional infection, return to preoperative heart abnormalities, or complications of surgical procedure, and reports to physician.
14. Client wears or carries medical identification at all times.
15. Client complies with follow-up physician and laboratory appointments.
16. Client participates in self-help or support groups, contacts community agencies for information, and utilizes nutritionist or sex therapist as needed.

Hypertension

Hypertension can be defined as sustained arterial blood pressure of over 140 mm Hg systolic and 90 mm Hg diastolic. It causes arterial walls to become thickened, lose elasticity, and resist blood flow, which results in decreased blood supply to tissue and increased cardiac workload. The etiology of essential, or primary, hypertension is unknown. It can be treated and controlled, not cured. Secondary hypertension is associated with disorders of the kidney, adrenal glands, central nervous system, or great vessels or with the use of medications. In the absence of complications, essential hypertension is asymptomatic. Clinical manifestations are nonspecific and result from vascular changes in the heart, brain, or kidneys.

Home care is primarily concerned with the teaching of medication regimens to control the condition and preventive measures to control complications and risk factors.

Nursing diagnosis

Knowledge deficit

Related factors: Lack of information about medical regimen

Defining characteristics: Request for information about medications, dietary and exercise program, disease and its effects and complications

OUTCOMES

Short-term

Adequate knowledge, as evidenced by client's ability to describe disease process and effects, signs and symptoms, risk factors, and life-style modification requirements; familiarity and compliance with medication regimen (3 to 7 days)

Long-term

Adequate knowledge, as evidenced by meeting requirements of modified life-style to control condition and achieve optimal health and functioning (expected within 2 weeks)

NURSING INTERVENTIONS/INSTRUCTIONS

1. Assess life-style, learning and adaptation abilities, interest level, and family participation and support (first visit).
2. Assess all systems for effect of long-term hypertension; note history for predisposing factors or disorders that relate to secondary hypertension (first visit).
3. Assess and instruct client in monitoring blood pressure and pulse (first visit).
4. Inform client of high-risk factors associated with condition, including smoking, obesity, high sodium, fat, and cholesterol intake, stress, and sedentary life-style, and include family members in teaching, since heredity plays a role in predisposition to increased blood pressure (first visit).
5. Advise client about life-style changes, methods of stress management, and dietary changes, and to have regular screening for blood pressure and circulatory and visual changes (first visit).
6. Instruct client to take blood pressure 3 times per week; emphasize sitting quietly for 5 minutes before taking pressure, using the right size of cuff, applying cuff smoothly and snugly and fastening securely, and positioning arm at heart level; instruct client to report repeated and unexplained elevations to physician (first visit and reinforce when needed).
7. Instruct client in administration of diuretics, antihypertensives, antilipidemics, potassium replacement, and vasodilators, including doses, route, frequency, side effects, and food, drug, or alcohol interactions; caution client not to alter doses or abruptly stop medication and to avoid OTC drugs unless

recommended by physician (first visit and reinforce second visit).

8. Encourage client to participate in full range of previous activity as long as blood pressure is controlled; include an exercise program of walking, swimming, and biking, with 8 hours of sleep per night (first visit).
9. Advise client about weight reduction if needed; instruct client to maintain a food diary for 1 week, and offer a list of foods to avoid (ones that are high in cholesterol and saturated fats); encourage a more liberal intake of fruits and vegetables, whole grains, fish, and poultry (first and second visits).
10. Instruct client in sodium restriction (usually 2 g/day); advise client not to add salt to foods, and to avoid cured, processed, or convenience foods, and suggest use of herbs and spices for flavoring (first visit).
11. Inform client about foods that are high in potassium with diuretic therapy, including a list of those to include and avoid, especially if potassium supplement not given (first visit).
12. Suggest that client reduce or stop smoking and limit or avoid alcohol intake and hot baths or hot tub (first visit).
13. Instruct client to rise slowly from lying position to avoid orthostatic hypotension (first visit).
14. Instruct client to carry or wear identification information about condition and medications (first visit).
15. Emphasize importance of keeping appointments with physician for monitoring condition and therapy changes if needed, as well as for laboratory testing (first visit).
16. Initiate referral to community agencies and groups for information and support or counseling, including American Heart Association and smoking and weight control groups.

CLIENT AND FAMILY/CAREGIVER INTERVENTIONS

1. Client monitors blood pressure as instructed and recommended and records in log to review with physician.
2. Client administers medications correctly and records any side effects.
3. Client participates in an exercise program that is ongoing and progressive as appropriate.
4. Client avoids alcohol and tobacco in excess; reduces frequency.

5. Client complies with dietary restriction of sodium, fat, and cholesterol.
6. Client monitors weight weekly if on reduction diet and adjusts caloric intake accordingly.
7. Client wears or carries identification information.
8. Client maintains laboratory and physician appointment schedules.
9. Client utilizes support groups and counseling services if needed.

Nursing diagnosis

Risk for injury

Related factors: Internal factor of complication of hypertension

Defining characteristics: Failure to comply with medical regimen; sustained elevated blood pressure; cardiovascular and central nervous system symptomatology (hypertensive crisis, heart attack, cerebrovascular accident)

OUTCOMES

Short-term

Absence of signs and symptoms of complication, as evidenced by compliance with medication regimen (expected within 1 week)

Long-term

Optimal cardiovascular, neurologic, and renal system function, as evidenced by life-style modification and ongoing compliance with medical regimen to achieve health and wellness without complications (expected within 1 month and ongoing).

NURSING INTERVENTIONS/INSTRUCTIONS

1. Assess for behaviors that indicate resistance to or inability to comply with prescribed treatment regimen (first visit).
2. Reinforce instruction in diet, exercise, and medication programs and limitations on stress, alcohol, tobacco, and weight gain (first visit).
3. Assess for markedly elevated blood pressure, headache, visual disturbance, nausea, vomiting, palpitations, restlessness, confusion, tachycardia, arrhythmias, chest pain, or dyspnea, and

instruct client in noting and reporting such signs and symptoms (each visit).
4. Encourage client to participate in plan and take control of care (each visit).
5. Assist client with compliance by writing out plan and expectations (first visit).
6. Encourage client to ask questions, seek information, and participate in discussions about condition; praise compliance and accomplishments (each visit).
7. Inform client of importance of life-style changes that maintain blood pressure status and prevent complications (each visit).

CLIENT AND FAMILY/CAREGIVER INTERVENTIONS

1. Client complies with life-style changes and medical regimen.
2. Client reports signs and symptoms of complications immediately to physician.
3. Client supports all attempts at management of care and prevention of complications.
4. Client secures and reads information about condition and consequences of poor control of hypertension.

Nursing diagnosis

Ineffective management of therapeutic regimen (individual)

Related factors: Complexity of therapeutic regimen

Defining characteristics: Inappropriate choices of daily living for meeting the goals of a treatment or prevention program; failure to achieve weight loss and lower cholesterol level; inaccurate medication administration; observed smoking; reduction in exercise program; verbalization that action not taken to reduce risk factors for prevention of complications

OUTCOMES

Short-term

Verbalization of and specific plans and behaviors for therapeutic regimen, as evidenced by intention of following recommended dietary, exercise, and medication regimens with commitment (expected within 1 week)

Long-term

Compliance with management of therapeutic regimen, as evidenced by active participation in therapy and by demonstration of behaviors consistent with goals of therapy to achieve optimal health and prevent complications (expected within 1 month and ongoing)

NURSING INTERVENTIONS/INSTRUCTIONS

1. Assess reasons for client's disregarding therapeutic regimen and which aspects are difficult to comply with (first visit).
2. Provide client with detailed written instructions and a plan for specific behaviors, such as medications regimen via oral route, and include a simplified method if several medications are taken per day; regimen should be tailored to client life-style in peak action and scheduling where possible (first and second visits).
3. Inform client of consequences of smoking, and assist him or her to develop a plan to quit smoking, cope with withdrawal symptoms, deal with the possibility of a relapse, and use available resources and community programs (first visit).
4. Assist client to plan realistic dietary modifications; inform client of the benefits of the diet and the effects of noncompliance (first and second visits).
5. Inform client that behavior changes take time, and suggest methods to reinforce behavior changes and environmental changes to accommodate daily routines (first visit).
6. Instruct client in monitoring behavior(s) regularly, recording for analysis, and the need for alternative behaviors or strengthening of existing behaviors (first and second visits).

CLIENT AND FAMILY/CAREGIVER INTERVENTIONS

1. Client demonstrates accurate performance of specific health behavior(s) consistent with goals of therapeutic regimen.
2. Client verbalizes and adheres to a plan to follow diet, quit smoking, follow exercise program, and take medications as prescribed.
3. Client establishes a system to administer medications accurately and to manage the medication regimen for optimal effects in accordance with life-style.
4. Client uses resources and support groups to assist with compliance.

5. Client modifies life-style to fit management of therapeutic regimen and changes when needed.

Myocardial Infarction (MI)

A myocardial infarction results from a partial or complete occlusion of a coronary artery. It is caused by atherosclerotic buildup in the artery, resulting in narrowing of the artery, a thrombus in the artery, or arterial spasm, leading to ischemia and necrosis of the heart tissue. The location of the infarct may vary, but most occur in the area of the left ventricle. Management is directed at preventing further damage, preventing recurrence or complications, and control of symptomatology.

Home care is primarily concerned with assessment and with the teaching of a medication regimen, control of risk factors to prevent recurrence, and measures to allow the heart to heal.

Nursing diagnosis

Pain

Related factors: Biologic injuring agents

Defining characteristics: Verbalization of pain descriptors (deep, crushing, squeezing chest pain in varying degrees of intensity); chest pain radiating to left arm, jaw, or neck (substernal or visceral); changes in vital signs; arrthymias; holding chest; dyspnea; nausea; vomiting; sense of impending doom; diaphoresis; restlessness

OUTCOMES

Short-term

Reduced pain, as evidenced by client's statement that pain has been relieved; relaxed facial expressions and posturing; and participation in ADL without pain (expected within 1 week)

Long-term

Absence of pain, as evidenced by progression to optimal level of health and performance of ADL without pain recurring (expected within 2 weeks)

NURSING INTERVENTIONS/INSTRUCTIONS

1. Assess pain location, severity, and type; precipitating factors; effect of medication on pain (each visit).
2. Instruct client in medication administration to relieve pain (nitrites) (first visit).
3. Instruct client to notify physician if pain returns or is not controlled and have emergency numbers available (first visit).
4. Instruct client to stay calm and to rest in semi-Fowler's position or with head elevated until emergency assistance arrives (first visit).

CLIENT AND FAMILY/CAREGIVER INTERVENTIONS

1. Client administers medications correctly and effectively.
2. Client reports complaints of pain to physician.
3. Client maintains calm environment and reduces stressors when pain occurs.
4. Client calls on emergency services if pain and associated symptoms occur indicating heart attack.

Nursing diagnosis

Activity intolerance

Related factors: Imbalance between oxygen supply and demand

Defining characteristics: Verbal report of fatigue or weakness; abnormal heart rate or blood pressure or dyspnea in response to activity; reduced energy and endurance level

OUTCOMES

Short-term

Increased activity and endurance, as evidenced by performance of ADL and other activities and by progressive moderate exercising and ambulation (expected within 2 to 3 weeks)

Long-term

Participation and independence in ADL and mobility to achieve optimal level of health and functioning with progressive increase in endurance (expected within 1 to 2 months)

NURSING INTERVENTIONS/INSTRUCTIONS

1. Review results of discharge treadmill exercise test if done (first visit).
2. Assess for and encourage participation in ADL and diversional activities (each visit).
3. Encourage gradual increase in an individualized daily exercise and/or walking program based on absence of symptoms, results of treadmill exercise test, and physician recommendation; relate activities to age, general condition, cardiac status, interests, and life-style (each visit).
4. Instruct client to rest before and after exercise program; to avoid heavy lifting, stress, large meals, extremes in temperature, and stimulants (caffeine) or any combination of these; and to avoid isometric exercises (first visit and reinforce on second visit).
5. Instruct client to cease activity and notify physician if activity intolerance occurs, including unwarranted fatigue, shortness of breath, diaphoresis, weakness, pulse not reverting to baseline within 5 minutes after rest, change in pulse trends, or chest pain (first visit).
6. Encourage client to enroll and participate in formal cardiac rehabilitation program with prescription from physician (first visit).
7. Refer HHA to assist in ADL.

CLIENT AND FAMILY/CAREGIVER INTERVENTIONS

1. Client participates in planned activities with progressive increases.
2. Client schedules rest periods with activities and plans diversional activities.
3. Client refrains from cardiac stressors and extreme exertion or activities.
4. Client adjusts work to activity tolerance.
5. Client reports new or recurrent symptoms of activity intolerance.

Nursing diagnosis

Decreased cardiac output

Related factors: Electrical factor of alteration in rate, rhythm, and conduction

Defining characteristics: Changes in hemodynamic readings; arrhythmias; ECG changes

OUTCOMES

Short-term

Adequate cardiac output, as evidenced by vital signs returning to baseline determinations (expected within 2 to 3 days)

Long-term

Cardiac output maintained, as evidenced by vital signs and cardiac status returning to level to achieve optimal functioning without complications (expected within 2 weeks)

NURSING INTERVENTIONS/INSTRUCTIONS

1. Assess circulatory status, noting blood pressure, PMI, pulse rate and rhythm, capillary refill time, skin color and temperature, presence of pain or edema, fatigue, weakness, nausea, vomiting, or unexplained restlessness or anxiety (see Cardiovascular System Assessment, p. 10, for guidelines) (first visit and ongoing).
2. Instruct client to monitor vital signs and record in a log, noting any changes to report to or ask physician about (first visit).
3. Instruct client in administration of and assessment of response to medications (vasodilators, β-adrenergic blocking agents, calcium channel blockers, antihypertensives, diuretics, inotropic agents, low-dose aspirin), including dose, route, frequency, side effects, food, drug, or alcohol interactions, and implications for self care; emphasize compliance with regimen and avoidance of OTC drugs, and caution against altering, omitting, or abruptly stopping any of the prescribed medications (first visit and reinforce on each visit).

CLIENT AND FAMILY/CAREGIVER INTERVENTIONS

1. Client administers all prescribed medications correctly and monitors for desired effects.

2. Client monitors vital signs daily as instructed, in different positions and at different times, and records; identifies changes to report.
3. Client reports signs and symptoms of reduced cardiac output.

Nursing diagnosis

Sexual dysfunction

Related factors: Altered body function caused by disease process

Defining characteristics: Verbalization of the problem; actual or perceived limitations imposed by disease; fear of heart attack and death

OUTCOMES

Short-term

Improved sexual adequacy, as evidenced by client's statement of awareness that sexual activity is allowed and that options with intimacies are being explored (expected within 1 week)

Long-term

Optimal sexual relationship with significant partner achieved with required adaptations (expected within 2 months)

NURSING INTERVENTIONS/INSTRUCTIONS

1. Assess sexual history, concerns, beliefs and attitude about sexual activity after MI; activity tolerance and results of treadmill exercise test and 2-flight stair-climb test; review drug profile and relate to persistent problems with decreased libido or impotence (first visit).
2. Provide written information about sexual activity after MI to client and partner (first visit).
3. Encourage expression of concerns and questions after initial assessment, and include partner in all discussions (each visit).
4. Encourage nonsexual activities that promote intimacy, including participating in activities together and talking together (first visit).
5. Advise client about sexual options that minimize cardiac workload (first visit):

   Rest before sexual activity, or engage in activity after a night's rest.

Take prophylactic nitrite, if prescribed, before activity.
Use side-to-side or less taxing positions.
Avoid activity after eating a large meal or drinking alcoholic beverages.
Avoid extremes of temperature, stress, and fatigue.
Avoid anal intercourse.

6. Instruct client to cease activity and to notify physician if intolerance to sexual activity occurs, including persistent increase in pulse and respirations after activity, chest pain at any time, or extreme protracted fatigue following activity (first visit).
7. Refer client to sex therapist if appropriate (any visit).

CLIENT AND FAMILY/CAREGIVER INTERVENTIONS

1. Client verbalizes concerns and inquires about sexual activity.
2. Client communicates concerns with partner.
3. Client promotes intimacy through nonsexual as well as sexual approaches.
4. Client structures sexual activity to minimize stressors and distractors.
5. Client verbalizes effect of fear and certain medications on sexual activity, desire, or performance.
6. Client sees therapist with partner if needed.

Nursing diagnosis

Knowledge deficit

Related factors: Lack of information about post-myocardial infarction medical regimen

Defining characteristics: Request for information about medications, dietary and fluid needs, need for life-style changes, and follow-up requirements; denial of condition

OUTCOMES

Short-term

Adequate knowledge, as evidenced by client's ability to describe signs and symptoms of condition, management of risk factors, and compliance with medical regimen (expected within 1 week)

Long-term

Adequate knowledge, as evidenced by client's meeting requirements of adapted life-style to achieve optimal health and functioning without complications (expected within 1 month)

NURSING INTERVENTIONS/INSTRUCTIONS

1. Assess life-style, ability to adapt, coping and learning abilities, and family participation and support (first visit).
2. Assess for precipitating or risk factors associated with the condition, including family history, previous MI, hypertension, diabetes mellitus, obesity, sedentary life-style, hyperlipidemia, and personality response to stress; adapt teaching to data (first visit).
3. Instruct client in circulatory assessment, to monitor resting pulse for 1 full minute daily, and to withhold inotropic agent if pulse is less than 60; inform client of signs and symptoms of cardiac complications to report, including changes in pulse or blood pressure, chest pain, edema, skin color change, fatigue, weakness, nausea, vomiting, or restlessness (first visit).
4. Instruct client in administration of medications (vasodilators, β-adrenergic blocking agents, calcium channel blockers, antihypertensives, diuretics, anticoagulants, antilipidemics, inotropic agents, low-dose aspirin), and prepare a written schedule with administration instructions for client (first visit).
5. Instruct client to weigh weekly on same scale, at same time of day, and wearing same clothing (first visit).
6. Assess nutritional status and caloric requirements, and instruct client in reduction diet to maintain ideal weight and in low-cholesterol, low-fat, sodium-restricted diet as prescribed (first visit and reinforce on second visit).
7. Instruct client to avoid smoking, stress, alcohol, and stimulating beverages (first visit).
8. Inform client of importance of compliance with exercise and cardiac rehabilitation program (each visit).
9. Instruct client in bowel program and to avoid straining at defecation (first visit).
10. Assist client in identifying stressors, and teach relaxation techniques and stress management (each visit).
11. Offer food list and sample menus of food and fluid inclusions and restrictions (first visit).

12. Instruct client to maintain fluid intake, to monitor intake and output for balance, and to compare with weight gains or losses and presence of edema (first visit).
13. Instruct client to avoid high altitudes; inform client of possible limitation of air travel (first visit).
14. Instruct client to notify physician of deteriorating condition or complications, including erratic pulse, dyspnea, unexplained anxiety, feelings of confusion or impending doom, persistent or recurrent chest pain, or fever (first visit).
15. Encourage client to comply with physician and laboratory appointments (first visit).
16. Advise client to carry or wear identification and information regarding health status (first visit).
17. Initiate referral to counseling, community agencies and groups for smoking cessation and weight loss, and the American Heart Association for literature and support (first visit).

CLIENT AND FAMILY/CAREGIVER INTERVENTIONS

1. Client administers all medications safely as instructed.
2. Client monitors vital signs and reports changes.
3. Client balances work, rest, exercise, and diversional activities.
4. Client avoids smoking, stressful situations, and alcohol.
5. Client maintains ideal weight.
6. Client prepares and consumes special diet of calculated calories, low in sodium, cholesterol, and fat.
7. Client maintains bowel pattern of soft, formed stool.
8. Client reports symptoms of condition change or inquires if unsure about changes to physician.
9. Client complies with physician and laboratory appointments.
10. Client wears medical identification at all times.
11. Client contacts support or self-help groups as needed.

Pacemaker Implantation

A permanent pacemaker is an electric device, inserted in the chest wall, that maintains a normal rhythm of myocardial contractions by delivering an electrical stimulus to the myocardium. A pacemaker may stimulate the heart at a constant and fixed rate (asynchronous, competitive), or it may deliver a stimulus on demand (synchronous, noncompetitive) when the heart does not contract at a set rate. A transvenous approach is frequently done, in which the electrode (lead) is inserted percutaneously through the right cephalic, jugular, or subclavian vein and positioned in the right ventricle. The distal end of the electrode is attached to the pulse generator (pacemaker), which is placed in a subcutaneous pocket in the upper chest. The pacemaker contains circuitry and battery programs for a heart rate generally between 50 and 100 beats/min. The pacemaker regulates the heart rate, which results in an adequate cardiac output. Permanent pacemakers are inserted in clients with heart block, arrhythmias, or conduction defects.

Home care is primarily concerned with the teaching of the medical regimen that is followed and the monitoring of pacemaker functioning and heart rate to prevent complications.

Nursing diagnosis

Risk for infection

Related factors: Invasive procedure of pacemaker insertion

Defining characteristics: Redness, swelling, pain, fluid collection at the site of insertion; temperature elevation

OUTCOMES

Short-term

Absence of infection, as evidenced by clean and dry insertion site, with healing in progress and edges of incision well approximated (expected within 3 days)

Long-term

Skin integrity maintained at incisional site, as evidenced by completely healed incision without irritation, discomfort, or disruption of skin (expected within 4 to 6 weeks)

NURSING INTERVENTIONS/INSTRUCTIONS

1. Assess, and instruct client to assess, vascular (cutdown) access and pacemaker insertion sites for local heat, erythema, edema,

tenderness or pain, drainage, or disruption of suture edges (each visit).

2. Instruct client in hand-washing technique and clean wound and skin care (first visit and reinforce on second visit).
3. Monitor temperature and instruct client in taking temperature and noting chilling or flushing and reporting these changes and elevations over 100° F to physician (first visit).
4. Instruct client in antibiotic prophylactic therapy if prescribed (first visit).

CLIENT AND FAMILY/CAREGIVER INTERVENTIONS

1. Client monitors temperature and condition of sites.
2. Client verbalizes signs and symptoms to report.
3. Client provides clean wound care; performs hand washing before giving any care to wounds.
4. Client administers antibiotic therapy.
5. Client utilizes positions that prevent pressure on sites and promote comfort.

Nursing diagnosis

Anxiety

Related factors: Change in health status; fear of death

Defining characteristics: Verbalization of fear of pacemaker malfunction and consequences; feeling of helplessness caused by dependence on pacemaker; increased apprehension and uncertainty

OUTCOMES

Short-term

Reduction in anxiety, as evidenced by client's statement that anxiety has decreased, that muscles and posturing have relaxed, and that pacemaker function and limitation imposed on life-style are understood (expected within 2 to 3 days)

Long-term

Anxiety controlled and managed, as evidenced by life-style changes made to achieve level of health commensurate with pacemaker and medical regimen (expected within 2 weeks)

NURSING INTERVENTIONS/INSTRUCTIONS

1. Assess mental and emotional status and effect of stress on pacemaker function (see Psychosocial Assessment, p. 48, for guidelines) (first visit).
2. Assess for inner personal resources, ability to cope, and responses to presence of pacemaker (first visit).
3. Provide an accepting environment, and allow for expression of fears and concerns regarding pacemaker function (each visit).
4. Instruct client in relaxation techniques, and help client to identify and avoid stressful situations (first and second visits).
5. Provide continuing information about condition, improvements, tests, and treatments, and answer all queries honestly and in understandable language (each visit).
6. Initiate referral for counseling for stress and anxiety reduction as indicated (any visit).

CLIENT AND FAMILY/CAREGIVER INTERVENTIONS

1. Client verbalizes and vents concerns regarding pacemaker, restrictions, and knowledge needed to prevent complications.
2. Client inquires about pacemaker and its function and about changes in life-style expected.
3. Client uses relaxation and diversional techniques to decrease anxiety.
4. Client consults physician if unable to control anxiety and if it affects daily activities.

Nursing diagnosis

Knowledge deficit

Related factors: Lack of knowledge about pacemaker

Defining characteristics: Request for information about pacemaker function, pacemaker monitoring, malfunction of pacemaker battery, failure to capture or sense, or malpositioning or malfunctioning of pacing catheter

OUTCOMES

Short-term

Adequate knowledge of pacemaker, as evidenced by client's ability to describe type of pacemaker, why it is needed, how it functions, and symptoms and signs of pacemaker failure or complications and consequences; pulse maintained at set rate and regularity (expected within 3 days)

Long-term

Adequate knowledge of safe, appropriate pacemaker functioning, as evidenced by meeting requirements of pacemaker monitoring and functioning and associated medical regimen to achieve optimal level of cardiac function and general health (expected within 2 to 4 weeks)

NURSING INTERVENTIONS/INSTRUCTIONS

1. Assess life-style, ADL abilities, ability to learn and adapt, interest in learning pacemaker functioning, and family participation and support (first visit).
2. Assess cardiovascular status; note blood pressure, pulse rate, and rhythm of apical and peripheral pulses (see Cardiovascular System Assessment, p. 10, for guidelines) (each visit).
3. Review pacemaker instruction manual and note implications for client teaching (first visit).
4. Instruct client in administration of medications for underlying conditions and cardiac medications prescribed (first visit).
5. Instruct client to take and record radial pulse daily; stress resting 5 minutes before taking pulse and monitoring pulse for 1 full minute; instruct client to report to physician any significant deviation from pacer setting or any change that reflects prepacemaker condition (first visit and reinforce on second visit).
6. Instruct client in normal function of the heart and how the pacemaker performs to maintain heart rate (first visit).
7. Monitor client for signs and symptoms of decreased cardiac output, including fatigue, vertigo, decreased blood pressure, slow or erratic pulse, shortness of breath, diminished peripheral pulses, altered mental status, or chest pain, and instruct client to notify physician if any occur (first visit).
8. Inform client of range of activities allowed or when they may be resumed, such as sexual activity, according to physician recommendations; instruct client to avoid contact sports, constrictive clothing around pacemaker, jerky or exaggerated movements on pacemaker side, or toying with insertion sites (first visit).

9. Inform client of sources of electromagnetic interference and implications for pacemaker (first visit).
   - Ground all home appliances (electric and battery operated) and maintain them in good working order.
   - Client may use light switches, radios, television, and most household convenience appliances as long as none are held over the insertion site.
   - Avoid proximity to microwave ovens (stay at least 6 feet away if in use); avoid large electrical generators.
   - Move away from any field that interferes with pacemaker function, and normal function will resume.
   - Always inform other professionals (dentist, technician, physician) about presence of pacemaker before having any procedure or testing done.
   - When travelling by air, inform security personnel before passing through metal detector, since pacemaker will trigger alarm.
10. Instruct client in telephone pacemaker check (done every 3 months) and to keep physician appointments for monitoring pacemaker and evaluation at least twice a year (first visit).
11. Inform client of need for battery change and unit replacement, and instruct client to schedule evaluation before and near "expiration date" (first visit).
12. Instruct client in range-of-motion (ROM) exercises on side of pacemaker if needed (first visit).
13. Instruct client to carry pacemaker history at all times with information that includes type, manufacturer, model and serial number, programmed rate, location of pulse generator, implant date, medications being taken, and name and number of attending physician (first visit and reinforce on second visit).
14. Instruct client to have emergency number at hand at all times (first visit).
15. Provide list of agencies and groups that can assist with information and support (first visit).

CLIENT AND FAMILY/CAREGIVER INTERVENTIONS

1. Client monitors pulse daily as instructed.
2. Client administers medications safely and effectively.
3. Client reports signs and symptoms of pacemaker malfunction to physician.

4. Client reports signs and symptoms indicating change in cardiac output as a result of malfunction to physician.
5. Client engages in full range of activities, with adaptations to minimize injury or electromagnetic interference.
6. Client monitors pacemaker function periodically by telephone or by clinic or hospital visit.
7. Client carries pacemaker information at all times.
8. Client complies with instruction to avoid complication of pacemaker dysfunction.
9. Client complies with appointments and schedules for evaluation and battery change.
10. Utilize community resources for information and support.

Peripheral Vascular Disease (PVD)

Peripheral vascular disease refers to a condition characterized by interference with blood flow to or from the extremities; the condition may involve either arteries or veins of the extremities. It may be caused by atherosclerosis or arteriosclerosis resulting in narrowing of the arteries, inflammation (as in thrombosis or thromboangiitis obliterans), or vasospasms (as in Raynaud's disease or varicose veins). Whether PVD is caused by inefficient cardiac pump actions or obstructed, damaged, inflamed, or infected vessels, the defining characteristic is a decreased peripheral blood flow resulting in ischemia.

Home care is primarily concerned with the teaching of a medical regimen that enhances circulatory status in the extremities and prevents complications associated with impaired peripheral circulation.

Nursing diagnosis

Altered peripheral tissue perfusion

Related factors: Interruption of arterial flow or venous congestion

Defining characteristics: Arterial flow—intermittent claudication, absent or weak peripheral pulses, decreased capillary filling time, cold feet, pallor on elevation, rubor when dependent, delayed healing, atrophy of skin, hair loss. Venous flow—aching; heavy sensation; Homan's sign; deep muscle tenderness and cramping pain; swelling, warmth, and increased pigmentation of area; prominent superficial veins; stasis ulcer

OUTCOMES

Short-term

Improved circulation to extremities, as evidenced by return to baseline lower-extremity color, temperature, size, and peripheral pulse; absence of discomfort in extremities (expected within 1 week)

Long-term

Adequate perfusion of extremities, as evidenced by return of circulation to baselines with optimal use and functional ability of extremities (expected within 1 to 2 months)

NURSING INTERVENTIONS/INSTRUCTIONS

1. Assess circulatory status and effect on extremities (see Cardiovascular System Assessment, p. 10, for guidelines) (first visit).
2. Review history for age at onset of circulatory problem, cardiac status, number of pregnancies, chronic disease, familial tendency toward circulatory problems, trauma, infections, use of tobacco and alcohol, or weight problem (first visit).
3. Differentiate between arterial and venous deficiency or dysfunction (first visit).
4. Assess peripheral pulses, capillary refill time, skin color and integrity, temperature, pain in extremities, paresthesia, degree of motion and sensation, and calf measurement (each visit).
5. Instruct client to protect extremities against chilling; to avoid use of constrictive hose or clothing and accessories; to avoid prolonged standing or leg crossing; and to avoid use of heating pad or hot water bottle (first visit).
6. Instruct client in a walking program and elevation of legs above heart level when sitting to reduce venous congestion (first visit and reinforce on second visit).

7. Instruct client in measures to increase arterial flow, including elevating head using a foam-rubber wedge, resting with legs below heart level, performing postural exercises, and walking as prescribed (first visit and reinforce on second visit).

CLIENT AND FAMILY/CAREGIVER INTERVENTIONS

1. Client protects extremities from temperature extremes or burns or trauma.
2. Client avoids application of heat, constriction of circulation to extremities, and prolonged sitting or standing.
3. Client rests and exercises daily as prescribed to promote circulation and prevent pain.
4. Client performs ROM, Buerger-Allen, and walking exercises as prescribed.

Nursing diagnosis

Risk for impaired skin integrity

Related factors: Internal factor of altered circulation

Defining characteristics: Skin discoloration, thickening, scarring; dermatitis; altered sensation; ischemic lesion; stasis ulcer

OUTCOMES

Short-term

Absence of skin breakdown, as evidenced by intact skin and absence of irritation, excoriation, and trauma (expected within 2 days)

Long-term

Skin integrity maintained, as evidenced by skin intact and circulation improved, allowing for optimal health and use of extremities (expected within 1 month)

NURSING INTERVENTIONS/INSTRUCTIONS

1. Assess skin for breakdown areas and deviations from baseline condition (see Integumentary System Assessment, p. 36, for guidelines) (first visit).
2. Instruct client to monitor skin on extremities for trauma or any disruptions and to notify physician of changes (first visit).

3. Instruct client to avoid injury (first visit).
   Avoid scratching or rubbing extremities.
   Wear sturdy, well-fitting shoes with clean, loose-fitting white cotton hose.
   Bathe in tepid water with a neutral soap and dry thoroughly.
   Trim nails straight across.
   Apply cream to skin on extremities.
4. Instruct client in application of antiembolic hose or elastic bandages (first visit and reinforce on second visit).
5. Inform client that bed cradle may be used to keep linens off extremities (first visit).
6. Apply Unna's boot or dressings on leg ulcer as ordered (any visit).
7. Refer to podiatrist or perform routine foot care to treat ingrown nails, corns, calluses (first visit).

CLIENT AND FAMILY/CAREGIVER INTERVENTIONS

1. Client monitors skin daily and reports abnormalities to physician.
2. Client avoids conditions or trauma that injure skin on extremities.
3. Client wears support hose and proper shoes and socks.
4. Client maintains skin integrity in presence of circulatory disorder.
5. Client utilizes podiatrist for foot care if needed.
6. Client provides daily foot and skin care on both extremities.

Nursing diagnosis

Knowledge deficit

Related factors: Lack of information about circulatory disorder

Defining characteristics: Request for information about disease and its effects, measures to prevent symptoms and complications of disorder, and mobility requirements and restrictions

OUTCOMES

Short-term

Adequate knowledge, as evidenced by client's statement of signs and symptoms of circulatory deficiency and escalating condition, compliance with medical regimen, and adaptive life-style behaviors (expected within 4 to 7 days)

Long-term

Adequate knowledge, as evidenced by client's meeting requirements to achieve optimal level of health and functioning within limitations imposed by chronic circulatory condition; absence of complications (expected within 1 to 2 months)

NURSING INTERVENTIONS/INSTRUCTIONS

1. Assess life-style, adapting abilities, learning interest and abilities, and family participation and support (first visit).
2. Assess mobility status, including ability to walk without pain or discomfort, claudication, or aching extremities with increased ambulation, and instruct client to rest when pain occurs (first visit).
3. Instruct client to cease or reduce smoking and give rationale (first visit).
4. Instruct client to reduce weight or to maintain desired body weight, and assist client to plan low-fat, low-cholesterol diet (first visit).
5. Instruct client in medication administration, including vasodilators, adrenergic blocking agents, and analgesics, and instruct client to avoid OTC drugs without physician advice (first visit and reinforce on second visit).
6. Assess client's knowledge of condition and its signs and symptoms, and instruct client to notify physician of deteriorating condition or worsening symptoms indicating complications, including severe pain with or without activity, decrease in or loss of sensory or motor function, and changes in skin appearance or temperature (first visit).
7. Instruct client to obtain adequate rest, including 8 hours' sleep per night, to maintain proper positioning of extremities based on arterial or venous insufficiency, to follow only the prescribed activity and exercise regimen, and to stop activity when pain occurs (first visit).
8. Instruct client in stress management techniques, or inform client of availability of assistance from counseling (any visit).
9. Refer client to support group for weight reduction or to stop smoking (first visit).

CLIENT AND FAMILY/CAREGIVER INTERVENTIONS

1. Client administers medications safely and monitors effects.
2. Client notifies physician if signs and symptoms of circulatory compromise are present.
3. Client participates in programs to reduce weight and stop smoking.
4. Client maintains weight reduction diet and restricts intake of fat and cholesterol.
5. Client maintains rest and exercise programs.
6. Client avoids stressful situations; practices stress-reducing exercises.
7. Client reconciles pain with activity needs.

Thrombophlebitis

Thrombophlebitis refers to a venous thrombus accompanied by venous inflammation, usually occurring in the lower extremity. Symptoms may vary; they depend in part on location and which vessels are affected. The causes of thrombophlebitis include venous stasis, venous trauma, and increased blood coagulation. The condition may be complicated by vessel obstruction by the clot or movement of the clot into the circulation (embolus).

Home care is primarily concerned with the control of factors that contribute to thrombus formation and the prevention of chronic venous insufficiency or pulmonary emboli by teaching the client the medical regimen and the importance of compliance with instruction.

Nursing diagnosis

Pain

Related factors: Biologic injuring agents

Defining characteristics: Verbalization of pain descriptors; pain, warmth, redness, edema of calf; Homan's sign; protective behavior of affected leg

OUTCOMES

Short-term

Decreased pain, as evidenced by client's statement of pain reduction; relaxed posture and absence of guarding behavior; decrease in inflammation of calf; and resumption of physical activity (expected within 1 week)

Long-term

Absence of pain, as evidenced by independence in ADL and by activity to achieve optimal level of health and functioning without discomfort (expected within 2 to 4 weeks)

NURSING INTERVENTIONS/INSTRUCTIONS

1. Assess pain, including type, location, severity, and influence of position and activity (each visit).
2. Encourage periods of rest with leg elevated and supported; perform ROM exercises as prescribed (active or passive) (each visit).
3. Instruct client to avoid any constriction of popliteal space on affected leg (first visit).
4. Apply warm soaks or compresses to affected leg, and teach client to perform procedure (first visit).
5. Encourage client to perform as many ADL as possible, and instruct client in ambulation as allowed (first visit).
6. Instruct client in application of antiembolic hose if prescribed (first visit).
7. Instruct client in administration of analgesics, and especially note any interactions with anticoagulant therapy (first visit).
8. Refer HHA to assist with ADL.

CLIENT AND FAMILY/CAREGIVER INTERVENTIONS

1. Client provides activity and rest with progressive increases daily.
2. Client administers medications and heat treatments as instructed.
3. Client uses aids in ambulation as needed.
4. Client participates in ADL, and progresses until independence is achieved.
5. Client reports return of pain to physician.
6. Client utilizes physical therapist if appropriate.

Nursing diagnosis

Knowledge deficit

Related factors: Lack of information about medical regimen and preventive measures

Defining characteristics: Request for information about risk factors for recurrence or complication of condition, activity and weight restrictions, and normal peripheral perfusion

OUTCOMES

Short-term

Adequate knowledge, as evidenced by client's statement of effects of activity and weight on condition; compliance with medication regimen; and adequate perfusion of extremity (expected within 2 to 3 days)

Long-term

Adequate knowledge, as evidenced by client's meeting requirements to achieve optimal functioning of extremity without complications or recurrence of condition (expected within 1 month)

NURSING INTERVENTIONS/INSTRUCTIONS

1. Assess for knowledge of disease and history or life-style that includes risk factors for the condition, including use of contraceptives, past surgeries and injuries, use of tobacco, tendency toward overweight, and blood pressure problems (first visit).
2. Assess extremies for integrity, color, warmth, size (take calf measurements bilaterally), motion, pain, presence of peripheral pulses, capillary refill time, and paresthesias (each visit).
3. Instruct client in calf assessment and to report asymmetry caused by edema (first visit).
4. Instruct client in weight reduction, including reducing calories in diet and following exercise program when appropriate (first visit and reinforce on second visit).
5. Instruct client in leg exercises, ROM exercises, and a progressive walking program with or without aids (each visit).
6. Suggest reduction in or cessation of smoking; refer client to support group for assistance (first visit).

7. Instruct client to avoid constricting clothing, prolonged sitting or standing, or crossing legs while sitting or resting; to elevate the legs above heart level when sitting; and to position the legs to avoid popliteal compression by use of pillows under the knees (first visit).
8. Measure and apply elastic antiembolic hose from toes to knees or to groin area smoothly; instruct client in application and how to avoid bunching or rolling down of hose and to remove for sleep (first visit).
9. Suggest use of bed cradle or other device to keep covers off leg (first visit).
10. Instruct client to avoid rubbing or massaging extremity (first visit).
11. Instruct client in administration of anticoagulants, including dose, frequency, side effects, and food, drug, or alcohol interactions; to avoid OTC drugs that contain aspirin or other drugs (nonsteroidal antiinflammatories) that interfere with platelet function; and to comply with laboratory testing for prothrombin time as prescribed (first visit and reinforce on second visit).
12. Instruct client in signs and symptoms of effects of anticoagulant therapy, including bleeding of gums, ecchymoses, epistaxis, and blood in urine or stool or sputum, and to report such incidents to physician (first visit).
13. Instruct client to report any change in skin integrity of extremity, such as stasis dermatitis or ulceration, and to report any signs and symptoms of pulmonary emboli, including anxiety, restlessness, breathlessness, syncope, increased pulse and respirations, cough, or pleuritic pain (first visit).
14. Instruct client to carry or wear identification indicating medications being taken (first visit).
15. Refer client to podiatrist if appropriate (any visit).

CLIENT AND FAMILY/CAREGIVER INTERVENTIONS

1. Client monitors extremities, including skin of extremities, daily for signs and symptoms to report.
2. Client complies with leg exercise, activity program, and dietary program as instructed.
3. Client avoids circulatory compromise in clothing, positioning, movement, pressure, or massage.
4. Client reduces smoking and alcohol and caffeine intake.

5. Client engages in weight-reduction program if needed.
6. Client wears antiembolic hose properly; removes every 8 hours for skin and leg assessment.
7. Client administers anticoagulant therapy correctly, based on periodic prothrombin time testing.
8. Client avoids trauma, medications, or straining that increases the risk of bleeding, and reports bleeding from any orifice, skin, or mucous membrane; reports the presence of blood in any excretions or secretions.
9. Client complies with laboratory testing and physician appointments.
10. Client wears identifying information.
11. Client utilizes podiatrist for foot care.

Neurologic system

Alzheimer's Disease

Alzheimer's disease is a degenerative disease of the brain. It is a progressive dementia type of disease characterized by a large loss of cells from the cerebral cortex and other areas. It results in behavior changes, memory loss, and impaired intellectual functioning. The brain changes include atrophy with wide sulci, senile plaques, and neurofibrillary tangles. The exact cause is unknown, but the disease is believed to be associated with genetic, viral, autoimmune disease, and choline O-acetyltransferase deficiency etiologies. The degree of severity of the dementia is a clinical judgment; diagnosis of Alzheimer's disease is made after years of evaluation of the presenting signs and symptoms.

Home care is primarily concerned with the teaching of safety and the medical regimen and with preservation of cognitive, social, physical, and psychological function.

Nursing diagnosis

Altered thought processes

Related factors: Physiologic changes

Defining characteristics: Cognitive dissonance; memory deficit or problems; impaired ability to make decisions, grasp ideas, solve problems, reason, and conceptualize; altered attention span; disorientation to time, place, person, circumstances, and events; hallucinations; inappropriate or nonreality-based thinking

OUTCOMES

Short-term

Preservation of cognitive and intellectual function, as evidenced by an ability to maintain reality within disease limitations (expected within 2 weeks, depending on stage of illness)

Long-term
Optimal cognitive and intellectual functioning within parameters established for the stage of the disease (expected ongoing)

NURSING INTERVENTIONS/INSTRUCTIONS

1. Assess short-term memory deficits; orientation to time, place, and person; effect of medications on cognitive function; reactions to stimulation; aggressive, abusive behavior (each visit).
2. Instruct family or caregiver to provide orientation-based stimulation, including clocks, calendars, and familiar objects within reach, and to repeat or correct misunderstood or confusing interactions (first visit).
3. Instruct family to approach client calmly and quietly, in a nonthreatening manner, to treat client with dignity and respect, and to avoid hostility and criticisms when behavior is unacceptable (first visit).
4. Instruct family to allow client time for accomplishing tasks, to set up a schedule for care and events, and to allow for time to respond to client's questions (first visit).
5. Instruct family to limit stimulation to what client can manage without confusion and agitation and to reduce environmental stimulation such as noise and excessive lighting (first visit).

CLIENT AND FAMILY/CAREGIVER INTERVENTIONS

1. Caregiver orients client to time, place, and person, and helps client maintain a realistic thought process when appropriate.
2. Caregiver modifies environment to enhance cognitive ability; permits hoarding, pictures of past life, and use of a telephone.
3. Caregiver maintains a supportive, nonjudgmental environment.
4. Caregiver allows client time to accomplish tasks, to communicate, and to process thinking in order to reduce frustration and agitation.
5. Caregiver avoids actions that cause overstimulation or sensory overload.

Nursing diagnosis

Risk for injury

Related factors: Internal biochemical regulatory function of brain

Defining characteristics: Integrative dysfunction; sensory dysfunction; wandering; unsafe environment; restlessness; balance and coordination problems; lack of awareness; disorientation; forgetfulness

OUTCOMES

Short-term

Reduction in risk for physical trauma, as evidenced by absence of environmental hazards and accidental injury (expected within 1 week)

Long-term

Absence of injury, as evidenced by adjustment of environment and provision of assistance necessary for safe ambulation and activities of daily living (ADL) practices (expected within 1 to 2 weeks and ongoing)

NURSING INTERVENTIONS/INSTRUCTIONS

1. Assess gait for instability, muscle weakness, and sensory-perceptual dysfunction; assess environment for hazards to be corrected (first visit).
2. Instruct family or caregiver in environmental changes to be made: clear pathways; remove or move furniture; remove small rugs; make slippery floors safe; remove matches from accessibility and remain with client when he or she is smoking; other adjustments, such as hand bars, assistive aids for walking (first visit).
3. Instruct family to secure and install a signaling device that will sound an alarm when client wanders past a certain point or out the door (first visit).
4. Provide assistance, and incorporate appropriate amount of assistance and appropriate frequency of ambulation into daily activity plan (first visit and reinforce on second visit).
5. Instruct family to reorient client to environment when necessary, to orient client to anything new in the immediate surroundings, to place articles for frequent use within reach, and to maintain same placement of articles and furniture (first visit).
6. Instruct family to avoid application of hot articles to the skin, offering food that is hot, or hot water for bathing; burns can result (first visit).

7. Instruct family to store medications in a safe, locked cabinet (first visit).
8. Inform family that low-heeled, nonskid shoes should be used by client for walking; instruct client to use a wide base when standing or ambulating (first visit).

CLIENT AND FAMILY/CAREGIVER INTERVENTIONS

1. Caregiver identifies and eliminates or controls hazards in the environment.
2. Caregiver prevents falls or other injuries or trauma.
3. Caregiver provides identification bracelet or alarm device to prevent wandering away and reduce risk for injury.
4. Caregiver assists and supervises activities on the basis of client's cognitive and mentation status.
5. Caregiver incorporates ambulation and diversional activities into client's daily schedule.

Nursing diagnosis

Self-care deficit (bathing/hygiene, dressing/grooming, feeding, toileting)

Related factors: Perceptual or cognitive impairment; motor deficits

Defining characteristics: Inability to perform ADL; inability to recognize need for daily personal care; inability to use articles or utensils; inability to distinguish what is appropriate from what is inappropriate in dressing, grooming, and toileting

OUTCOMES

Short-term

Self-care maintained within limitations imposed by disease, as evidenced by personal appearance and care being adequate and appropriate (expected within 1 to 2 weeks)

Long-term

Appropriate pattern of ADL achieved, as evidenced by cleanliness and adequate hygiene, grooming, dressing, eating, and toileting with or without assistance or assistive aids (expected within 1 month and ongoing)

NURSING INTERVENTIONS/INSTRUCTIONS

1. Assess areas of self-care deficits and causes for them, need for assistance or supervision, and need for assistive aids (see Functional Assessment, p. 57, for guidelines) (each visit).
2. Instruct family or caregiver to verbally remind or use cues for client to perform specific activity and to give only the assistance that is needed while avoiding expectations of task performance that may be frustrating (each visit).
3. Provide and instruct client and family in use of assistive aids and devices for eating, including large or padded handles on utensils, plate guard, placing food within view, and removing items not needed for meal (first visit).
4. Provide and instruct client and family in use of aids for toileting, including raised toilet seat, commode, hand bar for holding, and undergarments that are easy to remove and replace, offering toileting opportunity or remind to use toilet (first visit).
5. Provide and instruct client and family in use of aids for bathing, dressing, and grooming, including Velcro closures, zippers, large neck openings, elastic waists, articles within reach; suggest possibility of purchasing several articles of clothing that are the same if client likes to wear the same things every day; lay out clothing daily in order of application and demonstrate use of articles if needed (each visit).
6. Provide and instruct client in use of a stool in the shower or hand bars to get in and out of the tub; supervise client in regulating the water temperature (first visit).
7. Refer home health aide (HHA) to assist in ADL as needed.
8. Initiate referral to physical, recreational, and/or occupational therapy (any visit).

CLIENT AND FAMILY/CAREGIVER INTERVENTIONS

1. Caregiver assists in ADL as needed.
2. Caregiver supervises self-care activities without impinging on independence and causing frustration; avoids rushing client to complete a task.
3. Caregiver provides assistive aids to enhance self-care in ADL.
4. Caregiver recognizes client's capabilities and assists in areas of self-care deficits.
5. Client maintains adequate personal care, grooming, hygiene, and appearance.

Nursing diagnosis

Risk for violence directed at others

Related factors: Brain abnormalities

Defining characteristics: Restlessness; irritability; combative behavior; fear, bewilderment; agitation; outbursts when unable to complete tasks; lack of rest and sleep; frustration

OUTCOMES

Short-term

Minimal violence directed at others, as evidenced by reduction in agitation, frustration, and combative behavior (expected within 1 to 2 weeks)

Long-term

Absence of other-directed violence, as evidenced by lack of agitation, frustration, and combative behavior (expected ongoing)

NURSING INTERVENTIONS/INSTRUCTIONS

1. Assess possible sensory overload, reactions to events and precipitating factors, depression, coping mechanisms used, misinterpretation of environment, and sleep and rest patterns (each visit).
2. Note behaviors indicating suspiciousness, fear, irritability, agitation, or combativeness (each visit).
3. Provide for verbalization of feelings to avoid suppressed feelings that lead to frustrations; instruct family or caregivers to avoid assigning tasks or having expectations that cause frustrations (each visit).
4. Promote a calm environment, and instruct family or caregiver to reduce stimuli, to avoid distressing client, and to provide diversion to diffuse a situation that does distress client (first visit).
5. Instruct family or caregiver to approach slowly and in a calm manner, to use slow gestures, and to keep hands where client can see them (first visit).
6. Instruct family or caregiver (and reinforce regularly) to avoid giving care or bothering client when agitated; limit foods and

beverages containing caffeine (chocolate, coffee); face client when present during upsets or combative periods and protect self from possible injury from client (each visit).

7. Instruct family to avoid allowing client excessive napping and to offer daily activities; remind client when bedtime approaches, and fulfill rituals before sleep; if client is awakened during night, reassure him or her with a quiet, calm voice that it is night and time for sleep (first visit).

CLIENT AND FAMILY/CAREGIVER INTERVENTIONS

1. Caregiver identifies cause of agitation and combative behavior, and takes measures to prevent violence and frustration.
2. Caregiver responds to client's emotions and provides a calm, reassuring environment.
3. Caregiver allows for open expression of anxiety, frustrations, and feelings with an accepting attitude.
4. Caregiver allows client as much control over environment as possible.
5. Caregiver provides for rest and sleep needs as determined by previous patterns.
6. Caregiver eliminates or minimizes stimuli or expectations that agitate client.

Nursing diagnosis

Altered family processes

Related factors: Situational crisis of progressive degeneration of brain function of family member

Defining characteristics: Family system unable to meet physical and emotional needs of family and ill family member; family unable to express or accept feelings and security needs of members; family unable to accept change or deal with traumatic experience of caring for ill member

OUTCOMES

Short-term

Progressive adaptation to care of family member, as evidenced by family's statement of decreased anxiety and fatigue and by effective use of coping mechanisms (expected within 1 to 2 weeks)

Long-term

Optimal adjustment and adaptation to care of ill member, as evidenced by satisfactory physical, social, and psychological health of family members (expected within 1 month and ongoing)

NURSING INTERVENTIONS/INSTRUCTIONS

1. Assess family interventions, dynamics, supportive behaviors, past patterns of social and diversional activities, past roles, and overall health status of caregiver(s) (see Family Assessment, p. 55, for guidelines) (first visit).
2. Inform family that disorder is progressive, that no cures are available, and that care is supportive (first visit).
3. Include all family members or significant persons in all teaching and planning of care, with scheduling and incorporation into daily routines (each visit).
4. Discuss possible hired help or respite care to assist in care and supervision of client, day care program, or other useful programs to relieve family from constant attendance to client needs (any visit).
5. Inform and instruct family in relaxation and coping techniques and in strategies to manage own behavior caused by unrelieved responsibilities (first and second visits).
6. Instruct family or caregivers to monitor their own health needs, and help them to identify problem areas for referral and evaluation if needed; emphasize the need to maintain their physical and emotional health (first and second visit).
7. Inform family of the importance of continuing or maintaining social and diversional activities and of the availability of social supports to participate in care (first visit).
8. Discuss anxiety produced by role reversal and feeling of powerlessness in caring for parent (any visit).
9. Instruct family in, and encourage them to discuss, methods to deal with client behavior and reactions (first visit).
10. Refer family to social services for assistance with finances or consultation with legal advisor if needed for client who has changes in cognitive ability and competence (any visit).
11. Refer family or caregiver to family counseling or individual counseling as appropriate (any visit).
12. Suggest and discuss local and national resources, such as Alzheimer's Disease and Related Disorders Association and

Children of Aging Parents, for information and support (first visit).

13. Discuss the need for long-term placement in the future as disease progresses or if family resources become exhausted (any visit).

CLIENT AND FAMILY/CAREGIVER INTERVENTIONS

1. Family verbalizes feelings and concerns.
2. Family identifies problems in family and how family solves them together.
3. Family resolves life-style changes together.
4. Family seeks out and participates in support group activity.
5. Family utilizes respite day care assistance.
6. Family maintains family health: physical, emotional, and social.
7. Family consults with social worker, financial counselor, and legal advisor for assistance.
8. Family considers and begins to adapt to future long-term custodial care.

Nursing diagnosis

Caregiver role strain

Related factors: Unpredictable illness course or instability in care receiver's health; psychological or cognitive problems in care receiver; lack of respite for caregiver

Defining characteristics: Report of not having enough resources to provide care (emotional and physical strength, help from others); worry about the receiver's health and emotional state or about having to place care receiver in an institution; feeling that caregiving interferes with other roles

OUTCOMES

Short-term

Caregiver role strain identified, as evidenced by verbalization of difficulties encountered in performing care and concern about ability and conflicts in giving care and adapting to role (expected within 1 week)

Long-term

Adaptation to, and reduction of strain in, caregiver role, as evidenced by continued safe and appropriate care provided without compromise to caregiver's own physical and emotional needs (expected within 1 month and ongoing)

NURSING INTERVENTIONS/INSTRUCTIONS

1. Assess demands and care needs of receiver and ability and desire of caregiver to perform role; participation of family members in care (first visit).
2. Assess relationship between care receiver and caregiver before illness and stressors placed on the relationship by the progressive nature of the disorder (first visit).
3. Assist caregiver to monitor his or her continued ability to perform care and treatments and provide for day-to-day needs and how care receiver's behavior and needs change this ability; maintenance of routines; need for additional resources (aides, homemaker, respite care, friends, family) (each visit).
4. Discuss role performance and whether expectations are realistic; flexibility of role and decision-making process (first visit).
5. Initiate referral to HHA, social services, or psychological counseling, and suggest other community resources to contact for assistance with economic, mental health, or physical health needs (any visit).

CLIENT AND FAMILY/CAREGIVER INTERVENTIONS

1. Caregiver develops coping strategies for the caregiving role and flexibility in day-to-day functioning.
2. Caregiver explores financial, legal, and physical assistance sources and considers referral to these services.
3. Caregiver maintains own health and well-being in caregiver role.
4. Caregiver utilizes respite care and assistance from others for relief from stress of constant caregiving.
5. Caregiver maintains ongoing caregiving and treatment regimen.

Nursing diagnosis

Knowledge deficit

Related factors: Lack of information about disease and care

Defining characteristics: Expressed need for information about medication administration, measures to prevent acute or chronic illness, prognosis, and progression of disease

OUTCOMES

Short-term

Adequate knowledge, as evidenced by family or caregiver's statement of correct medication scheduling and administration and methods to identify health problems (expected within 1 week)

Long-term

Adequate knowledge, as evidenced by optimal health and function within disease limitations (expected ongoing)

NURSING INTERVENTIONS/INSTRUCTIONS

1. Instruct family or caregiver in assessment for presence of urinary tract infection, upper respiratory infection, or other physical manifestations that might arise when client is unable to communicate symptoms; instruct family in taking temperature and recognizing changes in vital signs or urine or stool characteristics or expressions (nonverbal) of pain in any area and to report them to the physician (each visit).
2. Instruct family in administration of tranquilizers, antidepressants, and sedatives, including dose, action, frequency, side effects to report, when to discontinue the drug, and food and drug interactions (first visit and reinforce second visit).
3. Inform family that it is important to prevent exposure to infections and that health maintenance measures are important to prevent hospitalization, which would be traumatic for the client and might hasten progression of the disease (first visit).
4. Instruct family in daily nutritional, fluid, and elimination needs, and provide written lists of high-calorie foods that can be managed successfully, even if finger foods; a daily intake of 8 glasses of fluid per day if appropriate; use of stool softeners or suppository to prevent constipation and fecal impaction; regularity in elimination pattern for urination and defecation (first visit).

CLIENT AND FAMILY/CAREGIVER INTERVENTIONS

1. Caregiver manages daily elimination needs; provides for basic nutritional and fluid needs.

2. Caregiver takes preventive measures to ensure health of client.
3. Caregiver correctly administers medications and reports untoward effects.
4. Caregiver assesses and reports changes in physical health status.

Amyotrophic Lateral Sclerosis (ALS)

Amyotrophic lateral sclerosis is a motor neuron disease with the presenting symptoms associated with the part of the nervous system most affected. It is characterized by progressive degeneration of the corticospinal tracts and the anterior horn cells or bulbar efferent neurons. This degeneration causes muscle weakness and atrophy, beginning in the hands and spreading to the forearms and legs, and may eventually become generalized. In some cases, chewing, talking, and swallowing are affected. Muscle fasciculations are also commonly apparent. The exact cause is unknown, and treatment is based on symptomatic relief.

Home care is primarily concerned with the maintenance and teaching aspects of preservation of muscle function and independence in and control of therapy and care.

Nursing diagnosis

Impaired physical mobility

Related factors: Neuromuscular impairment

Defining characteristics: Inability to purposefully move within physical environment, including bed mobility, transfer, and ambulation; decreased muscle strength, control, or mass

OUTCOMES

Short-term

Preservation of physical mobility, as evidenced by ambulation and participation in ADL within limitations imposed by disease (expected within 1 week and ongoing)

Long-term

Optimal continued ability to perform gross and fine motor activities to achieve and maintain functioning (expected ongoing)

NURSING INTERVENTIONS/INSTRUCTIONS

1. Assess degree of mobility, range of motion, weakness of upper extremities, muscle wasting, and fasciculations (see Musculoskeletal System Assessment, p. 29, for guidelines) (each visit).
2. Assess ability to wash body parts, put on or take off clothing, get to and use toilet, bring food from receptacle to mouth, and difficulty in chewing and swallowing (first visit).
3. Instruct client in strengthening exercises to maintain function for as long as possible (first and second visits).
4. Instruct client in use of assistive devices for ambulation and ADL, and help client to obtain necessary equipment to maintain independence, such as lift, hospital bed, wheelchair, and spring seats (first visit).
5. Instruct client in positioning, transfer, and turning techniques (first visit and reinforce as needed).
6. Initiate referral to physical and occupational therapists, if appropriate, to address above interventions (any visit).
7. Refer home health aide to assist in ADL.

CLIENT AND FAMILY/CAREGIVER INTERVENTIONS

1. As long as possible, client performs ADL and walking activities with or without use of assistive aids, as disease progression allows.
2. Client uses techniques to assist in turning, positioning, and transfer.
3. Client maintains function within disease limitations as long as possible, with as much independence as possible.
4. Client complies with physical and occupational therapy schedule and practices activities as instructed.

Nursing diagnosis

Ineffective individual coping

Related factors: Personal vulnerability; multiple life changes; consequences of fatal chronic illness

Defining characteristics: Verbalization of inability to cope or ask for help; chronic worry and anxiety; chronic fatigue; chronic depression; emotional tension; inability to meet basic needs and role expectations

OUTCOMES

Short-term

Adequate coping, as evidenced by client's statement of need for life-style changes, expectations of disease and prognosis, need for improved coping mechanisms (expected within 1 week)

Long-term

Adequate coping, as evidenced by progressive grieving throughout illness, with reduction in anxiety and worry about prognosis and debilitation (expected within 3 months and ongoing)

NURSING INTERVENTIONS/INSTRUCTIONS

1. Establish rapport; provide an accepting environment for expression of concerns and questions (each visit).
2. Assess mental status, ability to adapt, use of coping mechanisms, and internal resources, and explore with client the most effective coping mechanisms and selection of positive options (first visit).
3. Help client to identify goals and positive coping mechanisms (each visit).
4. Allow client to participate in and plan care and practice effective problem-solving skills (each visit).
5. Instruct client to avoid events that produce stress or prevent use of constructive coping mechanisms or behavior (first visit).
6. Instruct client in coping, communication, and problem-solving skills if able (first and second visits).
7. Instruct client in relaxation techniques, and in diversional techniques such as music, muscle relaxation, and reading (first visit).

CLIENT AND FAMILY/CAREGIVER INTERVENTIONS

1. Client develops effective use of coping mechanisms.
2. Client avoids stress-provoking events.
3. Client engages in relaxation and diversional activities.
4. Client requests assistance when needed.
5. Client reduces and/or controls anxiety level; expresses feelings and concerns.

6. Client adapts to change in life-style to comply with medical regimen.

Nursing diagnosis

Altered nutrition: less than body requirements

Related factors: Inability to ingest food

Defining characteristics: Dysphagia; decreased gag reflex; weight loss; muscle wasting; inability to chew food

OUTCOMES

Short-term

Adequate nutrition, as evidenced by intake of nutrients via mouth, nasogastric tube, or total parenteral nutrition (expected within 1 week)

Long-term

Adequate nutritional intake by appropriate method and route to maintain sustenance for as long as disease permits (expected ongoing)

NURSING INTERVENTIONS/INSTRUCTIONS

1. Assess nutritional status, caloric and vitamin and mineral needs, ability to chew and swallow, presence of choking episodes, weight loss, and ideal weight (see Gastrointestinal System Assessment, p. 20, for guidelines) (each visit).
2. Instruct client to weigh weekly at same time, on same scale, wearing the same clothing, and compare with ideal weight (first visit).
3. Assess for feeding method, presence of nasogastric tube, gastrostomy, esophagostomy, right atrial catheter and feeding provided (first and second visits).
4. Instruct caregiver to offer soft foods, as in casseroles, that can be easily managed for oral feeding; client should avoid liquids after chewing food (first visit).
5. Instruct caregiver to offer foods that are hot or cold to stimulate mouth receptors; avoid semisolid foods and milk (first visit).
6. Instruct client to position himself or herself upright with neck flexed during feedings or meals (first visit).

CLIENT AND FAMILY/CAREGIVER INTERVENTIONS

1. Client maintains nutritional status via oral, intravenous, or gastrostomy route.
2. Client maintains actual weight, or as close to it as possible with consideration of muscle wasting; weighs weekly.
3. Client calculates caloric intake and compares with weight loss.
4. Client minimizes the risk of choking and aspiration of food.
5. Client prepares and ingests foods that are easy to chew and swallow.

Nursing diagnosis

Knowledge deficit

Related factors: Lack of information about disease

Defining characteristics: Expressed need for information about medical regimen, safety precautions to prevent trauma, and measures to maintain function

OUTCOMES

Short-term

Adequate knowledge, as evidenced by client's ability to describe progressive characteristics of the disease, the medical regimen, and precautions to be taken to maintain function for as long as possible (expected within 1 week)

Long-term

Adequate knowledge, as evidenced by compliance with treatments for optimal preservation of abilities for functioning (expected ongoing based on disease progression)

NURSING INTERVENTIONS/INSTRUCTIONS

1. Assess life-style, ability to adapt, extent of disease and its effects, learning ability and interest, and family participation and support (first visit).
2. Inform client of disease process, prognosis, reason for loss of neuromuscular function, and the primary symptoms of the disease (first visit).

3. Inform client of and stress need for continuing activity and socialization; offer suggestions for diversional activities to support cognitive abilities; emphasize continuing need for self-care and independence for as long as possible (each visit).
4. Suggest use of a companion, ways to change life-style, and methods of stress and anxiety management (first visit).
5. Assist client with compliance with medical regimen by writing out plan of care and activities and realistic expectations (first visit and reinforce or revise on second visit).
6. Instruct client in medication administration, including dose, time, frequency, action of drug, side effects, and food and drug interactions (first visit).
7. Instruct client in skin care, massage and protective padding of bony areas, and importance of changing positions every 2 to 4 hours; report any breakdown or skin changes that do not disappear (first visit).
8. Refer client to speech pathologist if he or she is still able to speak, or if client is having a problem with swallowing; suggest a microphone for amplification or electrolarynx for phonation; if client is unable to speak, use environmental control system activated by pictures or slight movements (eye opening or closing) (first visit).
9. Instruct client that risk for infection is high, especially respiratory infection, and to avoid people with upper respiratory infections or other illnesses; dispose of tissues properly; instruct caregiver to use proper hand-washing technique before giving care; report any respiratory changes to the physician (first visit).
10. Inform client of, and instruct in and provide, mechanical ventilator assistance if client is at end stage and remaining at home and family or caregiver is able to manage this care (each visit).
11. Refer client and family to community agencies or social worker for assistance and support (any visit).

CLIENT AND FAMILY/CAREGIVER INTERVENTIONS

1. Client supports all care and treatments and prevents complications.
2. Client adapts to and complies with the medical regimen.
3. Client manages life-style changes and supports independence in functional activities.

4. Client maintains cognitive abilities with assistance and provides stimulation.
5. Client reports complications when appropriate.
6. Client secures assistance with physical, economic, or psychological referral as needed.

Cerebrovascular Accident (CVA)

Cerebrovascular accident is the cerebral inefficiency or hemorrhage resulting from blood flow disturbance caused by infarction or rupture of a blood vessel. The blood flow interruption may be caused by a thrombosis or an embolism, and the hemorrhage may be caused by a congenital aneurysm, trauma, or hypertension. Transient ischemic attacks (TIA) are temporary disturbances that may precede a CVA. Both types of CVA may have abrupt onsets, with the hemorrhagic type having the most acute and destructive onset. The extent of neurologic deficits and their permanence depend on the person's age and health status and on the site and size of the lesion.

The nature of the home care required depends on the severity and extent of the neurologic deficit; home care is primarily concerned with teaching the medical regimen that is used to treat the underlying condition and with rehabilitation and aftercare to maximize the health and wellness potential of the client.

Nursing diagnosis

Impaired physical mobility

Related factors: Neuromuscular impairment

Defining characteristics: Hemiplegia; hemiparesis; inability to purposely move within physical environment, including bed mobility, transfer, and ambulation; immobility

OUTCOMES

Short-term

Progressive return of physical mobility, as evidenced by ambulation within limitations imposed by condition (expected within 1 week)

Long-term

Optimal continued return of mobility, as evidenced by maximal level of ability to ambulate, transfer, and perform other activities (expected ongoing)

NURSING INTERVENTIONS/INSTRUCTIONS

1. Assess degree and type of mobility impairment, range of motion (ROM), ability to transfer and change positions, muscle flaccidity, spasticity, and reflexes (see Musculoskeletal System Assessment, p. 29, for guidelines) (each visit).
2. Perform and instruct client in passive ROM exercises, with progress to active ROM exercises as appropriate in affected extremities (each visit).
3. Instruct client to position affected extremities using pillows, trochanter roll (hip), or other aids (footboard); place affected side with joint at higher level than joint proximal to it (first visit).
4. Instruct client to support limbs when repositioning (first visit).
5. Instruct client to elevate head of bed 15 degrees when in supine position and to use hard devices to support hand and soft devices to support leg (first visit).
6. Instruct client to limit turning to and lying on affected side for 1 hour and to avoid allowing the affected arm to rest on chest when in side-lying position (first visit).
7. Instruct client in exercises and movements, such as sitting up in bed or at side of bed, using head and body supports to prevent falling out of bed, moving to sitting position from lying position, moving from bed to chair, and moving from sitting position to standing position (first visit and reinforce each visit).
8. Initiate referral to physical and/or occupational therapy, and inform client of importance of compliance with exercises taught and use of aids to maximize self-mobility (first visit).

CLIENT AND FAMILY/CAREGIVER INTERVENTIONS

1. Client performs exercises and ambulation with or without aids.
2. Client uses techniques to assist in turning, positioning, and transfer.
3. Client maintains ambulation within limitations.
4. Client prevents contractures, maintains circulation, and maintains tone of muscles.
5. Client complies with physical rehabilitation schedule, and practices activities as instructed.

Nursing diagnosis

Self-care deficit (bathing/hygiene, dressing/grooming, feeding, toileting)

Related factors: Perceptual impairment; paralysis; urinary and/or bowel incontinence

Defining characteristics: Inability to wash body parts, put on or take off clothes, get to and use toilet or be aware of urge to eliminate, bring food from receptacle to mouth; inadequate nutritional intake; inability to swallow

OUTCOMES

Short-term

Progressive return to self-care, as evidenced by participation in feeding, toileting, bathing, personal hygiene, dressing, and grooming (expected within 1 week)

Long-term

Optimal return of functional abilities, as evidenced by maximal level of ability to perform ADL with or without assistance or assistive aids (expected within 2 to 3 months and ongoing)

NURSING INTERVENTIONS/INSTRUCTIONS

1. Assess client's ability to perform self-care; ability to swallow and eat; ability to get on and off bedpan or use commode; ability to use one hand if hemiplegic; neurologic impairment (tactile, visual, auditory, kinesthetic) and response to stimuli (see Functional Assessment, p. 51, for guidelines) (each visit).

2. Instruct family or caregiver to provide assistance or supervision as needed for performance of ADL (first visit).
3. Provide and instruct client in use of assistive aids and devices for eating, including large, swivel, or padded handles on utensils; plate guard; placing food within view; and removing items not needed for meal (first visit).
4. Provide and instruct client in use of aids for toileting, including raised toilet seat, commode, hand bar, and undergarments that are easy to remove and replace (first visit).
5. Provide and instruct client in use of aids for bathing, dressing, and grooming, including Velcro closures, zippers, large neck openings, elastic waists, and articles that may be placed in a holder or stuck to wall or counter (first visit).
6. Initiate referral to occupational therapy for instruction and practice in ADL and suggestions for other assistive aids or performance of above interventions as appropriate (any visit).
7. Refer home health aide for assistance in ADL (first visit).

CLIENT AND FAMILY/CAREGIVER INTERVENTIONS

1. Caregiver assists with ADL while encouraging independence.
2. Client uses assistive aids and devices in performance of ADL.
3. Client maintains functional abilities in daily activities.
4. Client complies with occupational rehabilitation schedule and practices activities as instructed.

Nursing diagnosis

Impaired verbal communication

Related factors: Physical barrier of decreased circulation in brain

Defining characteristics: Inability to speak (aphasia); dysarthria

OUTCOMES

Short-term

Adequate communication, as evidenced by ability to communicate needs effectively (expected within 1 week)

Long-term

Return to communication patterns, as evidenced by optimal speech or development of an effective method of communication (expected within 2 to 3 months and ongoing)

NURSING INTERVENTIONS/INSTRUCTIONS

1. Determine communication deficits and remaining strengths or positive features (first visit).
2. Instruct family or caregiver to speak to client in short simple statements, to ask questions that need a yes or no answer, to speak slowly and in a normal tone, and to allow time for a response (first visit).
3. Instruct client to use gestures, paper and pencil, slate board, pictures, or cards and to reinforce established communication techniques if appropriate (first visit).
4. Instruct client in oral and facial exercises to improve muscular integrity (first and second visits).
5. Initiate referral to speech pathologist for therapy (any visit).

CLIENT AND FAMILY/CAREGIVER INTERVENTIONS

1. Caregiver speaks to client slowly and clearly and in a normal tone.
2. Caregiver avoids interruptions, forcing client to communicate, or criticism of his or her speech.
3. Client uses facial expressions or pantomime to communicate.
4. Client uses pencil and paper, slate board, pictures, cards, or any other effective method to communicate.
5. Caregiver maintains a quiet environment, positions speaker in front of client, and decreases distractions.
6. Caregiver anticipates needs if client is unable to express them.
7. Client complies with speech pathologist's schedules and instructions.

Nursing diagnosis

Risk for trauma

Related factors: Weakness; balancing difficulties; reduced temperature and/or tactile sensation; neurologic deficit

Defining characteristics: Hemiparesis; hemiplegia; loss of muscle tone; visual-spatial misperception; inability to orient self and movement in the environment; unsteady gait; lack of safety precautions in the environment; neurosensory impairment (tactile)

OUTCOMES

Short-term

Minimal possibility of trauma, as evidenced by absence of falls or injury, and by client's statement of safety precautions to take (expected within 1 week and ongoing)

Long-term

Absence of trauma, as evidenced by safe environment maintained to accommodate neurologic deficits (expected within 1 month and ongoing)

NURSING INTERVENTIONS/INSTRUCTIONS

1. Assess sensory perception of heat and cold, sharpness and dullness; awareness of body parts; visual or auditory deficits; presence and degree of paralysis and ability for ambulation and movement; disorientation or change in mentation (each visit).
2. Instruct client and family to adjust environment to reduce possibility of falls and trauma by arranging furniture for holding, providing clear pathways, removing a door to accommodate a wheelchair, removing small rugs, and providing proper lighting and to use assistive aids when walking or refer to occupational therapy for this assistance (first visit).
3. Provide, and instruct family or caregiver to provide, a consistent approach when assisting with ambulation and ADL (first visit).
4. Instruct client to turn head and scan environment; instruct caregiver to approach on affected side and to place objects on affected side if visual field impairment is present (first visit).
5. Instruct client to protect affected limbs from extremes of hot or cold or from hot or cold applications to limbs if tactile perception is affected (first visit).
6. Instruct family or caregiver to supervise all activities if judgment of position, distance, or rate of movement is impaired (first visit).
7. Instruct family or caregiver in skin care if tactile perception is affected, including assessment and protection and massage of pressure points, frequent changes of position (every 2 hours), cleansing, and application of an emollient to the skin (first and second visits).

CLIENT AND FAMILY/CAREGIVER INTERVENTIONS

1. Caregiver allows as much independence as possible.
2. Caregiver protects client from falls and from trauma to skin and affected limbs.
3. Caregiver promotes visual field enhancement.
4. Client and caregiver adapt environment to deficits and for safe mobility.

Nursing diagnosis

Knowledge deficit

Related factors: Lack of information about disease and treatments

Defining characteristics: Expressed need for information about medication, medical regimen, and rehabilitation program

OUTCOMES

Short-term

Adequate knowledge, as evidenced by client's statement of nutritional, fluid, elimination, and medication regimen and rehabilitation needs (expected within 3 days)

Long-term

Adequate knowledge, as evidenced by compliance with medical regimen and achievement of optimal health and functioning (expected within 1 to 3 months)

NURSING INTERVENTIONS/INSTRUCTIONS

1. Assess life-style, learning and adaptation abilities, interest level, and family participation and support (first visit).
2. Assess all systems for effect of long-term hypertension; note history for predisposing factors or disorders that relate to secondary hypertension (first visit).
3. Assess and instruct client in monitoring blood pressure and pulse (first visit).
4. Advise client about life-style changes, methods of stress management, and dietary changes; to have regular screening for blood pressure, circulatory, and visual changes; and to have

laboratory testing if warfarin sodium (Coumadin) therapy is prescribed (first visit).

5. Instruct client in administration of antihypertensives, anticoagulants, diuretics, stool softeners, and vitamin and/or mineral supplements, including dose, route, frequency, side effects, and food and drug interactions (first visit).
6. Instruct client in constipation program to include increased fluid intake (8 to 10 glasses/day), increased bulk in diet, and daily activity and exercise program (first visit).
7. Instruct client in dietary inclusion of foods of preference that are textured for easy swallowing; use of thickeners; placing foods on unaffected side of mouth and allowing plenty of time for meals; avoiding milk and foods that are too thin and smooth (first visit).
8. Instruct client in urinary bladder rehabilitation by offering elimination opportunity every 2 hours; scheduling voiding at certain times with fluid intake and temporary measures such as pads or waterproof undergarments (first and second visits).
9. Inform client of importance of compliance with physical, occupational, and speech therapy regimens (first visit).
10. Instruct client to report changes such as headache, vertigo, changes in mentation, or visual disturbances to the physician (first visit).
11. Inform client that emotional lability is not uncommon and of the possibility of becoming depressed and the need for counseling services if appropriate (any visit).
12. Inform client of agencies such as American Heart Association to contact for information, assistive devices, and support services (first visit).

CLIENT AND FAMILY/CAREGIVER INTERVENTIONS

1. Client adapts to life-style changes to accommodate medical regimen.
2. Client verbalizes nutritional, fluid, and elimination measures to ensure optimal function.
3. Client complies with medication and rehabilitation schedules and carries out safe interventions as instructed.
4. Client verbalizes signs and symptoms to report indicating possible recurrence of stroke.
5. Client utilizes community agencies for assistance and support.

Nursing diagnosis

Ineffective family coping: compromised

Related factors: Prolonged disease or disability that exhausts the supportive capacity of significant people

Defining characteristics: Expression of concern or complaint about client's health problem; lack of information about residual damage from stroke

OUTCOMES

Short-term

Improved coping, as evidenced by acknowledgement of disabling effects of disease and required life-style changes and by cooperation and participation in treatment regimen (expected within 1 week)

Long-term

Optimal level of participation and support by family members to facilitate changes in client's life-style and improvement in health status (expected within 1 to 2 months)

NURSING INTERVENTIONS/INSTRUCTIONS

1. Assess family interactions and coping abilities, strengths of individual members, level of participation and support, and resources available and utilized by family (see Family Assessment, p. 55, for guidelines) (first visit).
2. Provide accurate information to family about treatment regimen and deficits that cannot be changed; allow time for questions or clarifications (each visit).
3. Encourage family to discuss strengths and options for change and to identify coping mechanisms used (each visit).
4. Include family members in teaching and realistic planning of care (each visit).
5. Inform client and family that full or partial recovery may take a long time (first visit).
6. Inform client and family of government and community agencies available for support and assistance (first visit).
7. Initiate referral to social services, and encourage family to contact counselor if appropriate (any visit).

CLIENT AND FAMILY/CAREGIVER INTERVENTIONS

1. Family verbalizes concerns and feelings about burden of care of family member with chronic disorder.
2. Family seeks assistance if needed.
3. Family participates in planning and implementing care.
4. Family adapts to limitations of client and integrates them into family activity.
5. Family copes with client's response to the losses.
6. Family continues family activities and open communication.

Head Injury

Head injury is penetration of the skull or traumatic impact to the skull that damages the brain tissue at the point of impact. The injury may be a concussion, cerebral contusion, laceration, or brainstem trauma and may result in edema, hemorrhage, causing increased intracranial pressure, amnesia, hemiplegia, impaired consciousness, breathing impairment, or coma. Head injury is usually the result of an accident.

Home care depends on the extent and severity of the injury and is primarily concerned with teaching of the medical regimen and treatment of the residual effects to facilitate restoration of normal function.

Nursing diagnosis

Risk for injury

Related factors: Internal regulatory function; physical function; psychological function

Defining characteristics: Inability to purposefully move about; unsteady gait; sensory and/or perceptual deficits; disorientation; change in consciousness; visual disturbances; seizure activity

OUTCOMES

Short-term

Improved function within limitations imposed by condition, as evidenced by mental alertness; return of thought processes; orientation to time, place, and person; and resumption of mobility and ADL without injury (expected within 1 week or as practical)

Long-term

Progressive return to optimal health and functioning without injury, with awareness of residual deficits (expected within 3 to 6 months)

NURSING INTERVENTIONS/INSTRUCTIONS

1. Assess for presence of reflexes, mentation changes, changes in motor or sensory function, paralysis, visual impairment, and cognitive ability (each visit).
2. Inform client of possible changes in judgment, emotional control, and social restraint in association with this condition (first visit).
3. Instruct family or caregiver to adjust environment to prevent trauma from falls or other injury, to reorient client as needed, to provide supervision and/or assist with ambulation and ADL as needed, and to provide assistive aids as needed (each visit).
4. Instruct family or caregiver in measures to protect client from injury during seizure activity, including staying with client, turning client on side, avoiding restraining client, and placing pillow under head (first visit).
5. Refer home health aide to assist with ADL as needed.
6. Consult with home care rehabilitation specialist (any visit).

CLIENT AND FAMILY/CAREGIVER INTERVENTIONS

1. Caregiver provides assistance with ambulation and ADL with or without aids.
2. Caregiver maintains safe environment with clear pathways and lighted rooms; makes sure client has proper shoes and glasses.
3. Caregiver prevents injury during seizure activity with protective measures.
4. Caregiver notes and reports changes in mentation or behavior.

Nursing diagnosis

Knowledge deficit

Related factors: Lack of knowledge about consequences of injury

Defining characteristics: Expressed need for information about injury, effects, prognosis, and medication and rehabilitative regimens

OUTCOMES

Short-term

Adequate knowledge, as evidenced by client's ability to describe cause and effects of the injury and the medication and rehabilitative regimens (expected within 1 week)

Long-term

Adequate knowledge, as evidenced by compliance with medical regimen to achieve optimal health and functioning and progressive recovery (expected within 1 to 6 months)

NURSING INTERVENTIONS/INSTRUCTIONS

1. Assess life-style, ability to adapt, learning ability and interest, cognitive deficits, and family participation and support (first visit).
2. Inform family that time and patience are needed to deal with the deficits or problems and that the appearance of client may not be an indication of level of recovery if any (first visit).
3. Instruct family or caregiver in medication administration, usually anticonvulsants, anticoagulants, and muscle relaxants, including dose, action, frequency, side effects, and food and drug interactions, and not to skip doses or discontinue without advice of physician (first visit).
4. Instruct family or caregiver in doing neurologic checks and assessment of mentation and changes in consciousness to report (each visit).
5. Inform client that recovery may take 6 months, including rehabilitation to treat specific residual deficits of posttraumatic stage (first visit).
6. Instruct family in appropriate interaction patterns to avoid family dysfunction and that client should avoid alcohol, driving, use of hazardous equipment, and unsupervised smoking (first visit).
7. Inform family of importance of keeping appointments with rehabilitation team and with agencies that assist with economic, psychological, and physical support (any visit).

CLIENT AND FAMILY/CAREGIVER INTERVENTIONS

1. Client adapts to change in life-style to include rehabilitation.
2. Caregiver participates in and supports client's recovery from chronic problems and mental and emotional sequelae.
3. Client administers medications correctly and reports side effects or ineffective response from medications.
4. Caregiver provides a safe environment, including avoidance of alcohol, smoking alone, use of guns and hazardous machinery or appliances, driving a car, and use of over-the-counter (OTC) drugs.
5. Client maintains rehabilitation schedule as prescribed.

Multiple Sclerosis (MS)

Multiple sclerosis is a chronic, slowly progressive central nervous system disease causing demyelination in the brain and spinal cord. It is associated with an immunologic abnormality causing an inflammatory process that is responsible for the loss of the myelin sheath from the axon cylinders of the nerves, primarily in the white matter. The disease is characterized by remissions and exacerbations of symptoms, which include transient weakness, stiffness and fatigue of a limb, gait disturbances, vertigo, loss of bladder and bowel control, visual disturbances, emotional lability, and lack of judgment.

Home care is primarily concerned with the teaching of safety and the medical regimen and with the preservation of physical and mental function.

Nursing diagnosis

Self-esteem disturbance

Related factors: Biophysical, psychosocial factors

Defining characteristics: Verbal responses to change in body function; self-negating verbalizations; expression of shame (incontinence); inability to deal with illness; hestitancy to change life-style; inability to perform ADL; depression

OUTCOMES

Short-term

Improved self-esteem, as evidenced by client's statement of ability to cope with long-term debilitation and changes in life-style associated with dysfunction (expected within 1 week)

Long-term

Progressively more positive attitude about prolonged illness, with participation in treatment regimen to achieve optimal health and functioning within limitations of disease (expected within 2 to 3 months and ongoing)

NURSING INTERVENTIONS/INSTRUCTIONS

1. Assess client for behavioral changes and emotional status, including anxiety and depression, feelings of powerlessness, and use and effectiveness of coping mechanisms (each visit).
2. Focus on remaining abilities, and instruct family to maintain a positive attitude and support (each visit).
3. Discuss effect of illness on self-concept (any visit).
4. Encourage client to participate in treatments and ADL; instruct family to assist when needed but to allow for independence when possible (first visit).
5. Allow for expression of feelings and concerns about neurologic functioning and effect on life-style (each visit).
6. Refer client to counseling and social services if appropriate.

CLIENT AND FAMILY/CAREGIVER INTERVENTIONS

1. Client sets goals and participates in treatments.
2. Client identifies and uses coping mechanisms that are effective.
3. Client uses a planned program for entire day to deal with boredom and anxiety.
4. Client maintains independence and uses measures to reduce embarrassment caused by changes in function.
5. Client ventilates feelings during nurse's visits.
6. Client accepts and participates in counseling services if needed.

Nursing diagnosis

Altered patterns of urinary elimination

Related factors: Sensorimotor impairment

Defining characteristics: Urgency, frequency, dribbling, incontinence, retention, or spastic or flaccid bladder, depending on site of lesion

OUTCOMES

Short-term

Progressive absence of urinary elimination impairment, as evidenced by reduction in incontinence episodes and retention with residual less than 150 ml (expected within 1 to 2 weeks)

Long-term

Urinary continence and absence of retention, as evidenced by establishment of urinary elimination pattern for optimal functioning (expected within 2 to 3 months and ongoing)

NURSING INTERVENTIONS/INSTRUCTIONS

1. Assess for presence of spastic bladder (incontinence), flaccid bladder (retention), suprapubic distention, or cloudy, foul-smelling urine (first visit).
2. Instruct client and family in administration of cholinergic or anticholinergic medications to relieve bladder symptoms, including action, dose, frequency, side effects, precautions, and food and drug interactions (first visit).
3. Instruct client and family in fluid needs (8 to 10 glasses/day), and assess for possible urinary bladder infection if residual is present (first visit).
4. Perform Credé's maneuver or reflex stimulation manually, and instruct in use of these methods if retention is present (first and second visits).
5. Instruct client or family to perform catheterization on intermittent basis if ordered to treat retention (any visit).
6. Instruct client in protection methods to prevent embarrassment from incontinence.
7. Refer client to bladder training program if appropriate (any visit).

CLIENT AND FAMILY/CAREGIVER INTERVENTIONS

1. Client maintains fluid intake of 3000 ml/day.
2. Client participates in methods to stimulate or control urinary elimination.
3. Client administers medications correctly to relieve bladder symptoms.
4. Client monitors intake and output; assesses for presence of urinary tract infection.
5. Client utilizes garment protectors and waterproof underwear.
6. Client participates in bladder training program.

Nursing diagnosis

Impaired physical mobility

Related factors: Neuromuscular impairment

Defining characteristics: Inability to purposefully move within physical environment, including bed mobility, transfer, and ambulation; weakness; pain and spasms of muscles; unsteady gait; limb stiffness; vertigo; paresthesias; inability to perform ADL

OUTCOMES

Short-term

Adequate mobility and activity performance, as evidenced by preservation of ability to ambulate and participate in ADL within limitations imposed by disease (expected within 1 to 2 weeks)

Long-term

Optimal ability to perform gross and fine motor activities to achieve and maintain present functioning (expected within 1 to 2 months and ongoing)

NURSING INTERVENTIONS/INSTRUCTIONS

1. Assess mobility status; presence and duration of muscle spasms; risk for injury related to altered mobility, paralysis, or paresthesia; need for wheelchair (see Musculoskeletal System Assessment, p. 29, for guidelines) (each visit).
2. Instruct client and family in administration of antispasmodics to decrease spasticity, including dose, time, frequency, precautions, and side effects (first and second visits).

3. Emphasize and instruct client in daily exercises, including stretching and stride increasing by walking with feet farther apart (for gait training) (first visit).
4. Instruct client to apply ice to spastic muscle (or use warm bath) before exercising and to rest between exercises (first visit).
5. Instruct client in use of assistive devices for self-care, instruct family to assist while encouraging independence (each visit).
6. For a safe environment, and especially to prevent falls, instruct family to clear pathways, remove small rugs, and provide rails or assistive aids for ambulation (first visit).
7. Initiate referral to physical and occupational therapists as needed.
8. Refer client to HHA and homemaker services as needed.

CLIENT AND FAMILY/CAREGIVER INTERVENTIONS

1. Client administers medications correctly and reports side effects; avoids driving and hazardous activities, use of alcohol, and abrupt discontinuation of medications.
2. Client meets needs for ADL with or without assistance and use of aids.
3. Client relieves muscle spasticity, increases coordination, and uses nonaffected muscles for impaired ones if possible.
4. Client participates in physical therapy with water exercises, massage, and occupational therapy as needed.
5. Family provides safe environment for functioning.
6. Client utilizes HHA and homemaker services to assist with ADL, meal preparation, and shopping; utilizes any other services that are needed.

Nursing diagnosis

Knowledge deficit

Related factors: Lack of information about disease and manifestations

Defining characteristics: Expressed need for information about changes in life-style to promote functional maintenance and to maintain general health

OUTCOMES

Short-term

Adequate knowledge, as evidenced by client's statement of precautions and treatments to implement and methods to ensure health and functioning (expected within 1 week)

Long-term

Adequate knowledge, as evidenced by maintenance of general health and functioning and by compliance with medical regimen and instructions (expected within 1 to 2 months)

NURSING INTERVENTIONS/INSTRUCTIONS

1. Assess life-style, ability to adapt, learning ability and interest, and family participation and support (first visit).
2. Inform client and family of cause of disease and reason for neurosensory and neuromuscular dysfunction (first visit).
3. Inform client and family of, and stress need for, long-term physical therapy and maintenance of mobility and independent functioning (first visit).
4. Advise client to avoid fatigue, extremes of heat and cold, and any exposure to people with illness or infections; instruct client to balance rest and activity (first visit).
5. Instruct client to avoid constipation by increasing fiber and fluids in dietary intake, including items from the basic four food groups, and eating well-balanced, nutritious meals (first and second visits).
6. Inform client that tinnitus or decreased auditory acuity and visual changes such as blurred vision or patches of blindness are caused by central nervous system involvement; suggest large print and other aids available for visual or auditory deficits (first visit).
7. Instruct client and family in skin care if client is confined to wheelchair or bed.
8. Review and instruct client in administration of all medications, and instruct client to avoid OTC drugs unless advised by physician (first and second visits).
9. Inform client of eventual possible sexual dysfunction, impotence in males, decreased libido, and decreased vaginal lubrication in women and suggest resources (any visit).

10. Instruct client and family in grieving process and reason for behaviors that are normal and perhaps predictable as function is lost (each visit).
11. Inform client and family that signs and symptoms of disease and changes in behavior (anger, depression) may be initiated by fatigue, infection, or physical or emotional stress or trauma (any visit).
12. Refer client and family to National Multiple Sclerosis Society and local agencies for information and support (any visit).

CLIENT AND FAMILY/CAREGIVER INTERVENTIONS

1. Client describes health measures to prevent complications and maintain function.
2. Client avoids stress, fatigue, formation of contractures, and skin breakdown by compliance with physical therapy protocol.
3. Client participates in goal setting and decisions regarding care schedule.
4. Client maintains nutritional status needed for health and functioning; includes vitamins, fiber, and fluid intake of 3000 ml/day.
5. Client avoids exposure to or involvement in activities that predispose to infections.
6. Client seeks out assistance for sexual dysfunction by counseling or sex therapy and alternate sexual expression.
7. Client adapts to and complies with complete medical regimen safely and appropriately.
8. Client contacts and utilizes social services and community agencies for information and support.

Parkinson's Disease

Parkinson's disease is a chronic, progressive central nervous system disorder characterized by muscular rigidity, a slow decrease in movement, and tremors. It involves the degeneration of the brain centers that control movement and is associated with low concentrations of dopamine, which account for the symptoms of the disease. The incapacitation that occurs from this disease may take years to develop.

Home care is primarily concerned with teaching medication administration and self-care activities to ensure meeting basic needs, depending on symptomatic effects of the disease.

Nursing diagnosis

Impaired physical mobility

Related factors: Neuromuscular impairment; decreased strength and endurance

Defining characteristics: Inability to purposefully move within physical environment, including ambulation, bradykinesic tremor, contractures, deformities, unsteady gait, muscle rigidity

OUTCOMES

Short-term

Preservation of physical mobility, as evidenced by ambulation and participation in ADL within limitations imposed by disease (expected within 1 week and ongoing)

Long-term

Continued optimal ability to perform gross and fine motor activities to achieve or maintain present functioning throughout illness (expected ongoing)

NURSING INTERVENTIONS/INSTRUCTIONS

1. Assess degree of mobility, ROM, presence of contractures, bradykinesia, ability to stand from sitting position, need for assistive aids (see Musculoskeletal System Assessment, p. 29, for guidelines) (first visit).
2. Assess client's ability to wash body parts, put on or take off clothing or fasten clothing, bring food to mouth to feed self, and perform personal hygiene and grooming activities (see Functional Assessment, p. 51, for guidelines) (first visit).
3. Instruct client in daily ambulation and active or passive ROM and other exercises in all extremities, head, and neck; include stretching, stride increasing, and facial exercises (first and second visits).
4. Instruct client to use straight chair for sitting and how to get up using arm rests, to carry object in hand or place hand in

pocket to reduce tremors, to change positions to avoid resting tremor, to lift toes when stepping and step over imaginary or real lines, and to step backward once and forward with two steps to correct akinesia or freezing (first visit and when needed).

5. Instruct client in application of hot packs and use of massage to reduce muscle rigidity (first visit).
6. Encourage and instruct client in use of assistive aids for ADL, and provide assistance by home health aide referral when needed (any visit).
7. Initiate referral to physical and occupational therapists as appropriate (first visit).

CLIENT AND FAMILY/CAREGIVER INTERVENTIONS

1. Client performs ambulation and exercises, ADL, and other activities within limitations imposed by disease.
2. Client makes use of measures to facilitate mobility, reduce tremor, and change positions.
3. Client uses aids to facilitate ADL and maintain independence.
4. Client participates in physical and occupational therapy.
5. Client makes use of measures to reduce muscle rigidity.

Nursing diagnosis

Ineffective individual coping

Related factors: Personal vulnerability, multiple life changes

Defining characteristics: Verbalization of inability to cope, inability to meet basic needs, alteration in societal participation, change in usual communication patterns, chronic anxiety, depression, loss of control

OUTCOMES

Short-term

Adequate coping, as evidenced by progressive participation in treatment program and use of coping and problem-solving skills (expected within 1 week)

Long-term

Adequate coping, as evidenced by attitude and life-style changes indicating achievement of optimal physical and emotional functioning (expected within 3 months and ongoing)

NURSING INTERVENTIONS/INSTRUCTIONS

1. Assess for verbalization of behavioral changes indicating anxiety, lability, depression, social isolation, or body image disturbance; assess use and effectiveness of coping mechanisms (see Psychosocial Assessment, p. 48, for guidelines) (each visit).
2. Discuss self-concept, including appearance and loss of neurologic and musculoskeletal functioning (drooling, tremor, slurred speech); discuss adjustment to and acceptance of the disease (each visit).
3. Instruct client to use typewriter, slate, or paper and pencil to assist in communication (first visit).
4. Inform client and family of need for socialization and of agencies and groups in the community that perform services and provide information and support (first visit).
5. Assist client to establish realistic goals for functioning, and instruct client in coping and problem-solving skills to achieve these goals (first and second visits).
6. Initiate counseling as appropriate (any visit).

CLIENT AND FAMILY/CAREGIVER INTERVENTIONS

1. Client uses a planned program for entire day to deal with anxiety and depression.
2. Client identifies and uses coping skills that are effective.
3. Client sets realistic goals and participates in treatments.
4. Client maintains independence and uses measures to reduce embarrassment from changes in functioning.
5. Client ventilates feelings and concerns; accepts counseling if needed.
6. Client improves self-concept with adjustment to the disease and its problems.

Nursing diagnosis

Knowledge deficit

Related factors: Lack of information about disease

Defining characteristics: Expressed need for information about disease's cause, effects, and prognosis; medication administration; fluid, nutritional, and activity regimen; preservation of abilities; prevention of injury

OUTCOMES

Short-term

Adequate knowledge, as evidenced by client's description of disease's cause and progressive nature, medical regimen, and precautions for preventing complications (expected within 1 week)

Long-term

Adequate knowledge, as evidenced by compliance with medical regimen for optimal preservation of functional abilities (expected within 1 month and ongoing)

NURSING INTERVENTIONS/INSTRUCTIONS

1. Inform client of disease process and cause and of reason for loss of neurologic and musculoskeletal functioning (first visit).
2. Inform client of and stress need for continuing activity and socialization and need for self-care and independence in ADL to maintain functioning (first visit).
3. Instruct client to take frequent rest periods throughout the day (first visit).
4. Instruct client and family in nutritional needs, including small, frequent meals of high-calorie, protein food choices and a selection of high-fiber foods and fluid intake of up to 3000 ml/day to maintain nutrition and prevent constipation; inform client and family that accidents involving food and drinks are common and need to be ignored and treated with kindness; suggest eating slowly and chewing foods thoroughly (first and second visits).
5. Instruct client and family in administration of medications, including dose, action, frequency, side effects, precautions, and signs and symptoms to report to physician as a result of medication; discuss stool softeners, antiparkinsonian drugs (dopaminergic, anticholinergic, antihistamine), and antidepressants, and instruct client to avoid OTC drugs unless advised by physician (first visit and any visit as needed).
6. Instruct client and family in safety measures, including removal of small rugs and furniture from pathways and use of elevated chair and toilet seat (first visit).
7. Inform client that exercises to strengthen muscles used for speaking, chewing, and swallowing should be included in daily physical therapy and refer to speech pathologist if appropriate (first visit).
8. Inform of and direct client and family to community resources,

including American Parkinson's Disease Association, for information and support (first visit).

CLIENT AND FAMILY/CAREGIVER INTERVENTIONS

1. Client adapts to and complies with medical regimen.
2. Client administers medications correctly as prescribed and reports untoward effects.
3. Client participates in activity, rest, and fluid and nutritional program within limitations or restrictions imposed by disease.
4. Client establishes and maintains adequate bowel elimination, weight, and nutritional status.
5. Client and family institute measures to prevent falls and encourage independence.
6. Client and family contact and utilize community agencies for information and support.

Seizure Disorders

Seizures are recurrent paroxysmal disorders of cerebral function that are characterized by altered consciousness, sensory phenomena, motor activity, or changes in behavior. Any seizure pattern that is recurrent is known as epilepsy. Seizures are classified as partial or generalized and may be caused by cerebral or systemic disorders, such as acute infections (including central nervous system infections), cerebral hypoxia, cerebral fracture, brain lesions or tumors, toxic agents, congenital brain defects, cerebral edema, cerebral trauma, cerebral hemorrhage, cerebral infarct, and anaphylaxis. Seizure activity resulting from any cause may be transient and not recur after the disorder is corrected or ends.

Home care is primarily concerned with the teaching of medication administration to control seizures and with prevention of physical and psychological trauma that may result from seizure activity.

Nursing diagnosis

Risk for injury

Related factors: Internal regulatory function (sensory, integrative dysfunction)

Defining characteristics: Musculoskeletal trauma from falls; oral tissue trauma from biting; soft-tissue bruising; lack of safety precautions; uncontrolled movements

OUTCOMES

Short-term

Minimal injury or absence of injury, as evidenced by mouth, tongue, bone, or soft-tissue damage being controlled or absent during and following seizure activity (expected within time frame of seizure)

Long-term

Absence of injury, as evidenced by no breaks in skin or mucous membranes or bones as seizures are controlled (expected ongoing)

NURSING INTERVENTIONS/INSTRUCTIONS

1. Assess type and frequency of seizure activity, loss of consciousness, loss of muscle tone, tongue biting, falling to the floor, weakness or paralysis, presence of aura (first visit).
2. Instruct caregiver to allow client to slide to floor; place client in side-lying position; avoid restricting any movement, jerking, or stiffening; loosen constricting clothing (first visit and reinforce on second visit).
3. Instruct caregiver to remain with client during entire seizure and to place small pillow under head or place head in lap (first visit).
4. Instruct client and family to remove harmful objects from the immediate environment (first visit).
5. Instruct client and caregiver to note if aura is present, how seizure began, and how it progressed and lasted; presence of cyanosis, excessive saliva, incontinence, and sleep period to report (first visit).
6. Instruct client to prevent seizure activity by avoiding emotional and physical stress or stimulation that triggers seizure (noise, lights, drugs) (first visit).

CLIENT AND FAMILY/CAREGIVER INTERVENTIONS

1. Caregiver performs measures to prevent trauma during seizure activity.
2. Caregiver provides safe environment during seizure activity.

3. Caregiver assesses aspects of seizure activity and reports to physician for evaluation.
4. Caregiver remains and supports client during seizure activity.
5. Client avoids actions and stimuli that cause seizure activity.

Nursing diagnosis

Anxiety

Related factors: Threat to self-concept; threat of change in health status

Defining characteristics: Verbalized apprehension and uncertainty about unpredictable seizure activity; social withdrawal; feelings of inadequacy; stigma attached to presence of disorder

OUTCOMES

Short-term

Reduced anxiety, as evidenced by client's statement that anxiety is at manageable level, embarrassment controlled, and social and family interactions improved (expected within 1 to 2 weeks)

Long-term

Anxiety level at optimal level for achievement of health and functioning, with self-concept enhanced (expected within 2 to 3 months)

NURSING INTERVENTIONS/INSTRUCTIONS

1. Assess anxiety level; social interactions and how condition impacts life-style and self-esteem; perception of how others view disease (first visit and as needed).
2. Allow client to express feelings about diagnosis of epilepsy (each visit).
3. Assist client to develop coping strategies to reduce anxiety, and instruct client in relaxation techniques, including reading, music, imagery, and relaxation exercises (first and second visits).
4. Inform client of importance of maintaining social relationships and recreation and occupational activities (each visit).
5. Initiate referral to counseling if appropriate (any visit).

CLIENT AND FAMILY/CAREGIVER INTERVENTIONS

1. Client discusses feelings, anger, and anxiety regarding condition.
2. Client develops coping skills to reduce anxiety.
3. Client utilizes relaxation techniques to reduce anxiety.
4. Client maintains relationships and activities for optimal functioning.
5. Client adapts to life-style that includes stigma or misconception of the disease by others.
6. Client participates in counseling services if needed.

Nursing diagnosis

Knowledge deficit

Related factors: Lack of information about disorder

Defining characteristics: Expressed need for information about medication administration and compliance and about cause, treatment, and prognosis of disorder

OUTCOMES

Short-term

Adequate knowledge, as evidenced by client's ability to discuss cause, treatment, prognosis, and medication regimen (expected within 1 week)

Long-term

Adequate knowledge, as evidenced by compliance with medical regimen to achieve optimal health and functioning (expected within 1 month)

NURSING INTERVENTIONS/INSTRUCTIONS

1. Assess life-style, ability to adapt, learning ability and interest, and family participation and support (first visit).
2. Inform client of cause of seizure activity and of the importance of compliance with follow-up visits for laboratory testing and physician evaluation (first visit).
3. Instruct client in administration of anticonvulsant therapy, including dosage, route, action, and side effects to assess and report (gingival hypertrophy, visual disturbances, rashes, con-

fusion); food and drug interactions; not to discontinue medication without physician advice; and to avoid OTC drugs without physician advice (first and second visits).

4. Instruct client to have dental checkups every 6 months; instruct client in tooth care, including brushing and use of dental floss to prevent oral infection (first visit).
5. Instruct client to report fever, sore throat, fatigue, or weakness, which may indicate agranulocytosis, and inform client of need to have complete blood count done every 6 months if ordered (first visit).
6. Instruct client to avoid late-night television, alcohol, fatigue, and stimulants known to cause seizure activity (first visit).
7. Inform client of immediate actions to take at onset of seizure and when to notify emergency service (first visit).
8. Suggest wearing an identification bracelet or carrying a card in a purse or wallet indicating condition, medication, physician, and physician's telephone number (first visit).
9. Inform client of antidiscrimination laws affecting work and other activities (first visit).
10. Inform client of National Epilepsy League and other agencies available for support and of groups for people with the disorder (any visit).

CLIENT AND FAMILY/CAREGIVER INTERVENTIONS

1. Caregiver promotes independence and avoids overprotection.
2. Client complies with medication administration as instructed and maintains regimen unless advised to change by physician; keeps follow-up appointments.
3. Client manages life-style changes and adapts to changes brought about by disorder; utilizes resources available for information and support.
4. Client reports complications of condition when appropriate.
5. Client carries identification information.

Spinal Cord Injury

Spinal cord injury is the contusion, compression, hemorrhage, laceration, or transection of the spinal cord, causing loss of neurologic function. The injury may be acute, in which all sensation and reflex activity below the injury level are lost, or partial, in which some motor and sensory loss occurs, depending on the tracts affected. The injury is usually the result of car or sports accidents, falls, wounds from guns or implements of war, or diseases of the spinal cord.

Home care depends on the extent of the injury and is primarily concerned with teaching of the medical regimen and with rehabilitation and aftercare to maximize health and function.

Nursing diagnosis

Impaired physical mobility

Related factors: Neuromuscular impairment, perceptual impairment

Defining characteristics: Paraplegia, quadriplegia; immobility; inability to purposefully move within physical environment, including bed mobility, transfer, and ambulation; spasticity; muscle weakness

OUTCOMES

Short-term

Enhanced mobility, as evidenced by improved activity and movement, ability to transfer and change positions, and absence of contractures and muscle atrophy (expected within 1 to 2 weeks)

Long-term

Achievement of optimal mobility, movement, and activity for health and functioning within injury limitations (expected ongoing)

NURSING INTERVENTIONS/INSTRUCTIONS

1. Assess degree and type of injury and impairment; muscle strength; presence of spasticity, muscle wasting, and sensorimotor deficits (see Musculoskeletal System Assessment, p. 29, for guidelines) (each visit).
2. Perform and instruct client in passive, assistive, or active ROM exercises, to be done every 2 to 4 hours or as prescribed by physical therapist (first and second visits).
3. Instruct client in positioning and position changes and to provide any assistance needed; suggest prone position to relieve pressure on susceptible areas and use of fracture board under mattress to prevent sagging of mattress (first and second visits).

4. Instruct client in removal and application of hand or foot splints (or, for feet, to use tennis shoes with the toe cut out) to prevent contractures; avoid use of footboard, which may promote development of plantar flexion (first visit).
5. Instruct client, and support physical therapy instructions, in methods to move and turn in bed, and to transfer to chair, wheelchair, care, or elsewhere (any visit).
6. Instruct client to schedule rest periods to alternate with ROM and muscle strengthening exercises and activities.
7. Inform client of comfort resulting from warm baths and massage and their role in preventing spasticity (first visit).
8. Initiate referral to physical and/or occupational therapist for rehabilitation to maximize function remaining and to obtain special equipment for ambulation and other activities.
9. Provide information for securing bed with trapeze, Hoyer lift, transfer board, and other aids and protective devices (first visit).

CLIENT AND FAMILY/CAREGIVER INTERVENTIONS

1. Client performs exercises alternating with rest periods daily.
2. Client progresses in transfer techniques, movement, and activities, and improves in use of assistive aids and devices.
3. Client maintains optimal independence in mobility and activities within injury limitations.
4. Client secures necessary equipment and supplies for optimal movement.
5. Caregiver encourages and praises all attempts and accomplishments of client and goal achievement.
6. Client complies with rehabilitation regimen initiated by the physical therapist.
7. Client performs follow-up muscle and joint preservation measures.

Nursing diagnosis

Risk for impaired skin integrity

Related factors: External factors of pressure, physical immobilization, excretions from urine and bowel incontinence; internal factors of altered sensation and nutrition

Defining characteristics: Disruption of skin surface, redness at bony prominences, inability to change position

OUTCOMES

Short-term

Reduction in risk for breaks in skin integrity, as evidenced by intact skin and absence of reddened areas (expected within 1 week)

Long-term

Skin integrity maintained, as evidenced by absence of actual skin breakdown or injury or signs and symptoms of beginning breakdown (expected ongoing)

NURSING INTERVENTIONS/INSTRUCTIONS

1. Assess skin at pressure areas for redness and perineal area for irritation or excoriation if client is incontinent of urine and/or feces (see Integumentary System Assessment, p. 36, for guidelines) (each visit).
2. Instruct client in proper positioning and position changes to relieve pressure and shearing forces on skin (first visit).
3. Instruct client in massage technique using lotion for hands, feets, and bony prominences in particular (first visit).
4. Instruct client in perineal care following elimination or incontinence, including washing with mild soap, rinsing with warm water, patting dry, and applying skin protector (first visit).
5. Instruct client to eliminate any crumbs or debris in bed, chair, or other area that comes in contact with skin (first visit).
6. To prevent burns to areas deprived of sensation, instruct client to avoid use of hot water for bathing or application of heat or spilling hot foods (first visit).
7. Perform decubitus care if break in skin is noted, and instruct client to assess, to perform treatment appropriate for stage of pressure ulcer, and to report poor response to treatment (any visit).

CLIENT AND FAMILY/CAREGIVER INTERVENTIONS

1. Client assesses skin condition daily and performs measures to prevent breakdown.
2. Client uses aids to prevent skin pressure.
3. Client avoids excessive heat or cold in contact with paralyzed area.
4. Client eliminates pressure and shearing or mechanical forces that injure skin.

5. Client performs movements and transfers without skin trauma, with or without assistance.

Nursing diagnosis

Self-care deficit (bathing/hygiene, dressing/grooming, feeding, toileting)

Related factors: Neuromuscular impairment, impaired mobility status

Defining characteristics: Inability to wash body parts, put on or take off clothes, get to and use toilet or be aware of urge to eliminate, bring food from receptable to mouth; paralysis

OUTCOMES

Short-term

Ability to perform ADL, as evidenced by beginning participation in feeding, toileting, bathing, personal hygiene, dressing and grooming, within limitations imposed by injury (expected within 1 to 2 weeks)

Long-term

Optimal participation in self-care for ADL with or without assistive aids or devices to achieve independence (expected within 2 to 3 months and ongoing)

NURSING INTERVENTIONS/INSTRUCTIONS

1. Assess client's ability to perform self-care (paraplegic, quadriplegic), including ability to feed self; use bedpan, urinal, or commode; and bathe, groom, and clothe self (see Functional Assessment, p. 57, for guidelines) (each visit).
2. Provide assistance or supervision as needed for performance of ADL, and instruct client to ask for assistance when needed (each visit).
3. Instruct client in and suggest use of assistive aids and devices for eating, dressing, grooming, personal hygiene, and toileting, and inform client of clothing and utensils to purchase to enhance self-care (first visit).
4. Instruct client to allow time to perform activities without rushing, for best results (first visit).

5. Initiate referral to occupational therapist for instruction and support in ADL and for suggestions for other aids (any visit).
6. Refer HHA to assist with ADL as needed.

CLIENT AND FAMILY/CAREGIVER INTERVENTIONS

1. Client participates in ADL with progressive results, with or without the use of assistive aids or devices.
2. Client performs self-care independently with maximal rehabilitative potential.
3. Caregiver assists client to maintain functional abilities in daily activities.
4. Client complies with occupational rehabilitation schedule and practices activities as instructed.

Nursing diagnosis

Ineffective individual coping

Related factors: Multiple life changes; inadequate coping method

Defining characteristics: Inability to cope, meet role expectations, meet basic needs; chronic anxiety; poor self-esteem; fear and feelings of grief; negative feelings about body; change in sexual function; feelings of dependence, helplessness

OUTCOMES

Short-term

Improved individual coping, as evidenced by client's statement of realization of life-style changes that need to be made and willingness to adapt and learn effective coping mechanisms (expected within 1 to 2 weeks)

Long-term

Effective coping and adaptation to changed self-concept, as evidenced by achievement of requirements for optimal health and functioning within injury limitations, returning to employment, and retraining in sexual function and other life changes (expected within 3 months and ongoing)

NURSING INTERVENTIONS/INSTRUCTIONS

1. Assess for anxiety; depression; feelings about appearance and loss of neurologic functioning and effect on self-concept and

body image; use and effectiveness of coping mechanisms; and behavioral and emotional changes and reasons for them (each visit).

2. Instruct client in development of new coping skills while maintaining current skills that are successful; assist client with problem-solving skills (first and second visits).
3. Include client in setting realistic goals for functioning and in developing the treatment plan and methods to evaluate progress (each visit).
4. Instruct client to avoid emotional and physical stress (first visit).
5. Show care, concern, and willingness to assist in coping with life-style changes (each visit).
6. Allow for expressions of feelings, concerns, and fears about the future, and inform client that this is acceptable behavior (each visit).
7. Refrain from using words such as "quad" or "cripple"; use words such as "disabled" or "handicapped" (each visit).
8. Initiate referral to social services, psychotherapy, sex counseling, occupational retraining, and rehabilitation as needed (any visit).

CLIENT AND FAMILY/CAREGIVER INTERVENTIONS

1. Client uses planned program during the entire day to meet goals and prevent depression, boredom, and fatigue.
2. Client ventilates feelings and grief as needed.
3. Client identifies and uses coping mechanisms that work; tries alternative methods to cope.
4. Client seeks counseling from appropriate referrals and rehabilitation resources; joins groups whose members have had similar experiences.

Nursing diagnosis

Bowel incontinence

Related factors: Neuromuscular involvement

Defining characteristics: Involuntary passage of stool, constipation, loss of voluntary function and urge to defecate

OUTCOMES

Short-term

Adequate elimination, as evidenced by reestablishment of regular, soft, formed stool pattern (expected within 1 to 2 weeks)

Long-term

Establishment of bowel elimination pattern without incontinence of stool or constipation (expected ongoing)

NURSING INTERVENTIONS/INSTRUCTIONS

1. Instruct client to have bowel evacuation at same time each day; instruct client to use gentle pressure on abdomen, gentle digital anal stimulation, and Valsalva maneuver to promote bowel movement (first and second visits).
2. Instruct client to drink 8 to 10 glasses of fluid per day and prune juice at bedtime (first visit).
3. Instruct client to add fiber to daily diet and suggest foods to include (first visit).
4. Instruct client to administer suppository 30 minutes before scheduled elimination during training for stool continence (first visit and reinforce on second visit).
5. Review and reinforce a total bowel regimen that includes fluids, diet, scheduling, stool softener, suppository, and digital stimulation (each visit).

CLIENT AND FAMILY/CAREGIVER INTERVENTIONS

1. Client maintains daily or every-other-day bowel evacuation regimen.
2. Client prepares and ingests high-fiber diet and maintains fluid intake as instructed.
3. Client administers medication as appropriate to enhance elimination at scheduled times.

Nursing diagnosis

Reflex incontinence

Related factors: Neurologic impairment (spinal cord injury)

Defining characteristics: No awareness of bladder filling or fullness; no urge to void; uninhibited bladder contraction or spasm;

neurogenic bladder; bladder distention; frequent voiding in small amounts; constant dribbling

OUTCOMES

Short-term

Improved bladder function, as evidenced by reduction in incontinence episodes with use of catheter or training program (expected within 1 to 2 weeks)

Long-term

Ability to maintain bladder function, with absence of infection, to achieve optimal urinary continence (expected ongoing)

NURSING INTERVENTIONS/INSTRUCTIONS

1. Instruct client in noting and reporting cloudy, foul-smelling urine (first visit).
2. Instruct client to increase fluid intake to 10 glasses/day, and suggest acid-ash juices such as cranberry juice (first visit).
3. Instruct client in use of indwelling catheter, if present, noting patency and using sterile technique in catheter and meatal care (first and second visits).
4. Instruct client in application and care of condom catheter if used (first visit).
5. Instruct client or family member in intermittent catheterization using sterile technique and care of catheters if procedure is appropriate (first and second visits).
6. Inform client of training program and instruct client in scheduling voiding and in performing Credé's technique if bladder is not distended, or refer client to a rehabilitation program if rehabilitation is possible (first visit).
7. Initiate referral to enterostomal therapist, if appropriate (any visit).

CLIENT AND FAMILY/CAREGIVER INTERVENTIONS

1. Perform assessment for urinary bladder infection whether catheter is used or not.
2. Perform intermittent catheterization using sterile or clean technique as appropriate.
3. Maintain catheter patency and catheter care or condom catheter procedures.
4. Participate in urinary control rehabilitation program if appropriate.

Nursing diagnosis

Knowledge deficit

Related factors: Lack of information about disability

Defining characteristics: Expressed need for information about medical and rehabilitative regimen and prevention of trauma or injury

OUTCOMES

Short-term

Adequate knowledge, as evidenced by client's statement of treatment regimen and potential for injury or complications (expected within 1 week)

Long-term

Adequate knowledge, as evidenced by achievement of requirements for optimal health and functioning within limitations imposed by injury (expected within 1 to 2 months and ongoing)

NURSING INTERVENTIONS/INSTRUCTIONS

1. Assess life-style and ability to adapt, learning abilities and interest, and family participation and support (first visit).
2. Include all family members and care providers in instructions (each visit).
3. Assist client to write plan incorporating medical regimen and rehabilitation schedules and instruction, and revise daily as needed (each visit).
4. Instruct client to modify environment to prevent falls, to provide space needed for use of assistive aids such as a wheelchair, and to secure supplies and equipment that will ensure a safe home environment for ADL and other activities (first visit).
5. Instruct client to protect affected areas from excessively hot or cold applications or from trauma resulting from decreased sensory perception and motor deficits (first visit).
6. Instruct client in need to maintain fluid intake of up to 3 L/day and a diet high in calories, protein, and carbohydrates, and offer food lists and sample menus to assist in planning meals (first visit).

7. Instruct client in signs and symptoms of respiratory infection and to report change in respiration, yellow or other color change in sputum, or temperature elevation (first visit).
8. Inform client of possible autonomic dysreflexia and actions to take to prevent this condition (first and second visits).
9. Inform client of importance of compliance with physical, occupational, psychologic, and other therapy if applicable and to comply with scheduled visits to physician (first visit).
10. Inform client of stages of grieving and behavioral changes that can be expected to achieve stage of adjustment (each visit).

CLIENT AND FAMILY/CAREGIVER INTERVENTIONS

1. Client identifies hazards and eliminates or modifies them.
2. Client uses assistive and supplemental aids.
3. Client maintains open communication during grieving process.
4. Client assesses for and reports complications.
5. Client maintains scheduled appointments for rehabilitative therapy.
6. Client utilizes agencies for assistance in transportation, information, support, food services, housekeeping services, and others.
7. Client complies with fluid, nutritional, rest, activity, and other regimens included in medical regimen with as much independence as possible.

Nursing diagnosis

Risk for caregiver role strain

Related factors: Inexperience with caregiving; complexity or amount of caregiving tasks; duration of caregiving required; inadequate physical environment for providing care (housing, transportation, equipment, accessibility)

Defining characteristics: Report of not having enough resources to provide care (emotional and physical strength, help from others); difficulty in performing specific caregiving activities (bathing, cleaning up after urinary or bowel incontinence, moving and transferring, catheterization, managing discomforts and total care needs)

OUTCOMES

Short-term

Identification of potential for caregiver role strain, as evidenced by caregiver's verbalization of difficulties encountered in performing care and concern about ability and conflicts in giving care (expected within 1 week)

Long-term

Prevention of caregiver role strain, as evidenced by caregiver's providing of continued, progressive, and safe care without compromise to own physical and emotional needs (expected within 1 month and ongoing)

NURSING INTERVENTIONS/INSTRUCTIONS

1. Assess severity of disability and care needs of the receiver of care and ability of caregiver to perform role (first visit).
2. Assess relationship between care receiver and caregiver before the illness and stressors placed on the relationship by the complexity of needs caused by the illness (first visit).
3. Assist caregiver to monitor continued ability to perform care and treatments, day-to-day needs that may need to be changed or learned, changes in stressors and strains, maintenance of routines, and need for additional resources (aides, friends, family) (first visit).
4. Discuss role performance, whether expectations are realistic, and flexibility of role and decision-making process (first visit).
5. Initiate referral to HHA, social services, or psychologic counseling to assist with economic or mental or physical health needs (any visit).

CLIENT AND FAMILY/CAREGIVER INTERVENTIONS

1. Caregiver develops ability to cope with caregiver role; incorporates flexibility into day-to-day functioning.
2. Caregiver explores financial, legal, and physical assistance sources, and considers a referral to these services.
3. Caregiver maintains own health and well-being in caregiver role.
4. Caregiver maintains ongoing care and treatment regimen for care receiver.

Gastrointestinal system

Cirrhosis of Liver

Cirrhosis of the liver is a chronic disease characterized by structural and degenerative changes causing liver dysfunction and possible liver failure. Changes include the destruction of the liver parenchyma with the development of fibrous tissue that surrounds the hepatocytes and separates the lobules and, finally, the formation of nodules as the liver attempts to regenerate itself. Cirrhosis may be caused by chronic alcoholism, long-standing right-sided heart failure, alterations in the immune system, stasis of bile in the liver, or hepatic or other infections.

Home care is primarily concerned with ongoing assessment of the chronic symptomatology of the disease, elimination of the underlying cause if possible, and the teaching involved in promoting maintenance of health status and prevention of further liver damage and complications.

Nursing diagnosis

Altered nutrition: less than body requirements

Related factors: Inability to ingest food because of biologic factors; inability to digest foods because of biologic factors

Defining characteristics: Anorexia; nausea; vomiting; inability to metabolize fats, proteins, and carbohydrates and store nutrients; diarrhea or constipation; excessive fluid losses; weight loss; abdominal pain

OUTCOMES

Short-term

Adequate nutritional intake, as evidenced by compliance with a diet that facilitates appropriate weight maintenance for size, age, and frame; client's verbalization of foods to be included in a high-carbohydrate, moderately high protein diet; abstinence from alcohol (expected within 3 days)

Long-term

Adequate nutrition, as evidenced by food consumption and weight within expected requirements; continued abstinence from alcohol; achievement of optimal health and functioning within limitations imposed by disease (expected within 1 to 3 months and ongoing)

NURSING INTERVENTIONS/INSTRUCTIONS

1. Assess nutritional status and dietary inclusions and restrictions needed in presence of disease and in accordance with stage and symptoms of the disease (see Gastrointestinal System Assessment, p. 20, for guidelines) (first visit).
2. Instruct client to maintain a log of types and amounts of food eaten, likes and dislikes; review intake and use data as a basis for teaching diet; coordinate with dietitian (first, second, and third visits).
3. Assess alcohol intake and provide client with the rationale for avoiding all alcoholic beverages (each visit).
4. Assess for presence of anorexia, nausea, vomiting, malaise, fatigue, muscle wasting; suggest a period of rest before meals (first visit).
5. Measure height and weight and calculate weight requirements (first visit).
6. Measure abdominal girth (each visit).
7. Assist client in planning and selecting foods for high-carbohydrate and moderate protein diet totaling about 2000 to 3000 calories per day; suggest supplemental feedings if needed (first visit and reinforce on second visit).
8. Instruct client to restrict fluids in presence of edema or ascites (any visit).
9. Instruct client to avoid salty and convenience foods and to restrict sodium intake to 200 to 500 mg/day in presence of edema or ascites; instruct client in how to read labels on foods to determine sodium content (first visit).
10. Instruct client in administration of vitamins and minerals, antiemetics, and other prescribed drugs; instruct client to avoid over-the-counter (OTC) drugs unless advised by physician (first visit).

11. Instruct client to eat smaller, more frequent meals rather than three large meals (first visit).
12. Advise client to perform oral hygiene after meals and to use hard candy or sips of carbonated beverages or dry foods for nausea (first visit).
13. Initiate referral to nutritionist.
14. Refer home health aide (HHA) to assist with activities of daily living (ADL) and food preparation.

CLIENT AND FAMILY/CAREGIVER INTERVENTIONS

1. Client adheres to prescribed diet as instructed; maintains food diary.
2. Client limits sodium, fluids, or protein if indicated.
3. Client avoids alcohol.
4. Client weighs daily and report any significant gains or losses.
5. Client administers medications and vitamin supplement.
6. Client eats six times per day in small amounts; adjusts intake if nausea or vomiting is present.
7. Client provides pleasant environment for meals.
8. Client maintains oral hygiene.
9. Client consults with nutritionist if needed.

Nursing diagnosis

Risk for infection

Related factors: Inadequate secondary defenses; malnutrition

Defining characteristics: Leukopenia; chronic inadequate nutritional intake and metabolism; elevated temperature; changes in breathing, urine characteristics, or any part of body

OUTCOMES

Short-term

Reduced risk for infection development, as evidenced by temperature and white blood count within normal ranges, lung fields clear, and skin intact (expected within 3 days)

Long-term

Absence of signs and symptoms of infection in any organ system (expected within 2 weeks)

NURSING INTERVENTIONS/INSTRUCTIONS

1. Assess skin for jaundice, pruritis, and evidence of scratches or excoriation (first visit).
2. Instruct client in relief measures for pruritis, including cool compresses, emollient baths, patting instead of rubbing skin dry, and use of mild soap and soft towel (first visit).
3. Instruct client to avoid scratching itchy areas and to keep fingernails short and clean and well filed for smoothness (first visit).
4. Assess lungs for decreased breath sounds, cough, adventitious sounds, or change in respiratory rate, depth, or ease (first visit).
5. Instruct client to take temperature and notify physician of elevations or of changes in respiratory pattern or airway clearance (first visit).
6. Instruct client to avoid exposure to persons with infections (first visit).
7. Instruct client in antibiotic administration as prescribed (first visit).
8. Refer HHA when necessary to assist.

CLIENT AND FAMILY/CAREGIVER INTERVENTIONS

1. Client maintains personal hygiene; adjusts bathing, grooming, and dressing to enhance body image and protect jaundiced skin.
2. Client administers medications as instructed.
3. Client reports signs and symptoms of infection to physician if present.
4. Client monitors temperature if symptoms appear.
5. Client maintains absence of infection of skin, lungs, or any other organ.

Nursing diagnosis

Altered protection

Related factors: Abnormal blood profile

Defining characteristics: Inability of liver to convert ammonia to urea, to produce coagulation factors, and to absorb vitamin K; leukopenia; ecchymoses; petechiae; bleeding from gums, mucous membranes

OUTCOME CRITERIA

Short-term

Control of bleeding tendency, as evidenced by absence of bleeding from any site (expected within 3 days)

Long-term

Maintenance of blood profile within normal ranges within limitations imposed by severity of disease (expected within 2 to 4 weeks)

NURSING INTERVENTIONS/INSTRUCTIONS

1. Assess for bleeding, including petechiae, ecchymoses, oozing or frank bleeding from any orifice or skin site; check hemoglobin and hematocrit levels if available; instruct client to report any bleeding to physician (each visit).
2. Instruct client to avoid trauma and constrictive clothing and to protect vulnerable areas from injury (first visit).
3. Instruct client in administration of vitamin K if appropriate (first visit).
4. Instruct caregiver or HHA to avoid toothbrushing (use swabs instead) and rectal temperatures.

CLIENT AND FAMILY/CAREGIVER INTERVENTIONS

1. Client identifies and reports signs and symptoms of bleeding.
2. Client administers prescribed medications.

Nursing diagnosis

Altered thought processes

Related factors: Physiologic changes

Defining characteristics: Confusion, memory deficit, disorientation, lethargy

OUTCOMES

Short-term

Improvement in neurologic function and mentation, as evidenced by stability in orientation and mental functioning (expected within 1 week)

Long-term

Appropriate level of mental function within limitations imposed by disease status (expected within 2 to 4 weeks)

NURSING INTERVENTIONS/INSTRUCTIONS

1. Assess mentation, including confusion, lethargy, irritability, depression, personality and behavioral changes, slurred speech, and psychotic ideations, and instruct client to report any of these conditions to physician (each visit).
2. Encourage client to participate in interactions with others and to use clock, calendar, newspaper, radio, and other stimulation that may be preferred (first visit).
3. Inform client of reason for mental changes if they occur (first visit).
4. Refer client to psychological counseling if appropriate (any visit).
5. Refer HHA to assist with ADL.

CLIENT AND FAMILY/CAREGIVER INTERVENTIONS

1. Client identifies and reports mental and emotional changes.
2. Client provides stimulation and reality reinforcement.
3. Client administers medications if prescribed.

Nursing diagnosis

Body image disturbance

Related factors: Biophysical factors caused by disease process

Defining characteristics: Jaundice; pruritis; skin irritation from scratching; chronic fatigue; estrogen-androgen imbalance; ascites; edema

OUTCOMES

Short-term

Improvement in self-image, as evidenced by participation in care and interest in appearance and by some resumption of outside activities or interactions (expected within 3 to 7 days)

Long-term

Adaptation to temporary and permanent changes in body image, as evidenced by resumption of self-care activities and social and work activities to achieve optimal level of function within disease limitations (expected within 1 to 3 months)

NURSING INTERVENTIONS/INSTRUCTIONS

1. Assess ability of client and family to cope and adapt (first visit).
2. Allow time for and acceptance of expressions of concern and negative comments about appearance (each visit).
3. Assess behavioral and emotional trends and changes, and integrate them into clinical profile for disease progression and encephalopathy (each visit).
4. Assess and discuss appearance and measures to minimize the effects of edema, jaundice, weight changes, loss of hair, menstrual irregularities, impotence, and changes in sex characteristics (first visit and reinforce as needed).
5. Initiate referral to counseling or support group.

CLIENT AND FAMILY/CAREGIVER INTERVENTIONS

1. Client expresses concerns and feelings about changes.
2. Client supports and adapts to physical changes.
3. Client participates in daily care and utilizes measures to conceal body changes and appearance.
4. Client reports signs and symptoms of hormonal imbalance or central nervous system dysfunction.
5. Client seeks counseling if needed, occupational retraining if appropriate.

Nursing diagnosis

Knowledge deficit

Related factors: Lack of information about disease and care

Defining characteristics: Request for information about disease process, causes, treatments, preventive measures, and medical regimen; denial as result of absence of symptoms or alcohol abuse

OUTCOMES

Short-term

Adequate knowledge, as evidenced by client's statement of status of disease and symptoms of worsening condition and of need for compliance in medication and activity regimens and alcoholism rehabilitation (expected within 1 week)

Long-term

Adequate knowledge, as evidenced by compliance with requirements to maintain liver function and obtain optimal level of health (expected within 2 to 3 months)

NURSING INTERVENTIONS/INSTRUCTIONS

1. Assess life-style, abilities to learn and adapt to treatments, interests and diversional activities, family participation and support, and presence of alcoholism (first visit).
2. Perform abdominal assessment, including measurement for changes in abdominal girth indicating ascites, splenomegaly, hepatic level and hardness, and abdominal discomfort, and instruct client in performing this assessment (first visit and ongoing).
3. Assess complaints of nausea, vomiting, anorexia, weight loss or gain, constipation or diarrhea, fatigue, or pruritis, and instruct client to report these conditions to physician if they occur (each visit).
4. Assess for history of alcohol abuse, use of hepatotoxic drugs, exposure to chemicals, or gastrointestinal surgery (first visit).
5. Discuss and reinforce importance of alcohol abstinence (first visit and reinforce when needed).
6. Instruct client to schedule 6 to 8 hours of sleep per 24 hours and to schedule rest hours around meals and activities (first visit).
7. Instruct client to report any signs or symptoms of complications or worsening condition, including fever, bleeding, shortness of breath, increase in abdominal girth, weight or urinary output changes, edema, confusion or personality changes, abdominal pain, or jaundice (first week).
8. Instruct client to avoid exposure to toxic agents, medications, or environments and to possible infection (first visit).
9. Instruct client in medication administration, including vitamins, antipruritics, stool softeners, diuretics, electrolyte replacement, aldosterone-blocking agents, digestive enzymes, and others as ordered; inform client of dose, frequency, route, side effects, and food, drug, and alcohol interactions (first visit and reinforce on second visit).

10. Advise client of importance of keeping appointments with physician and laboratory (first visit).
11. Provide information about community agencies and groups, such as Alcoholics Anonymous (AA), for support, counseling, or educational materials (first visit).

CLIENT AND FAMILY/CAREGIVER INTERVENTIONS

1. Client complies with medical regimen and changes life-style if needed.
2. Client reports signs and symptoms of complications.
3. Client avoids alcohol and other substances toxic to liver.
4. Client administers medications correctly and safely.
5. Client avoids stressful situations; seeks counseling if needed.
6. Client schedules adequate rest and sleep and promotes as part of daily routine.
7. Client maintains physician and laboratory appointments.
8. Client contacts AA or other support groups for assistance.
9. Client returns to work and activities within limitations.

Hepatitis

Hepatitis is the inflammation of the liver as the result of alcohol, drugs, or viruses. Viral hepatitis may be classified as hepatitis A, hepatitis B, or non-A, non-B hepatitis, depending on the viral strain. Hepatitis A is transmitted by the oral or fecal route, hepatitis B is transmitted by the parenteral route, and non-A, non-B hepatitis is transmitted through transfusions. The disease varies in severity, which determines the degree of liver cell injury and scarring and resolution or chronicity of the condition.

Home care is primarily concerned with proper testing and treatment necessary to prevent transmission and increased incidence of the disease in the community and with the teaching involved in the care and treatment of the acute stage of the disease and prevention of permanent liver damage.

Nursing diagnosis

Altered nutrition: less than body requirements

Related factors: Inability to ingest food; inability to digest foods because of biologic factors

Defining characteristics: Nausea; vomiting; anorexia; abdominal diarrhea; inability to store nutrients; inability to metabolize fats, proteins, and carbohydrates; excessive fluid losses; tenderness; weight loss

OUTCOMES

Short-term

Adequate nutrition, as evidenced by consumption of increased carbohydrates and increased calories and by prescribed protein intake (expected within 3 days)

Long-term

Nutritional status optimal, as evidenced by intake of prescribed diet and by weight maintenance for health and functioning during course of disease (expected within 1 to 2 months)

NURSING INTERVENTIONS/INSTRUCTIONS

1. Assess nutritional and gastrointestinal status, taking into consideration dietary preferences and restrictions or inclusions (see Gastrointestinal System Assessment, p. 20, for guidelines) (first visit).
2. Take height and weight and calculate weight requirements (first visit).
3. Measure abdominal girth, and determine weight on same scale, at same time of day with client wearing similar clothing (each visit).
4. Instruct client to keep food diary that includes types, portions, and preparation method of foods consumed (first visit).
5. Using these data as a basis for diet teaching, assist client in food selection for a high-carbohydrate, high-calorie diet; also should be high in protein in absence of edema (first visit and reinforce on second visit).
6. Instruct client to eat smaller, more frequent meals rather than three large meals; advise client to eat larger amounts during the day rather than in the evening (first visit).

7. Instruct client to drink 3000 ml of fluids per day (in absence of edema) and to estimate adequacy of output (first visit).
8. Suggest hard candy, sips of carbonated beverages, or dry food for nausea (first visit).
9. Instruct client in administration of prescribed antiemetic ½ hour before meals (first visit).

CLIENT AND FAMILY/CAREGIVER INTERVENTIONS

1. Client maintains a food and fluid diary.
2. Client takes and records weight, daily or as needed.
3. Client maintains prescribed carbohydrate and caloric intake.
4. Client spreads meals over entire day, with most eaten early in the day, and intersperses meals with fluid intake.
5. Client administers antiemetic before meals.
6. Client performs oral care as needed.
7. Client uses hard candy and other dietary aids to control nausea.
8. Client limits protein and fluids if edema is present.

Nursing diagnosis

Risk for impaired skin integrity

Related factors: Internal factor of altered pigmentation

Defining characteristics: Jaundice, pruritis, dry skin, scratches or disruptions on skin

OUTCOMES

Short-term

Skin intact and free from irritation, as evidenced by absence of rash, abrasions, excoriations, or disruptions (expected within 1 week)

Long-term

Skin integrity maintained, with optimal comfort and health achieved (expected within 1 month)

NURSING INTERVENTIONS/INSTRUCTIONS

1. Assess skin for color, temperature, integrity, and sensation; assess for presence of jaundice or pruritis and for evidence of scratching (see Integumentary System Assessment, p. 36, for guidelines) (each visit).

2. Instruct client in relief measures, such as cool warm shower or cool compresses to area, mild soap for bathing, patting instead of rubbing dry, diversional methods, and use of emollients in water and topically (first visit).
3. Instruct client to maintain clean, short nails and to apply pressure to itchy areas instead of scratching (first visit).
4. Instruct client in use of antipruritics and antihistamine, including dose, time, frequency, and side effects; inform client of drug or alcohol interactions (first visit).
5. Inform client to wear loose clothing and to avoid tight, restrictive types of clothing, which might increase itching (first visit).

CLIENT AND FAMILY/CAREGIVER INTERVENTIONS

1. Client administers medications for relief of itching.
2. Client uses other relief measures to control pruritis.
3. Client avoids scratching.
4. Client notifies physician if symptoms are not relieved or if breaks appear on skin.

Nursing diagnosis

Impaired social interaction

Related factors: Therapeutic isolation; body image disturbance

Defining characteristics: Verbalized discomfort in social participation, jaundiced appearance, fear of transmitting disease to others, stated lack of diversional activity and interactions

OUTCOMES

Short-term

Minimal boredom, loneliness, and impaired body image, as evidenced by client's statement that body image is improving as condition resolves and by participation in activities to provide stimulation (expected within 1 week)

Long-term

Adaptation to temporary restrictions in social relationships to prevent transmission of disease and sensory deficits and by maintenance of optimal level of health and functioning (expected within 1 month)

NURSING INTERVENTIONS/INSTRUCTIONS

1. Instruct client in reasons for isolation precautions and length of time restrictions must be observed (first visit).
2. Instruct family to provide separate room and bathroom for client if possible (first visit).
3. Instruct family to spend time with client at intervals during day (first visit).
4. Inform client and family of precautions to take to prevent transmission, including hand washing, care of utensils and articles used for meals, and bowel elimination (first visit).
5. Encourage family to provide for diversional activities, such as books, cards, television, radio, newspaper, and telephone (first visit).
6. Inform client that jaundice is not permanent and disappears as disease is resolved (first visit).
7. Remove mirrors and cover body parts to preserve body image if jaundice is present (first visit).
8. Note negative attitudes and comments regarding skin color and pruritis, and provide support (each visit).

CLIENT AND FAMILY/CAREGIVER INTERVENTIONS

1. Client encourages visits from friends.
2. Client maintains precautions to prevent transmission of disease.
3. Family provides diversional activities when client is confined to room.
4. Family promotes and supports positive attitude about temporary jaundice.

Nursing diagnosis

Knowledge deficit

Related factors: Lack of information about disease

Defining characteristics: Verbalization of need for information about disease and its transmission and about prevention of complications or relapse or recurrence

OUTCOMES

Short-term

Adequate knowledge, as evidenced by client's stating methods of disease transmission, treatment, and prevention of complications and by client's compliance with diet, activity, and hygiene and sanitation regimens (expected within 3 days)

Long-term

Adequate knowledge, as evidenced by client's meeting requirements to achieve optimal level of liver function and absence of symptoms and complications or transmittal of disease to others (expected within 1 to 2 months)

NURSING INTERVENTIONS/INSTRUCTIONS

1. Assess life-style, ability and interest to learn, ability to adapt, and family participation and support (first visit).
2. Review history of flulike symptoms: nausea, vomiting, anorexia, weight loss, fatigue, malaise, headache, myalgia, constipation or diarrhea; note also recent travel, transfusions, injections or sharing of needles, or exposure to toxins or to carriers (first visit).
3. Perform abdominal assessment (see Gastrointestinal System Assessment, p. 20, for guidelines) and note liver size and tenderness, enlarged nodes, presence of dark urine, clay colored stools, scleral icterus, jaundice (each visit).
4. Instruct client in causes, transmission, signs and symptoms, and treatment of disease (first visit).
5. Instruct client in hand-washing and isolation protocols, and emphasize washing hands especially after toileting (first visit).
6. Instruct client to avoid tiring self and to participate only in activity that is tolerated (first visit).
7. Instruct client to report edema in extremities or abdomen, unexplained weight gain, changes in personality or behavior, or evidence of bleeding (first visit).
8. Instruct client to avoid alcohol or toxins; review drug profile for hepatotoxic drugs (first visit).
9. Instruct client not to donate blood (first visit).
10. Instruct client to avoid sexual contact temporarily (first visit).
11. Instruct client to keep appointments with physician and for laboratory testing, and monitor laboratory results as available (each visit).

12. Initiate referral to appropriate health care facility for possible prophylactic care of household contacts and regular sexual partners (first visit).
13. Provide information on community agencies and groups, such as drug rehabilitation or counseling groups, for educational literature and support (first visit).

CLIENT AND FAMILY/CAREGIVER INTERVENTIONS

1. Client avoids transmission of disease by:
   - Proper hand washing
   - Proper disinfection of food utensils, clothing, and linens
   - Avoiding sharing of food, utensils, personal grooming items, toilet, clothing, or linens
   - Proper disposal of tissues
2. Client states cause, transmission, signs and symptoms, and treatment of disease.
3. Client avoids alcohol, hepatotoxic drugs, and exposure to toxins.
4. Client avoids sexual contact.
5. Client refrains from donating blood.
6. Client avoids stressful situations; sets aside rest periods during day.
7. Client reports signs and symptoms to physician as instructed.
8. Client reports for physician and laboratory appointments.
9. Client has contacts report for prophylactic therapy.
10. Client reports pregnancy status to all health workers.
11. Client contacts support groups or counselor for assistance if appropriate.

Peptic Ulcer

A peptic ulcer is a sharp, circumscribed ulceration of the mucous membrane of the stomach (gastric: usually at the lesser curvature) or the duodenum (duodenal: usually at the point where the stomach contents enters the small intestine). The condition may be acute or chronic and may be caused by the effect on the mucosal barrier of drug ingestion, high levels of hydrochloric acid and enzyme secretions, prolonged illness, trauma or stress, or autoimmune disorders.

Home care is primarily concerned with the teaching involved in the healing of the ulcer and prevention of factors that are associated with chronicity or recurrence.

Nursing diagnosis

Pain

Related factors: Biologic, chemical, or psychologic injuring agents

Defining characteristics: Communication of pain descriptors (epigastric pain, burning, gnawing, aching, sore, occurs before or during eating); heartburn; indigestion; weight loss or gain; high level of stress; ingestion of drugs (steriods, antiinflammatories, antihypertensives)

OUTCOMES

Short-term

Increased comfort, as evidenced by client stating that he or she feels better, that pain is decreased or absent (expected within 2 to 3 days)

Long-term

Absence of or minimal pain with decreased incidence of recurrence or relapse and achievement of optimal health and functioning (expected within 2 to 3 months)

NURSING INTERVENTIONS/INSTRUCTIONS

1. Assess abdomen (see Gastrointestinal System Assessment, p. 20, for guidelines); note vital signs, including temperature; type, intensity, and location of pain; radiation; bowel sounds; precipitating and alleviating factors (each visit).
2. Instruct client in administration of medications that will assist in relieving pain, such as antacids, sedatives, and histamine (H_2) blockers, if ordered (first visit).
3. When pain is minimal or relieved, review health regimen to include diet, rest and activity, and avoidance of stressors (each visit).

CLIENT AND FAMILY/CAREGIVER INTERVENTIONS

1. Client administers medications for pain correctly as instructed.
2. Client avoids stressors and stressful situations.
3. Client reports new, increased, or uncontrolled pain to physician.

Nursing diagnosis

Knowledge deficit

Related factors: Lack of information about disorder

Defining characteristics: Verbalization of need for information about disease, causes, treatment (diet and medications), and importance of compliance

OUTCOMES

Short-term

Adequate knowledge, as evidenced by client stating signs and symptoms of deteriorating condition or complication; diet, activity, and medication regimens; and life-style adaptations (expected within 3 days)

Long-term

Adequate knowledge, as evidenced by client meeting requirements to achieve optimal level of health and functioning (expected within 2 weeks)

NURSING INTERVENTIONS/INSTRUCTIONS

1. Assess nutritional status, food preferences, and cultural or religious restrictions (first visit).
2. Assess height and weight and calculate desired weight; instruct client to take and record weight weekly (first visit).
3. Instruct client on nutritionally adequate diet and prescribed modifications (first visit and reinforce on second visit).
   - Bland meals; eliminate food distressors such as black pepper; chili powder; raw, spicy, or fatty foods; fruit juices; and beverages containing caffeine
   - Smaller, more frequent meals (five or six per day), including a bedtime snack; include protein source at each meal
   - Use skim rather than whole milk

4. Suggest that client rest before meals and that environment be quiet and pleasant during meals (first visit).
5. Instruct client to restrict alcohol and refrain from smoking (first visit and reinforce on second visit).
6. Instruct client in administration of antacids (tablet or liquid), sedatives, antianxiety agents, and histamine antagonists; include dose, route, frequency, side effects, and food, drug and alcohol interactions, and instruct client to avoid OTC drugs, especially aspirin or aspirin-containing drugs (first visit).
7. Assist client to identify and to explore sources of emotional stress and to develop methods to minimize or eliminate them (first and second visits).
8. Inform client of importance of compliance with treatment regimen and expected effects (first visit).
9. Instruct client to notify physician immediately if hemorrhage occurs (weakness, apprehension, restlessness, vertigo/syncope, thirst, diaphoresis, dyspnea, tarry or bloody stools, vomiting with frank blood or coffee-ground appearance) (first visit).
10. Instruct client to notify physician immediately if obstruction occurs (bloated feeling after meals, fullness after meals, absence of bowel elimination, anorexia, weight loss, vomiting large amounts, projectile vomiting, dehydration) (first visit).
11. Instruct client to call ambulance and go to emergency room if perforation occurs (sudden sharp epigastric or abdominal pain, pain radiation to shoulders, abdominal rigidity, diaphoresis, fever, rapid and shallow respirations, increased pulse rate) (first visit).
12. Encourage modification rather than complete life-style changes to increase compliance (first visit).
13. Suggest community resources and groups for smoking and stress and dietary counseling and support (first visit).
14. Encourage client to keep appointments with physician and for laboratory tests (first visit).
15. Instruct client to avoid aspirin and aspirin products.

CLIENT AND FAMILY/CAREGIVER INTERVENTIONS

1. Client eats a well-balanced, bland diet in small and frequent meals; avoids dietary stressors.
2. Client avoids alcohol, tobacco, and caffeine.

3. Client avoids stress in environment, relationships and situations that may create stress.
4. Client administers medications correctly and as instructed; avoids aspirin and nonsteroidal antiinflammatories.
5. Client notifies physician of signs and symptoms of complications if they occur.
6. Client asks questions and clarifies information when needed.
7. Client seeks out reinforcement and support in community groups that might be helpful.
8. Client keeps appointments with physician for follow-up care.

Nursing diagnosis

Anxiety

Related factors: Threat to or change in health status

Defining characteristics: Increased tension and apprehension about change in health and life-style, client's verbalization of inability to manage stress and symptoms of the disease

OUTCOMES

Short-term

Decreased anxiety, as evidenced by more relaxed posture and facial expression, statements that anxiety has decreased and has been controlled, and decrease in symptoms as a result of compliance with health regimen (expected within 3 to 7 days)

Long-term

Anxiety minimal or controlled, as evidenced by client's acceptance of changes in life-style to achieve optimal health and functioning (expected within 4 weeks)

NURSING INTERVENTIONS/INSTRUCTIONS

1. Assess mental and emotional status (see Psychosocial Assessment, p. 48, for guidelines) (first visit).
2. Explore with client historical coping patterns and problem-solving ability; relate them to condition and pain episodes (first visit).
3. Assist client to develop effective coping and stress-reducing mechanisms (first visit and reinforce on second visit).

4. Include client in all aspects of planning care at home (each visit).
5. Provide continuing information about condition and progress (each visit).
6. Suggest counseling and/or relaxation techniques to reduce anxiety if chronic (first visit).

CLIENT AND FAMILY/CAREGIVER INTERVENTIONS

1. Client identifies current coping mechanisms and explores options for improved coping and stress control.
2. Client participates in planning of care, including adherence to dietary, activity, and medication regimens.
3. Client performs relaxation exercises when feeling anxious.
4. Client consults physician if unable to control anxiety.

Ulcerative Colitis/Crohn's Disease

Inflammatory bowel diseases include ulcerative colitis, involving the large intestine, and Crohn's disease, involving any part of the intestinal tract but most usually the terminal ileum. Ulcerative colitis affects the mucous membranes, causing purulent exudate and bleeding. Segments or the entire colon may be affected, with periods of remission and exacerbation of inflammation. The disease may be confused with Crohn's disease. Crohn's disease affects all layers of the mucous membranes, and segments separated by normal bowel may be inflamed. Both diseases exhibit extracolonic manifestations as well as affect absorption of nutrients. Complications include intestinal obstruction, anemia, and nutritional and fluid and electrolyte imbalances.

Home care is primarily concerned with the teaching aspects of care and treatment for the disease and preventive measures to maintain health and avoid exacerbation.

Nursing diagnosis

Chronic pain

Related factors: Biologic injuring agents of inflammatory disease

Defining characteristics: Verbalization of pain descriptors, groaning, abdominal guarding, restlessness, abdominal cramping

OUTCOMES

Short-term

Pain controlled, as evidenced by client's statement that pain has subsided, relaxed posture and facial expressions, and participation in ADL and other activities (expected within 3 to 4 days)

Long-term

Pain controlled, as evidenced by return to normal gastrointestinal function; achieved as a result of compliance with medical regimen (expected within 2 to 4 weeks)

NURSING INTERVENTIONS/INSTRUCTIONS

1. Assess pain type, location, characteristics, duration, intensity, and relationship to diet, activity, and elimination (first visit).
2. Instruct client in medication administration, including analgesics and antiinflammatories prescribed (first visit).
3. Instruct client in relaxation exercises and guided imagery and to practice these techniques between episodes (first visit).
4. Instruct client to notify physician if pain is not relieved or increases in severity and if bloating, distention, vomiting, or abdominal rigidity is associated with increasing pain (first visit).

CLIENT AND FAMILY/CAREGIVER INTERVENTIONS

1. Client administers medication for optimal effects.
2. Client practices diversional activities for relaxation and pain reduction.
3. Client notifies physician if pain persists or escalates or if new symptoms develop.

Nursing diagnosis

Altered nutrition: less than body requirements

Related factors: Inability to ingest or absorb nutrients because of biologic factors

Defining characteristics: Weight loss; inadequate intake of nutrients; anorexia; diarrhea; nausea

OUTCOMES

Short-term

Adequate nutrition, as evidenced by client's statement of compliance with dietary requirements and regimen and by stabilization of weight (expected within 1 week)

Long-term

Adequate nutritional status, as evidenced by intake of required nutrients for optimal health and functioning (expected within 1 month and ongoing)

NURSING INTERVENTIONS/INSTRUCTIONS

1. Assess nutritional status, including food preferences, cultural and religious restrictions, and effect of different foods on illness (first visit).
2. Calculate ideal weight for size, sex, frame, and height (first visit).
3. Assess for nausea, vomiting, anorexia, weight loss, fatigue, malaise, and reactions to meals (each visit).
4. Instruct client to schedule rest periods after meals and to have 6 to 8 hours of sleep per night (first visit).
5. Inform client of measures that facilitate eating, including eliminating odors, providing a relaxed atmosphere and a quiet environment, eating smaller, more frequent meals, and taking antiemetics ½ hour before meals (first visit).
6. Include client in planning a bland, high-protein, reduced-fiber, low-residue, and possibly high-calorie diet, avoiding highly seasoned foods, raw fruits and vegetables, foods containing coarse cereals, bran, seeds, or nuts, milk, and fatty or fried foods (first visit).

7. Administer iron preparation intramuscularly as prescribed (any visit).
8. Initiate referral to nutritionist if indicated.

CLIENT AND FAMILY/CAREGIVER INTERVENTIONS

1. Client maintains or gains weight as determined.
2. Client participates in planning and ingestion of a well-balanced diet with restrictions as determined.
3. Client promotes pleasant environment and dietary pattern that enhances intake.
4. Client maintains rest and sleep schedule.
5. Client avoids stress and irritants during meals.
6. Client includes increased calories and protein in diet plans.

Nursing diagnosis

Diarrhea

Related factors: Inflammation, irritation, or malabsorption of bowel

Defining characteristics: Abdominal pain; cramping; increased frequency; loose, liquid stools; urgency; mucus in stool; increased frequency of bowel sounds

OUTCOMES

Short-term

Return of baseline bowel pattern, as evidenced by decrease in the frequency of bowel eliminations and by stool characteristics within baseline parameters (expected within 1 week)

Long-term

Minimal or absence of diarrheal bowel eliminations, as evidenced by soft, formed stools eliminated according to baseline pattern (expected within 2 weeks)

NURSING INTERVENTIONS/INSTRUCTIONS

1. Assess bowel elimination patterns and stool characteristics (see Gastrointestinal System Assessment, p. 20, for guidelines) (first visit).

2. Instruct client to maintain a record of bowel movements, including number and when they occur and characteristics such as color, amount, consistency, odor, and presence of mucus, blood, or pus (first visit).
3. Monitor medication administration and instruct client in antidiarrheals, anticholinergics, corticosteroids, antiinfectives (each visit).
4. Instruct client to notify physician if diarrhea becomes more severe or frequent, if bleeding is noted, or if fatigue or weakness is noted (first visit).

CLIENT AND FAMILY/CAREGIVER INTERVENTIONS

1. Client monitors and records bowel elimination.
2. Client administers medications correctly and as instructed.
3. Client notifies physician if diarrhea becomes worse and condition deteriorates or complications occur.

Nursing diagnosis

Risk for impaired skin integrity

Related factors: Excretions and secretions

Defining characteristics: Diarrhea; irritation, redness, or disruption of perianal area; perianal pain

OUTCOMES

Short-term

Minimized risk for skin breakdown, as evidenced by appropriate care of perianal area, which should be free of maceration or excoriation caused by excretions (expected within 3 to 4 days)

Long-term

Skin integrity maintained, as evidenced by perianal area free of any irritation or breaks (expected within 1 week and ongoing)

NURSING INTERVENTIONS/INSTRUCTIONS

1. Assess perianal area for tissue integrity, color, and odor, and note presence of drainage, excoriation, maceration, abscess, fistula, or fissure formation (each visit).

2. Instruct client in perianal care to be done every morning and possibly after every bowel elimination, including sitz bath, cleansing with agent dispensed in a Peri-bottle, and application of protective ointment; advise client to continue care during periods of remission (first visit and reinforce on second visit).
3. Instruct client to notify physician if irritation is unrelieved and bleeding or drainage is noted (first visit).

CLIENT AND FAMILY/CAREGIVER INTERVENTIONS

1. Client provides perianal care daily or as needed.
2. Client protects perianal area from irritation.
3. Client maintains intact perianal tissue integrity.
4. Client notifies physician of severe excoriation or breakdown of perianal area.

Nursing diagnosis

Risk for fluid volume deficit

Related factors: Active fluid loss

Defining characteristics: Diarrhea, vomiting; diaphoresis; decreased urine output in relation to intake; dry skin and mucous membranes; weight loss; electrolyte imbalance (sodium, potassium)

OUTCOMES

Short-term

Adequate fluid and electrolyte balance, as evidenced by absence of signs and symptoms of dehydration, balanced intake and output, and electrolyte levels within normal ranges (expected within 1 week)

Long-term

Fluid and electrolytes within balance, with optimal health and functioning achieved whether during remission or during exacerbation of disease (expected within 2 weeks and ongoing)

NURSING INTERVENTIONS/INSTRUCTIONS

1. Assess fluid needs according to age, weight, and estimated fluid losses (each visit).

2. Monitor for dehydration, including thirst, decreased urinary output, poor skin turgor, dry mucous membranes, and furrowed tongue (each visit).
3. Instruct client to take and record daily weights and estimated intake and output (first visit).
4. Instruct client to drink 8 to 10 glasses of fluid per day in small, spaced servings and to avoid fluids that are too hot or cold (first visit).
5. Instruct client in administration of potassium supplements and intake of foods containing potassium, including bananas, citrus juices, and dried fruits (first visit).
6. Monitor for electrolyte imbalance and instruct client in recognition of signs and symptoms, including muscle weakness, cramping, twitching, confusion, paresthesias, and pulse irregularities (first visit).
7. Monitor laboratory values for potassium, sodium, calcium, chloride, magnesium, hemoglobin, and hematocrit if available (any visit).

CLIENT AND FAMILY/CAREGIVER INTERVENTIONS

1. Client maintains fluid intake according to calculated needs and fluid losses.
2. Client administers or increases intake of potassium replacement.
3. Client weighs daily, compares intake and output of fluids in relation to diarrhea.
4. Client reports any signs and symptoms of dehydration or electrolyte decreases.

Nursing diagnosis

Ineffective individual coping

Related factors: Multiple life changes; chronic illness

Defining characteristics: Verbalization of inability to cope or ask for or seek out help; inability to solve problems and use defense mechanisms effectively; exacerbation of symptoms; chronic anxiety; depression

OUTCOMES

Short-term

Improved coping ability, as evidenced by client's statement that recognizing and adapting to need for changes in life-style are necessary (expected within 1 week)

Long-term

Effective coping, as evidenced by compliance with treatment regimen and by changes in life-style to adapt to illness and to requirements for optimal health achievement (expected within 1 to 2 months and ongoing)

NURSING INTERVENTIONS/INSTRUCTIONS

1. Assess for developmental level and dependency needs, behavioral and emotional changes, use of defense mechanisms and their effectiveness, and ability to solve problems (first visit).
2. Establish a trusting relationship, and facilitate an open discussion to explore options and develop skills in coping and problem solving (each visit).
3. Identify coping skills that work, and encourage positive feeling about success of any adaptation or changes (each visit).
4. Include client in all planning and formulation of realistic goals; assist if requested to do so (each visit).
5. Encourage expression of fears about possible surgery and threat to life.

CLIENT AND FAMILY/CAREGIVER INTERVENTIONS

1. Client shares feelings, fears, and concerns with caretaker or family.
2. Client plans and participates in own care and health promotion.
3. Client sets goals and strategies for remissions and exacerbations.
4. Client participates in support group with persons who have similar condition.

Nursing diagnosis

Knowledge deficit

Related factors: Lack of information about disease and treatments

Defining characteristics: Request for information about disease, causes, signs and symptoms, medications, and need for compliance and for prevention of exacerbations

OUTCOMES

Short-term

Adequate knowledge, as evidenced by client's statement of precipitating, aggravating, and alleviating factors in symptomatology and signs and symptoms of exacerbation or worsening condition (expected within 3 days)

Long-term

Adequate knowledge, as evidenced by client's meeting requirements to achieve optimal health and gastrointestinal functioning with reduction in exacerbations (expected within 1 to 2 months and ongoing)

NURSING INTERVENTIONS/INSTRUCTIONS

1. Assess client's life-style, learning and coping abilities, interests, and family participation and support (first visit).
2. Instruct client to maintain log of ADL that includes food diary, fluid intake, and descriptions of gastrointestinal episodes (first visit).
3. Assist client to identify characteristic trends and influencing factors that precipitate or alleviate symptoms; use data as a physiologic and psychologic baseline and a basis for teaching (first visit).
4. Instruct client to notify physician of any change in condition that indicates complications or exacerbation (first visit).
5. Instruct client in correct medication administration, including vitamins, electrolyte replacement, antiemetics, antidiarrheals, steroids, immunosuppressants, antibiotics, and others prescribed; emphasize dosage, frequency, side effects, expected results, and interactions and to avoid OTC drugs without physician recommendation (first visit).
6. Instruct client to maintain scheduled physician appointments (first visit).
7. Provide information about agencies or groups for educational material, support or counseling, or new trends (first visit).

CLIENT AND FAMILY/CAREGIVER INTERVENTIONS

1. Client maintains log of progress and changes.
2. Client monitors for influences of diet, fluids, activity, and stress.
3. Client administers medications safely and correctly.
4. Client notifies physician of unremitting or escalating symptoms.
5. Client participates in educational and support programs.
6. Client carries out measures to prevent exacerbation.

Endocrine system

Diabetes Mellitus

Diabetes mellitus is characterized by absence or inadequate production of insulin by the pancreas to meet body needs for carbohydrate, fat, and protein metabolism. Long-term effects include vascular changes, retinopathy, and neuropathy. The most common type found in adults is non-insulin dependent, or type II (NIDDM). A second type is insulin dependent, or type I (IDDM).

Home care is primarily concerned with the teaching aspects of medication regimens, monitoring glucose levels, and the measures to take for control of the disease to prevent complications.

Nursing diagnosis

Ineffective individual coping

Related factors: Multiple life changes; chronic illness and consequences

Defining characteristics: Chronic worry, anxiety, and complaints; tension; inability to cope with necessary life-style changes

OUTCOMES

Short-term

Improvement in use of coping skills, as evidenced by use of coping mechanisms effectively and by verbalization of need to change life-style and request assistance when needed to meet needs (expected within 1 week)

Long-term

Effective coping with chronic illness, as evidenced by acceptable level of anxiety and concern and by adaptation to life-style changes (expected within 2 to 3 months)

NURSING INTERVENTIONS/INSTRUCTIONS

1. Assess for appropriate use of coping mechanisms, ability to solve problems, inner resources to manage anxiety and stress and support system (each visit).
2. Provide accepting, nonjudgmental attitude and environment when teaching and discussing needs and changes to be made in life-style (each visit).
3. Instruct to avoid events that produce stress or prevent use of constructive coping mechanisms or behavior (first visit).
4. Instruct client in coping, communication, and problem-solving skills (first and second visits).
5. Instruct client in relaxation and diversional techniques, such as music, muscle relaxation, and reading (first visit).
6. Encourage expression of concerns and mutual goal setting.

CLIENT AND FAMILY/CAREGIVER INTERVENTIONS

1. Client develops effective use of coping mechanisms.
2. Client avoids stress-provoking events.
3. Client engages in relaxation and diversional activities.
4. Client requests assistance when needed.
5. Client reduces and/or controls anxiety level.
6. Client adapts to change in life-style to comply with medical regimen.

Nursing diagnosis

Altered nutrition: less than body requirements

Related factors: Inability to metabolize nutrients

Defining characteristics: Hyperglycemia; hypoglycemia; noncompliance with dietary, activity, and insulin regimens in controlling condition

OUTCOMES

Short-term

Adequate nutrition, as evidenced by compliance with recommended American Diabetic Association (ADA) diet and absence of hyperglycemic or hypoglycemic states (expected within 1 week)

Long-term

Adequate nutritional intake and metabolic process, as evidenced by appropriate dietary planning and intake in relation to insulin production or administration and by blood and urinary glucose levels that are within normal ranges (expected within 1 month and ongoing)

NURSING INTERVENTIONS/INSTRUCTIONS

1. Assess nutritional status, including food preferences, religious and cultural restrictions, emotional factors related to food and eating, and actual and desired weight levels (first visit).
2. Instruct client to keep a diary of all foods consumed, amounts and methods of preparation, and weekly weights (first visit).
3. Instruct client about and review diabetic exchange lists and prescribed diet; use diary as a guide and make changes as needed; provide written instructions and information about diet (first visit and reinforce on second visit).
4. Instruct in ADA diets as prescribed, with reduced calories, sodium, and fat and cholesterol content if necessary; include avoidance of simple sugars (use sugar substitutes) and concentrated sweets and the importance of evenly spaced, regular meals and scheduled snacks; instruct client to eat all of meals and to avoid skipping or delaying a meal or bunching required foods in one meal to another (first visit and reinforce each visit).
5. Inform client of early signs and symptoms of hypoglycemia, including hunger, shakiness, palpitations, headache, weakness, irritability, nervousness, and visual disturbances (first visit).
6. Instruct client to carry candy or sugar at all times and, at first sign of hypoglycemic attack, to take milk (preferred) or fruit juice (sweetened), soft drink, or 4 teaspoons sugar or 4 or 5 pieces of hard candy or rub sugar preparation from a tube on gums (first visit and reinforce after any hypoglycemic episodes).
7. Inform client of signs and symptoms of hyperglycemia and possible ketoacidosis, including fatigue, malaise, flushed face, nausea and vomiting, marked thirst, fruity (acetone) breath, hyperpnea, or changes in mentation (first visit).

8. Instruct client to notify physician if diet is not tolerated or foods cannot be retained or at first onset of any sign or symptom of high or low glucose levels or presence of ketones in urine (first visit).
9. Refer client to nutritionist for assistance in ADA diet and exchanges if needed (first visit).
10. Review activity and exercise in relation to prescribed diet.

CLIENT AND FAMILY/CAREGIVER INTERVENTIONS

1. Client maintains record of foods and weekly weight and incidence of dietary changes to accommodate test results of blood and urine.
2. Client formulates meal menus and planning of dietary inclusions and restrictions.
3. Client eats regularly scheduled meals following prescribed ADA diet and exchange lists.
4. Client carries emergency sugar supply at all times.
5. Client identifies signs and symptoms of hypoglycemia and hyperglycemia.
6. Client takes extra nutrition before engaging in strenuous activities.

Nursing diagnosis

Knowledge deficit

Related factors: Request for information and instruction about disease and procedures to control disease and prevent complications

Defining characteristics: Verbalization of unfamiliarity with medication administration, dietary and exercise inclusions and restrictions, foot care, blood and urine testing for glucose, care of skin, teeth, and eyes, signs and symptoms of hyperglycemia and hypoglycemia, and measures to take to treat these conditions

OUTCOMES

Short-term

Adequate knowledge, as evidenced by client verbalizations of medication administration; blood and urine testing; activity regimen; care of feet, skin, and eyes; signs and symptoms of altered glycemic states; and treatment (expected within 4 to 7 days)

Long-term

Adequate knowledge, as evidenced by absence of complications following daily compliance with treatment regimen (expected within 1 month and thereafter)

NURSING INTERVENTIONS/INSTRUCTIONS

1. Assess all body systems for baselines; assess history of drug and hormone use and alcohol use (first visit).
2. Instruct client in and demonstrate self-administration of insulin, noting technique; rotation of sites; onset, peak, duration of action, and expected results of the insulin(s); possibility of local reaction to injection; and use and care of pump if applicable (first and second visits and ongoing as needed).
3. Instruct client in administration of oral hypoglycemics, noting dose, frequency, side effects, food, drug, and alcohol interactions, and expected action and results (first visit).
4. Instruct client in and demonstrate blood collection and testing for glucose and use of glucometer; relate to insulin administration and diet; instruct client in urinary glucose and ketone testing to be done if blood glucose reaches a predetermined level (first visit and reinforce on second visit).
5. Assess activities of daily living and exercise pattern, and instruct client to exercise daily, implementing a consistent routine; instruct client in actions to take if exercise is increased (first visit).
6. Encourage client to stop smoking; suggest support groups (first visit).
7. Inform client of importance of complying with medication, exercise, and diet regimens to maintain glucose level within normal range, and instruct client to notify physician of continuous signs and symptoms of hypoglycemia or hyperglycemia (first visit).
8. Impress on client the importance of notifying physician if stress, trauma, or infection is present (first visit).
9. Instruct client in meticulous care of feet, with daily bathing in tepid water; rinse well and pat dry, especially between toes; see podiatrist for foot care; apply cream to lower extremities; wear well-fitting shoes and cotton socks; check feet for cuts, scratches or blisters, ulcers, or delayed healing, and reduced sensation (first visit and reinforce on second visit).

10. Discuss sexual concerns (impotence, family planning) as appropriate (first visit).
11. Instruct client to inform all caregivers of diagnosis (dentist, surgeon) (first visit).
12. Instruct client to wear and/or carry identification indicating condition and medications (first visit).

CLIENT AND FAMILY/CAREGIVER INTERVENTIONS

1. Client administers insulin or hypoglycemic correctly and in timely manner.
2. Client uses insulin pump effectively if prescribed.
3. Client tests blood and urine at appropriate times, and analyzes results for proper actions to take.
4. Client exercises daily and maintains constant day-to-day program.
5. Client ceases smoking or joins support group for assistance.
6. Client states signs and symptoms of hypoglycemia and hyperglycemia and appropriate actions to take.
7. Client states signs and symptoms of infection to report to physician.
8. Client reports any visual disturbances; participates in periodic eye examinations.
9. Client notes neuropathies and reports any trauma to physician.
10. Client performs consistent, meticulous foot care.
11. Client follows up on sexual concerns to make informed decisions as indicated.
12. Client wears or carries identification information.
13. Client consults podiatrist, ophthamologist, and dentist for specific care.

Nursing diagnosis

Noncompliance

Related factors: Health beliefs and practices

Defining characteristics: Failure to adhere to medical regimen, with resulting development of complications or exacerbation of symptoms; failure to keep appointments or report to physician

OUTCOMES

Short-term

Compliance with medical regimen, as evidenced by client identifying and performing dietary and activity modifications, medication regimen, blood and urine testing, and foot and skin care (expected within 1 week)

Long-term

Optimal and effective compliance, as evidenced by participation in all aspects of care, absence of complications, and functioning at a well level (expected within 2 to 3 months)

NURSING INTERVENTIONS/INSTRUCTIONS

1. Establish rapport and provide a nonthreatening, accepting environment for care and teaching (each visit).
2. Assess coping and learning abilities, developmental level and achieved tasks, economic level, support system; note perceived implications of disorder for life-style (each visit).
3. Evaluate knowledge and performance of dietary, activity, medication, and testing procedures and modifications (first visit).
4. Include client and significant others in planning and teaching of health care (each visit).
5. Help client to modify life-style with as few changes as possible; explore options and praise efforts and successes (each visit).
6. Suggest counseling or support groups such as the American Diabetic Association for information, supplies, and support.
7. Encourage expression of perception of disease.

CLIENT AND FAMILY/CAREGIVER INTERVENTIONS

1. Client participates in all aspects of health care; complies with requirements.
2. Client accepts support from family, friends, and agencies.
3. Client demonstrates facility in performance of all procedures and planning of care for optimal health and functioning.

Hematologic system

Acquired Immunodeficiency Syndrome (AIDS)

Acquired immunodeficiency syndrome is characterized by extreme immunosuppression, allowing for the development of malignancies and opportunistic infections caused by viruses, bacteria, fungi, and protozoa. It is a life-threatening illness whose cause is unknown. The disease demonstrates suppression of T helper cells and an increase in T suppressor cells, both of which decrease the body's ability to respond to an acute inflammatory reaction and depress a defensive response. AIDS is transmitted by administration of contaminated blood or blood products, sexual contact, use of contaminated needles, syringes, or instruments, or accidental exposure to contaminated blood through breaks in the skin or mucous membranes; perinatal transmission also occurs.

Home care is primarily concerned with the care and teaching aspects of infection prevention, activities of daily living, the medication regimen, and transmission prevention.

Nursing diagnosis

Anxiety

Related factors: Threat of death; change in health status

Defining characteristics: Presence of human immunodeficiency virus (HIV); presence of AIDS-related complex (ARC); apprehension and increased helplessness; absence of any effective treatment; fear of transmission to others.

OUTCOMES

Short-term

Decreased anxiety, as evidenced by client's statement of reduced fear and apprehension about change in health status and possible early death (expected within 1 week)

Long-term

Management or control of anxiety level, as evidenced by compliance with and acceptance of treatment regimen and change in life-style to prevent transmission of the disease to others (expected within 1 to 2 months and ongoing)

NURSING INTERVENTIONS/INSTRUCTIONS

1. Assess client's mental and emotional status in relation to life-threatening illness and associated stigma (see Psychosocial Assessment, p. 48, for guidelines) (first visit).
2. Encourage expression of fears and concerns in a supportive and nonjudgmental environment; instruct client in relaxation techniques (each visit).
3. Assist client to identify needed changes in life-style and methods to make necessary changes (first visit and thereafter as needed).
4. Inform client about activities allowed, treatments and tests to expect, and testing of contacts (first visit).
5. Initiate referral to counseling, support groups, or agencies that may assist with legal, economic, and health care needs (first visit).
6. Encourage expression of concerns and mutual goal setting.

CLIENT AND FAMILY/CAREGIVER INTERVENTIONS

1. Develop coping for long-term treatment and possible outcome.
2. Maintain manageable level of anxiety.
3. Seek information that will reduce anxiety.
4. Express fears and concerns about necessary changes in life-style.
5. Contact and consult with support services available.

Nursing diagnosis

Risk for infection

Related factors: Inadequate secondary defenses

Defining characteristics: Immunodeficiency; potential for opportunistic infection, hyperthermia, prostration, change in breathing pattern (*Pneumocystis* pneumonia), change in thought process (cytomegalovirus) with dementia

OUTCOMES

Short-term

Absence of infection, as evidenced by temperature and blood tests within normal ranges and by freedom from signs and symptoms of any opportunistic infection (expectation dependent on immune system status)

Long-term

Absence of infection with optimal functioning of all systems (expected as an ongoing finding)

NURSING INTERVENTIONS/INSTRUCTIONS

1. Perform complete physical assessment for database and note any signs and symptoms associated with the disease (first visit).
2. Instruct client to monitor for and report presence of fever, malaise, night sweats, cough, dyspnea, headache, enlarged glands, epigastric or abdominal pain, vomiting or diarrhea, skin lesions, rashes, weakness, joint pain, or sensory or intellectual deficits (first visit).
3. Instruct client in preventive measures regarding infections, including hand washing, personal hygiene, and avoidance of crowds and persons with infection or who are ill (first visit).
4. Instruct client in administration of antiinfectives and specific preventive drugs for disease and to avoid any immunosuppressive drugs (first visit).
5. Encourage health promotion, including rest, nutritious diet, and stress management (each visit).

CLIENT AND FAMILY/CAREGIVER INTERVENTIONS

1. Bathe daily and inspect for and report rashes, skin lesions or vesicles, or skin disruptions.
2. Perform hand washing after toileting, before meals, and before any procedures.
3. Take temperature if any symptoms appear, and report elevation.
4. Monitor for and report signs and symptoms of infection in any system.
5. Administer medications as instructed.
6. Avoid exposure to persons with infections.
7. Maintain healthy life-style that includes nutritious meals, 6 to 8 hours of sleep per night, and social and diversional activities.

Nursing diagnosis

Activity intolerance

Related factors: Generalized weakness

Defining characteristics: Verbalization of fatigue and weakness, inability to perform activities of daily living (ADL) and ambulate, repeated infections, malnutrition, wasting, lack of sleep

OUTCOMES

Short-term

Increased activity and energy, as evidenced by performance of ADL and utilization of energy-conservation techniques (expected within 1 week)

Long-term

Adequate activity within disease limitations, as evidenced by achievement of optimal level of self-care and general functioning (expected within 2 to 3 months as realistic)

NURSING INTERVENTIONS/INSTRUCTIONS

1. Assess client's ability to carry out ADL and energy and endurance levels; note strength, gait, posture, balance, presence of fatigue, general weakness, and sensory deficits (each visit).
2. Encourage rest after activity and at least 6 to 8 hours of sleep per night (first visit).

3. Assist client to identify activities that need pacing and in setting limits (first visit and reinforce on second visit).
4. Inform client of available energy-conserving aids to assist in dressing, bathing, grooming, toileting, and eating (first visit).
5. Assess support system; include support system in care planning and in care (first visit).
6. Coordinate social services and community resources for assistance and support (first visit).
7. Refer home health aide (HHA) to assist with ADL.

CLIENT AND FAMILY/CAREGIVER INTERVENTIONS

1. Client bases rest and sleep on individual needs and condition.
2. Client participates in activities within set limits.
3. Client uses energy-saving devices in ADL.
4. Caregiver assists with any activity requiring support.
5. Client utilizes private and public resources for assistance.

Nursing diagnosis

Altered nutrition: less than body requirements

Related factors: Inability to ingest food and absorb nutrients

Defining characteristics: Anorexia, infection of oroesophageal tract, gastroenteritis, diarrhea, weight loss, wasting

OUTCOMES

Short-term

Adequate nutrition, as evidenced by intake of nutritious and high-calorie foods and stable weight pattern (expected within 1 week)

Long-term

Optimal nutritional status, as evidenced by weight stability and by absence of disease manifestations that affect food intake necessary to maintain health and functioning (expected within 1 month and ongoing)

NURSING INTERVENTIONS/INSTRUCTIONS

1. Assess nutritional status, including height, actual and ideal weight, food preferences, and cultural and religious restrictions (first visit).

2. Perform gastrointestinal assessment (see Gastrointestinal System Assessment, p. 20, for guidelines); note presence of anorexia, nausea, vomiting, weight loss, persistent diarrhea, oroesophageal inflammation or lesions, and temperature elevation, and cross-reference signs and symptoms with drug profile (each visit).
3. Instruct client in regular, scrupulous oral hygiene and in use of soft toothbrush, topical antifungal agents, mouthwashes, and topical anesthetics as prescribed in presence of oral inflammation or lesions (first visit).
4. Instruct client to eat high-calorie, well-balanced diet and to include foods that will prevent or minimize distressing manifestations (first visit).
5. Instruct client to eat smaller, more frequent meals that include commercially prepared supplements (first visit).
6. If nausea is present, suggest use of toast or dry crackers, choosing foods that are less aromatic and less strong in taste, and drinking beverages ½ hour before meals rather than with meals (first visit).
7. Instruct client to eat when rested and to rest ½ hour after meals with head elevated (first visit).
8. Instruct client to administer vitamin and mineral supplements daily (first visit).
9. Instruct client in administration of antidiarrheals and antiemetics if prescribed (first visit).
10. Inform client of alternative feeding methods such as tube feedings or total parenteral nutrition (TPN), and instruct client in procedures if implemented (applicable visit with reinforcement).
11. Initiate referral to nutritionist for consultation and to community resources for food preparation and delivery if needed (first visit).

CLIENT AND FAMILY/CAREGIVER INTERVENTIONS

1. Client performs and records daily weight and reports any significant, progressive losses.
2. Client eats small, frequent, high-calorie meals that include preferences and nutritional requirements.
3. Client performs mouth care after meals and if oral mucous membrane is impaired and protects oral cavity from further trauma.

4. Client treats nausea with dry foods and timely intake of fluids.
5. Client supplements meals with foods and beverages of high nutrient value.
6. Client administers vitamin and mineral supplements, antidiarrheals, antifungals, antibiotics, and topical anesthetics as instructed.
7. Client monitors tube feedings or TPN if present and performs procedures for administration and care of these methods of feeding if capable of managing them.
8. Client consults with nutritionist.
9. Client utilizes community resources for food service.

Nursing diagnosis

Impaired social interaction

Related factors: Therapeutic isolation; inability to engage in satisfying personal relationship

Defining characteristics: Stigma associated with AIDS and unaccepted social behavior (drug abuse, sexual preference), fear of transmission of disease, fear of loss of confidentiality and loss of or rejection by significant others and community as result of diagnosis

OUTCOMES

Short-term

Involvement in social interaction, as evidenced by verbalization of behaviors resulting from isolation and of options to reverse these and to adapt to requirements for meaningful relationships (expected within 1 week)

Long-term

Optimal social relationships, as evidenced by participation in social activities with significant others and support group (expected within 1 month)

NURSING INTERVENTIONS/INSTRUCTIONS

1. Provide continuity of care by providing same professional caregiver for treatment and care (each visit).
2. Use therapeutic communication, including touch (each visit).

3. Identify type and amount of support available in home and community (first visit).
4. Provide an understanding, nonjudgmental environment (each visit).
5. Facilitate individual and group interaction; note that behavior or personality changes may be the result of neurologic dysfunction (each visit).
6. Provide a range of diversional options, including books, games, collecting, and visits from friends (first visit).
7. Refer to AIDS support group or counseling as needed (any visit).

CLIENT AND FAMILY/CAREGIVER INTERVENTIONS

1. Client occupies time with diversional activities.
2. Client accepts visits from friends.
3. Client verbalizes understanding of social fears and lack of knowledge regarding disease.
4. Client interacts with support groups and services.
5. Client consults counseling or agencies for assistance.

Nursing diagnosis

Anticipatory grieving

Related factors: Perceived potential loss of physiopsychosocial well-being

Defining characteristics: Expression of distress at potential loss; anger; guilt; denial of potential loss; sorrow; choked feelings; changes in sleep, eating, and activity patterns

OUTCOMES

Short-term

Progress in grieving, as evidenced by attitude and behavior changes manifested by stage in process (expected within days)

Long-term

Grief process resolving, as evidenced by resumption of life-style with or without changes as needed and by integration of grieving stage into life-style and activities (expected within 2 to 3 months and ongoing)

NURSING INTERVENTIONS/INSTRUCTIONS

1. Assess degree and stage of grief (each visit).
2. Inform client of stages of grieving process and that behavior is acceptable for specific stage and that acceptance will be final stage (first visit).
3. Allow expression of feelings and perceptions about disabilities and potential loss and death in a nonjudgmental environment (each visit).
4. Initiate referral for psychological and spiritual counseling and hospice care as appropriate (any visit).

CLIENT AND FAMILY/CAREGIVER INTERVENTIONS

1. Client progresses through grief process to acceptance.
2. Client seeks counseling as needed.
3. Client verbalizes stages and behaviors during grief process.

Nursing diagnosis

Knowledge deficit

Related factors: Lack of exposure to information

Defining characteristics: Request for information about change in sexual patterns and social behavior necessary to prevent transmission of disease, legal and medical rights and assistance, and community resources available

OUTCOMES

Short-term

Adequate knowledge, as evidenced by client's statements regarding disease progression and transmission and treatments (expected within 3 days)

Long-term

Adequate knowledge, as evidenced by compliance in meeting requirements of changed life-style, with limitations imposed by condition, to achieve optimal level of functioning (expected within 1 month)

NURSING INTERVENTIONS/INSTRUCTIONS

1. Carry out Centers for Disease Control (CDC) universal precautions in all aspects of nursing care (each visit).

2. Include significant others in instruction; allow for active participation in care planning (each visit).
3. Assess for and instruct client in recognition of opportunistic infection, recurrence, reinfections, neoplasms, and neurologic manifestations and in treatment available for these conditions (each visit).
4. Instruct client in transmission modes, and stress that disease is not transmitted by casual contact or living with others but by sexual contact, exchange of needles in drug use, administration of blood or blood products, or sharing of razors or other items that might contain the virus (first visit).
5. Instruct client in general cleaning and disinfection methods; bleach solution (1:10) may be used to clean contaminated materials (first visit).
6. Advise client of need for testing sexual contacts or high-risk contacts in addition to concurrent counseling about transmission (first visit).
7. Instruct client in options for sexual activity, including abstinence, use of latex condom lubricated with nonoxynol 9, and birth control planning (first visit and reinforce second visit).
8. Encourage rehabilitation of intravenous drug users; instruct them not to share needles or paraphernalia and to wash syringes with soap and water and then cleanse with bleach and rinse thoroughly after each use (each visit).
9. Instruct client in administration of zidovudine, pentamidine, antibiotics and antiinfectives, psychotropics, anticonvulsants, immunomodulators, analgesics, antipyretics, and chemotherapy as prescribed, including dose, route, frequency, side effects, and interactions; inform client of possible resources for medications (first visit and reinforce as needed).
10. Instruct client not to donate blood or organs (first visit).
11. Instruct client to inform all nursing, medical, dental, and laboratory personnel of condition (first visit).
12. Assist client in organizing health care information; provide written instructions and reminders for care, medications and schedules, and resource and emergency telephone numbers (first visit).
13. Inform client of importance of follow-up with physician and laboratory visits (first visit).
14. Refer client to community groups, resources, and organizations for support, information, and financial and legal needs (first visit).

CLIENT AND FAMILY/CAREGIVER INTERVENTIONS

1. Client monitors and reports any signs and symptoms of opportunistic infections.
2. Client prevents transmission to others.
3. Client reports contacts to be tested.
4. Client administers medications as prescribed and instructed; utilizes a written plan and schedule.
5. Client avoids activities that will spread disease and verbalizes how disease is transmitted and measures to take to protect others from disease.
6. Client informs those who need to know diagnosis, with assurance of confidentiality.
7. Client seeks out support services available for persons with AIDS.

Nursing diagnosis

Risk for caregiver role strain

Related factors: Severity of illness of the care receiver; complexity and number of caregiving tasks

Defining characteristics: Caregiver's report of not having enough resources to provide care (emotional and physical strength; help from others) and of difficulty in performing specific caregiving activities (bathing, cleaning up after incontinence, managing client's weakened condition and discomforts)

OUTCOMES

Short-term

Potential for caregiver role strain identified, as evidenced by caregiver's verbalization of difficulties encountered in performing care and concern about ability and conflicts in giving care (expected within 1 week)

Long-term

Prevention of caregiver role strain, as evidenced by continued safe and appropriate care provided without compromise to own physical and emotional needs (expected within 1 month and ongoing)

NURSING INTERVENTIONS/INSTRUCTIONS

1. Assess severity of illness and care needs of the receiver of care and ability of caregiver to perform role (first visit).
2. Assess relationship between care receiver and caregiver before illness and stressors placed on the relationship by the illness (first visit).
3. Assist caregiver to monitor continued ability to perform care and treatments, changes in day-to-day needs, changes in stressors and strains, maintenance of routines, and need for additional resources (aides, homemaker, respite care, friends, family) (first visit).
4. Discuss role performance and whether expectations are realistic, flexibility of role, and decision-making process (first visit).
5. Initiate referral to HHA, social worker, or psychological counseling to assist with economic and mental or physical health needs (any visit).

CLIENT AND FAMILY/CAREGIVER INTERVENTIONS

1. Caregiver develops ability to cope with caregiver role and flexibility in day-to-day functioning.
2. Caregiver explores financial, legal, and physical assistance sources, and considers a referral to these services.
3. Caregiver maintains own health and well-being in caregiver role.
4. Caregiver maintains ongoing care and treatment regimen.

Anemia

Anemia is a condition characterized by decreases in red blood cell, hemoglobin, and hematocrit levels. It may be caused by excessive blood loss (hypovolemic), a decrease in production of red blood cells by bone marrow (aplastic), a decrease in production of red blood cells from inadequate intake of iron and folic acid (iron deficiency), a decrease in the development of red blood cells because of the lack of the instrinsic factor needed for vitamin B_{12} absorption (pernicious), or the destruction of red blood cells (hemolytic). Whatever the type, the decrease in red blood cells affects the transport of oxygen in the body, with severity dependent on the degree of decrease.

Home care is primarily concerned with iron deficiency and pernicious anemias and the teaching aspects for compliance with the medical regimen to control the disorder and prevent relapses.

Nursing diagnosis

Altered nutrition: less than body requirements

Related factors: Inadequate intake of iron and folic acid

Defining characteristics: Reduced intake of food containing iron and folic acid, weight loss, weakness, anorexia, nausea, vomiting, glossy red tongue, lesions on oral mucosa, shortness of breath, pallor, headaches, irritability, dysphagia, fissures at angles of tongue

OUTCOMES

Short-term

Adequate nutrition, as evidenced by consumption of a well-balanced diet, with necessary supplementation, and maintenance of appropriate weight for height, frame, and age (expected within 4 days)

Long-term

Adequate nutritional status achieved, as evidenced by daily requirements and supplemental therapy maintained, with optimal level of health and physiologic functioning (expected within 1 month)

NURSING INTERVENTIONS/INSTRUCTIONS

1. Review history and focus on source and remediation of deficiency, including increased iron requirements, inadequate intake, decreased or inadequate absorption, or chronic blood loss (first visit).
2. Assess hematologic, cardiovascular, neurologic, integumentary, gastrointestinal, and endocrine systems for status and

effect of anemic condition on them (see specific system assessments for guidelines) (first visit).

3. Assess nutritional status, including food preferences and cultural or religious and medical restrictions (first visit).
4. Instruct client to take and record weights weekly (first visit).
5. Instruct client to maintain a food diary for 1 week that includes all foods consumed and amounts and methods of preparation; use data as a basis for dietary teaching (first visit).
6. Instruct client in a well-balanced diet that includes snacks and foods that will supply deficiency; inform client that more frequent, smaller meals are recommended if nausea, vomiting, or fatigue interferes with intake (first visit and reinforce on second visit).
7. Instruct client (and supply list) in sources of dietary iron, including red meat, organ meats, egg yolk, green leafy vegetables, dried legumes, enriched breads and cereals, and dried fruits (first visit).
8. Instruct client in good oral hygiene, especially after meals and if mouth is sore (first visit).
9. Instruct client in administration of iron preparation and vitamin C, and inform client that stools may turn dark green or black and that milk and antacids will decrease absorption of iron (first visit).
10. Suggest bland diet and to avoid irritating, hot, spicy foods if tongue is sore or in presence of gingival or mouth irritation or lesions (first visit).
11. Refer client to nutritionist or counselor if needed (any visit, based on evaluation).

CLIENT AND FAMILY/CAREGIVER INTERVENTIONS

1. Client takes and records weekly weight using same scale and clothing at same time of day.
2. Client maintains daily log of intake and reviews each week for possible changes.
3. Client eats a well-balanced diet that includes sources of iron and folic acid.
4. Client maintains oral hygiene; applies lubricant to lips if needed.
5. Client administers medications safely and as instructed.
6. Client modifies diet if oral discomfort occurs.
7. Client consults with nutritionist if needed.

Nursing diagnosis

Activity intolerance

Related factors: Generalized weakness; imbalance between oxygen supply and demand

Defining characteristics: Decreased red blood cells and hemoglobin; hypoxia; fatigue; inability to carry out ADL; decreased stamina; weakness; loss of positional and vibratory senses; numbness and tingling of extremities

OUTCOMES

Short-term

Tolerance and endurance improved, as evidenced by modification of ADL and increased participation in activities (expected within 1 week)

Long-term

Optimal activity tolerance, as evidenced by increased energy and endurance and independence in ADL and mobility for optimal or higher level of health and functioning (expected within 1 month)

NURSING INTERVENTIONS/INSTRUCTIONS

1. Assess client's ability to perform ADL by having client demonstrate several typical activities and noting vital signs afterwards for increases in pulse or dyspnea (first visit).
2. Instruct client to personalize and pace activities and to schedule rest periods between these activities; include work as well as home schedules (first visit).
3. Instruct client to change position slowly and to sit down if dizzy (first visit).
4. Instruct client to request assistance in ADL and ambulation if needed, especially if there are sensory changes in extremities (first visit).
5. Encourage self-care with use of aids if they promote independence (first visit).
6. Instruct client to elevate head of bed to facilitate respirations and to administer supplemental oxygen if needed, with instructions about hazards associated with this therapy (first visit).
7. Refer home health aide to assist with ADL as needed.

CLIENT AND FAMILY/CAREGIVER INTERVENTIONS

1. Client follows plan for rest and activity.
2. Client performs ADL independently with increasing endurance.
3. Client obtains assistance or aids as needed.
4. Client administers supplemental oxygen as instructed.
5. Client sleeps with head elevated; takes steps to eliminate dyspnea associated with activity by resting.

Nursing diagnosis

Knowledge deficit

Related factors: Lack of exposure to information

Defining characteristics: Request for information about medical regimen, maintenance therapy, and prevention of recurrence of signs and symptoms of anemia

OUTCOMES

Short-term

Adequate knowledge, as evidenced by client stating precautions needed for specific anemia being treated, medication regimen and implications, course of disease and treatment, and complications if not treated (expected within 3 days)

Long-term

Adequate knowledge, as evidenced by compliance with medication, dietary, and activity regimens and other treatment to prevent recurrence of anemia and complications (expected within 1 month)

NURSING INTERVENTIONS/INSTRUCTIONS

1. Instruct client to inform all physicians and dentists of disorder (first visit).
2. Inform client that, for pernicious anemia, parenteral vitamin B_{12} must be administered monthly for life, and instruct client in administration if warranted (first and second visit).
3. Instruct client to avoid infections by hand washing, good personal hygiene, and avoiding exposure to persons with upper

respiratory infections; encourage client to update immunizations (first visit).

4. Instruct client to report any presence of infection with fever to physician; any recurrence of skin color changes (pallor), changes in motor or sensory responses in extremities, presence of dizziness, or dyspnea should also be reported (first visit).
5. Instruct client to keep warm with extra clothing and blankets, if needed, and to avoid heating pads and hot water bottles (first visit).
6. Instruct client in skin care, including use of mild soap, gentle massage, and use of emollients; note pressure points for erythema and reduced sensation (first visit).
7. Inform client of measures to avoid trauma to skin if vasomotor disturbance or peripheral neuropathies exist (first visit).
8. Inform client that diet inclusions and several medications may be used for anemia, including iron, pyridoxine, vitamin B_{12}, and folic acid, and to avoid all OTC medications unless approved by physician (first visit).
9. Instruct client to keep physician and laboratory appointments, and emphasize need for compliance as symptoms decrease (first visit).

CLIENT AND FAMILY/CAREGIVER INTERVENTIONS

1. Client maintains dietary and medication regimens for specific anemia.
2. Client follows personal hygiene practice; avoids contact with possible infection; maintains immunizations.
3. Client maintains warmth and avoids injury to skin and dry, irritated skin.
4. Client notifies physician of signs and symptoms of infection or recurrence of condition.
5. Client complies with physician and laboratory visits for injection of vitamin B_{12} and assessment of condition.
6. Client wears clothes and shoes that maintain warmth and prevent trauma to extremities.
7. Client states cause of disorder and reason for treatment regimen.

Musculoskeletal system

Amputation

An amputation is the surgical removal of all or part of an extremity. The procedure may be performed at a joint or in the middle of a limb to treat a malignancy, severe infectious process, circulatory impairment, traumatic event or injury, or congenital defect. Care management includes the use of a prosthesis as part of the rehabilitative program as well as treatment for the underlying condition that is associated with the amputation.

Home care is primarily concerned with the teaching aspects of stump care, prosthesis care, and compliance with the rehabilitative phase of the medical regimen.

Nursing diagnosis

Impaired physical mobility

Related factors: Intolerance to activity; musculoskeletal impairment (lower extremity amputation)

Defining characteristics: Inability to purposefully move within physical environment; reluctance to attempt movement and ambulation; improper prosthesis fit; inadequate healing and conditioning of stump

OUTCOMES

Short-term

Adequate mobility, as evidenced by progressive independence in ambulation with prosthesis without falls or trauma (expected within 1 week)

Long-term

Adequate mobility achieved, as evidenced by effective use of prosthesis for ambulation and activities of daily living (ADL) with independence and optimal functioning (expected within 2 to 3 months)

NURSING INTERVENTIONS/INSTRUCTIONS

1. Assess client's mobility and activity status, effectiveness of use of prosthesis for ambulation, balancing difficulties, and use of assistive aids for walking (see Musculoskeletal System Assessment, p. 20, for guidelines) (first visit and each visit as needed).
2. Assess prosthesis fit, healing and conditioning of stump, and presense of pain when client is using prosthesis (each visit).
3. Instruct client in use of crutches, cane, or walker with or without prosthesis as appropriate (first visit).
4. Instruct client to balance on one leg without support and to ambulate with extension of stump (first visit).
5. Instruct client to ambulate with proper gait, using prosthesis as taught (first visit).
6. Provide and instruct in range-of-motion (ROM) exercises for unaffected joints (first visit).
7. Instruct client in exercises to tighten gluteal and abdominal muscles and to transfer from bed to sitting or standing position and back to bed (first and second visits).
8. Instruct client in prescribed exercises to legs, using weights, push-ups, knee bends, and standing or walking with one foot (each visit).
9. Instruct client to progress in ambulation from 5-minute periods to daily increases as tolerated and within restrictions; advise client to have assistance until stability and coordination are achieved (first visit).
10. Instruct client in arranging pathways and in furniture arrangement that promotes support in ambulation and prevents accidents from bumping or falling and injuring operative or other site (first visit).
11. Inform client of resources for purchasing or renting supplies and equipment (first visit).
12. Initiate or reinforce physical therapy (any visit).
13. Refer home health aide (HHA) for assistance in mobility and ADL.

CLIENT AND FAMILY/CAREGIVER INTERVENTIONS

1. Client performs daily progressive muscle and joint exercises.
2. Client ambulates safely with or without use of prosthesis.
3. Client provides safe environment for ambulation without trauma.

4. Client uses aids such as crutches, cane, and walker as needed.
5. Client performs prescribed physical rehabilitation as instructed by therapist.
6. Client avoids strain, fatigue, and falls while using prosthesis.
7. Client achieves independence in mobility with use of prosthesis, including transfer and position changes.
8. Client complies with appointments for physical therapy.

Nursing diagnosis

Self-care deficit (bathing/hygiene, dressing/grooming, feeding, toileting)

Related factors: Impaired mobility and activity ability (upper or lower extremity amputation)

Defining characteristics: Inability to wash body parts, put on or take off clothing, maintain appearance, bring food to mouth for ingestion, use toilet or commode, and carry out toilet hygiene

OUTCOMES

Short-term

Adequate participation in ADL, as evidenced by progressive independence in daily activities with use of prosthesis (expected within 1 week)

Long-term

Adequate participation in ADL achieved, as evidenced by effective use of prosthesis for all personal care, with optimal functioning and independence (expected within 2 to 3 months)

NURSING INTERVENTIONS/INSTRUCTIONS

1. Assess client's activity status, ability to perform ADL with or without prosthesis, and ability to use assistive aids for bathing, grooming, dressing, toileting, and eating (see Functional Assessment, p. 51, for guidelines) (first visit).
2. Assess prosthesis fit (artificial arm, hook, cosmetic hand) and healing and condition of stump (any visit).
3. Instruct client in use of one arm or hand and aids for cooking, personal care, and other activity needs (each visit).

4. Instruct in ROM exercises for unaffected joints and prescribed exercises for arm and shoulder, including frequency, length of time, and progressive increases (first and second visits).
5. Initiate or reinforce physical and/or occupational therapy (any visit).
6. Refer HHA to assist with ADL as needed (first visit).

CLIENT AND FAMILY/CAREGIVER INTERVENTIONS

1. Client performs daily progressive ADL with or without prosthesis.
2. Client uses aids to assist with toileting, eating, bathing, dressing, grooming, cooking, working in home, and returning to occupation.
3. Client avoids accidents and fatigue during use of prosthesis for ADL.
4. Client performs prescribed physical and occupational rehabilitation as instructed by therapists.
5. Client achieves independence in ADL with use of prosthesis.
6. Client complies with appointments for occupational therapy.

Nursing diagnosis

Risk for impaired skin integrity

Related factors: External mechanical factor of pressure

Defining characteristics: Weight bearing on stump; improper fit of prosthesis; improper care of stump and improper conditioning; redness, pain, edema, and irritation at stump site

OUTCOMES

Short-term

Preservation of skin integrity, as evidenced by intactness at stump surgical site and by absence of irritation, pain, or edema (expected within 1 week and after prosthesis use)

Long-term

Absence of skin damage or breakdown, as evidenced by maintenance of optimal skin integrity for health and prosthesis use (expected ongoing)

NURSING INTERVENTIONS/INSTRUCTIONS

1. Assess stump site for redness, tenderness, irritation, edema, flabbiness, fit of prosthesis, and pressure against stump (see Integumentary System Assessment, p. 36, for guidelines) (first visit and each visit thereafter).
2. Instruct client to assess stump and report changes to physician or prosthetist (first visit).
3. Instruct client in cleansing and gentle drying of stump and in massaging and exposing to air for 20 minutes (first visit).
4. Instruct client in removal and reapplication of dressing or bandage, with proper wrapping (first and second visits).
5. Instruct client to avoid use of powders or lotions on stump; instruct client in application of stump sock after cleansing and drying and to change daily (first visit).
6. Instruct client to pad pressure areas on skin and stump (first visit).
7. Instruct client to discontinue use of prosthesis if skin is red or irritated and to have prosthesis checked for fit if this occurs (first visit).
8. Advise client to seek assistance from prosthetist for problems of fit or use of prosthesis, whether for arm or leg (first visit).

CLIENT AND FAMILY/CAREGIVER INTERVENTIONS

1. Client maintains integrity and cleanliness of stump skin.
2. Client protects stump from pressure of prosthesis.
3. Client avoids skin damage from improper fit of prosthesis.
4. Client uses proper stump sock, mild soap and warm water, and thorough drying in stump care.
5. Client bandages or wraps stump properly.
6. Client secures services of prosthetist when needed.

Nursing diagnosis

Body image disturbance

Related factors: Biophysical factor of amputation procedure

Defining characteristics: Verbal response to change in structure and function of body part or to loss of body part; negative feelings about body; feelings of helplessness or powerlessness; change in social involvement

OUTCOMES

Short-term

Improved body image adaptation, as evidenced by statement of feelings and concerns about changes in appearance and limitations imposed by loss of body part and need to change life-style (expected within 1 week)

Long-term

Optimal adaptation to body image, as evidenced by improvement in role performance and interpersonal relationships and by willingness to change functional patterns and integrate them into life-style (expected within 2 to 3 months)

NURSING INTERVENTIONS/INSTRUCTIONS

1. Assess client's life-style, roles, and ability to adapt to changes (first visit).
2. Allow client to express fears and concerns about ability to resume normal life (each visit).
3. Allow time for questions and clarifications; provide accepting, nonjudgmental environment (each visit).
4. Instruct client to encourage visits from friends, clergy, and other amputees (any visit).
5. Encourage client to express strengths, and inform client of options for life-style changes, including sexual activity, ADL, social and occupational interactions, and recreational and leisure activities (any visit).
6. Inform client of and refer to sex therapist, occupational rehabilitation, counseling services, and driving instruction (first visit).
7. Inform client of clothing that deemphasizes lost limb (first visit).

CLIENT AND FAMILY/CAREGIVER INTERVENTIONS

1. Client verbalizes concerns and feelings about loss.
2. Client allows for grieving over loss.
3. Client participates in all aspects of care independently.
4. Client returns to work or enters vocational rehabilitation.

5. Client adapts to limitations imposed by loss of limb.
6. Client resumes close relationships with others and activities, interests, and social interactions with others.

Nursing diagnosis

Knowledge deficit

Related factors: Lack of information about condition and care

Defining characteristics: Request for information about prosthesis care, medical regimen for progressive rehabilitation, and signs and symptoms of complications

OUTCOMES

Short-term

Adequate knowledge, as evidenced by client's statement of treatment regimen, care of prosthesis, and signs and symptoms to report (expected within 4 days)

Long-term

Adequate knowledge, as evidenced by compliance with medical regimen and prevention of complications to achieve optimal level of health and functioning (expected within 2 to 3 months)

NURSING INTERVENTIONS/INSTRUCTIONS

1. Assess life-style changes, ability to adapt, learning ability and interest in learning, and family participation and support (first visit).
2. Instruct client to assess for complications, including swelling, color change, pain, purulent drainage from stump site, temperature elevation, and pulse and respiration changes, and to report these signs and symptoms to the physician (first visit).
3. Inform client that pain in the amputated limb (phantom pain) is a normal response (first visit).
4. Instruct client in washing and drying socket of prosthesis, application of prosthesis, wearing proper shoes with prosthesis for proper gait, and having prosthesis checked for fit or adjustment as needed (first visit and each visit thereafter as needed).

5. If medication is prescribed, instruct client in administration, including dose, frequency, time, food and drug interactions, and side effects (first visit).
6. Instruct client to keep all appointments with physician, laboratory, prosthetist, and therapists (first visit).
7. Inform client of community agencies and support groups for information and securing equipment and supplies (any visit).

CLIENT AND FAMILY/CAREGIVER INTERVENTIONS

1. Client assesses and monitors stump and remaining limbs for signs and symptoms of complications, and reports to physician.
2. Client cleans stump and prosthesis, and applies prosthesis correctly.
3. Client administers medications correctly and safely, with desired results.
4. Client adapts to change in life-style.
5. Client complies with medical regimen, and keeps appointments with interdisciplinary professionals.
6. Client contacts agencies, clubs, and groups for assistance, equipment, information, and support.

Osteoarthritis and Rheumatoid Arthritis

Arthritis includes conditions that affect and cause damage to joints, cartilage, and connective tissue and result in activity and mobility limitations. Osteoarthritis is a chronic degenerative disease that is localized and progressive; it results in cartilage erosion and most commonly affects weight-bearing joints. Rheumatoid arthritis is a chronic inflammatory disease; it is systemic and progressive and affects the synovial joints and related structures.

Home care is primarily concerned with the care of the involved joints and with teaching aspects of the medical regimen, prevention of injury to the joints, and progression of the disease.

Nursing diagnosis

Chronic pain

Related factors: Chronic physical disability

Defining characteristics: Verbal report of pain experienced for more than 6 months; fear of reinjury; altered ability to continue previous activities; guarded movement; physical and social withdrawal; depression

OUTCOMES

Short-term

Minimal pain or reduction in pain, as evidenced by client's statements that pain medication and measures to increase comfort are effective in controlling pain (expected within 3 days)

Long-term

Absence or control of pain, as evidenced by optimal mobility and activity necessary for functioning, socialization, and performing ADL independently (expected within 2 to 3 weeks)

NURSING INTERVENTIONS/INSTRUCTIONS

1. Assess pain and characteristics, including remissions and exacerbations or, if the pain is continuous, factors that relieve or precipitate pain (each visit).
2. Instruct client in administration of analgesics, antirheumatics, and steroid and nonsteroidal antiinflammatories, including dose, action of drug, times, frequency, side effects (especially steroids), to take drugs continuously regardless of improvement, and to avoid abrupt discontinuation of steroid therapy (first visit).
3. Instruct client to coordinate medication for pain with activities and to avoid overwork or activities that cause stress to joints (first visit).
4. Instruct client to avoid stressful situations, damp, moist environments, or extremes in environmental temperatures (first visit).
5. Instruct client to avoid prolonged activities, including walking, standing, and sitting, as well as sudden movements (first visit).

6. Instruct client in use of bed cradle, footboard, and bed board (first visit).
7. Instruct client in application of heat treatments, including warm baths and showers, electric blanket, and warm, wet compresses, and inform client of possible paraffin application during physical therapy session (first visit and reinforce on second visit).
8. Instruct client in application of splints to reduce pain by immobilization of the joints, including when to remove and reapply them (first visit).
9. Suggest relaxation techniques, methods of distraction, and use of transcutaneous electrical nerve stimulator (TENS) (first visit).

CLIENT AND FAMILY/CAREGIVER INTERVENTIONS

1. Client assesses and administers analgesic for pain.
2. Client places affected joints in position of comfort.
3. Client applies heat treatments as instructed.
4. Client administers medications as instructed; observes and reports side effects.
5. Client applies splints, footboard, soft linens, pillows, bed cradle, or other devices as appropriate to control pain and support joints.
6. Client employs relaxation and diversional activities during painful episodes.
7. Client avoids overactivity, stress, and environmental changes that affect joints.
8. Client applies and use TENS correctly and safely.
9. Client reports time, intensity, duration, and site(s) of pain.

Nursing diagnosis

Impaired physical mobility

Related factors: Pain and discomfort; musculoskeletal impairment

Defining characteristics: Reluctance to attempt movement, inability to purposefully move within physical environment, limited range of motion, imposed restrictions of movement

OUTCOMES

Short-term

Adequate activity and mobility, as evidenced by progressive ambulation and movement, within restrictions or limitations imposed by the disease process, and participation in ADL (expected within 1 week)

Long-term

Optimal achievement of physical mobility, as evidenced by ability to maintain health and functioning and by performance of ADL within restrictions without complications (expected within 1 to 2 months)

NURSING INTERVENTIONS/INSTRUCTIONS

1. Assess ability to ambulate and to participate in ADL, limitations of joint movement, presence of pain on movement, and need for assistive aids (see Musculoskeletal System Assessment, p. 29, for guidelines) (first visit).
2. Instruct client in prescribed limitations in use of joints, 1-hour rest periods throughout day to rest affected parts, and scheduling of activities to avoid fatigue and joint injury (first and second visits).
3. Instruct client to allow plenty of time to perform all activities and to take pain medication prior to exercises if drug is not too potent (first visit).
4. Instruct client in correct body alignment and in body mechanics for transferring, lifting, reaching, stooping, bending, pushing, and ambulating as well as in resting position (first visit and reinforce on second visit).
5. Instruct client in use of assistive aids and supportive devices, such as crutches, braces, corrective shoes, cane, walker, and wheelchair, and in use of helps to perform ADL, such as long-handled pickups, Velcro closures, holders for mirrors, books, etc., and zippered clothing (first visit).
6. Instruct client in exercises for involved and uninvolved joints, including type and frequency of ROM and muscle-setting exercises (each visit as needed).
7. Instruct client in joint protection during activities and in the use of immobilization aids to rest joints when needed (first visit).

8. Encourage client to participate in ADL and diversional activities within restrictions (first visit and as needed).
9. Instruct client in skin protection for areas under splints and at enlarged joint areas since these are susceptible to breakdown (each visit).
10. Initiate referral to physical therapist for exercise regimen and occupational therapist for ADL and fine-motor exercises (any visit).
11. Refer home health aide to assist with ADL as needed.

CLIENT AND FAMILY/CAREGIVER INTERVENTIONS

1. Client performs planned exercises and activities, with progressive increases daily or weekly.
2. Client performs ambulation, transferring, reaching, and position changes using proper body mechanics and maintaining body alignment.
3. Client participates in ADL as able, with progress until independence is achieved.
4. Client provides rest periods throughout day as needed to avoid overactivity.
5. Client uses assistive and supportive aids for joint protection.
6. Client adjusts work hours according to activity tolerance.
7. Client uses assistive aids for ADL, toilet seat, eating aids, reaching aids, and dressing and grooming aids as needed.
8. Client reports to physician any prolonged pain that is not controlled and that limits activity and exercise.
9. Client maintains physical and occupational therapy regimens with changes as indicated.
10. Client administers analgesic prior to activity or ambulation as appropriate.

Nursing diagnosis

Ineffective individual coping

Related factors: Personal vulnerability, multiple life changes

Defining characteristics: Verbalization of inability to cope with chronic illness or ask for help; inability to meet basic needs and role expectations; chronic worry and anxiety; chronic fatigue; inability to solve problems; immobility; chronic pain; social isolation

OUTCOMES

Short-term

Improved coping skills, as evidenced by client's statement of chronic nature of the disease and knowledge of need to develop new coping and problem-solving skills for compliance with long-term treatments (expected within 1 week)

Long-term

Positive coping with chronic illness, as evidenced by optimal participation in care and willingness to adapt to life-style changes to achieve maximum health and functioning status (expected within 2 months)

NURSING INTERVENTIONS/INSTRUCTIONS

1. Assess mental and emotional status, ability to adapt, level of anxiety, and coping mechanisms used and their effect (first visit).
2. Provide accepting environment, and allow expressions of fears, concerns, and feelings regarding deformity and effect on body image (each visit).
3. Allow client to control planning of care and to make decisions for mutual goal setting (each visit).
4. Assist client to identify desires and ways to change life-style, as well as which coping mechanisms work and which are destructive (each visit).
5. Instruct client in methods to develop new coping skills and to try changes without fear of failing (first visit).
6. Initiate psychotherapy, support group assistance, or counseling if indicated (any visit).
7. Refer to social worker if social services and mental health assistance are needed (any visit).

CLIENT AND FAMILY/CAREGIVER INTERVENTIONS

1. Client develops coping and problem-solving skills that are effective.
2. Client verbalizes feelings and concerns about body image and long-term disability with family members, and requests assistance when needed.
3. Client identifies negative and positive behaviors, and maintains productive coping methods.

4. Client utilizes significant others, groups, and agencies for help and support.
5. Client joins and participates in the Arthritis Foundation.
6. Client manages own care effectively, and maintains a positive attitude.

Nursing diagnosis

Knowledge deficit

Related factors: Lack of information about care and preventive measures

Defining characteristics: Request for information about disease process, cause, and treatment; risk of falls or injury in an unsafe environment; signs and symptoms of complications; need to modify life-style

OUTCOMES

Short-term

Adequate knowledge, as evidenced by client's statement of cause, treatment, measures to prevent injury or trauma, signs and symptoms to report, and medication regimen (expected within 1 week)

Long-term

Adequate knowledge, as evidenced by client's complying with medical regimen and meeting requirements of modified life-style necessary to achieve optimal health and musculoskeletal functioning (expected within 1 to 2 months)

NURSING INTERVENTIONS/INSTRUCTIONS

1. Assess life-style, ability to adapt to change and disabilities, learning ability and interest, and family participation and support (first visit).
2. Inform client of cause and chronicity of disease, remissions and exacerbations; need for long-term consistent therapy; and progressive joint weakness and instability (first visit).
3. Instruct client in fluid, nutritional, and rest plan and in need to avoid weight gain (first and second visits).
4. Instruct client in signs and symptoms of complications to report, including uncontrolled pain, redness, swelling, and inability to move joint (first visit).

5. Inform client of prevalence of advertised quack cures and misinformation (first visit).
6. Inform client of alternative timing and positioning for sexual closeness (any visit).
7. Instruct client to provide safe environment to reduce injury from falls, including removal of small rugs, use of night-lights and hand rails, use of cane or walker, wearing well-fitting, sturdy shoes, and clearing all pathways (first visit).
8. Instruct client fully in medication administration, including analgesics, steroids, salicylates, and gold injections, with action, dosage, frequency, side effects, results to expect, and food and drug interactions (first visit and reinforce each visit thereafter).
9. Inform client of need for and importance of all physical therapy recommendations and of need to keep appointments for laboratory work and with physician (first visit).
10. Instruct client to adjust daily schedules and change activities that are not tolerated well and to take 1-hour rest periods frequently during the day (first and each visit as needed).
11. Initiate referral to community agencies and support groups, such as the Arthritis Foundation, for literature and for places to acquire supplies and equipment (any visit).

CLIENT AND FAMILY/CAREGIVER INTERVENTIONS

1. Client states cause, prescribed treatments, fluid and dietary requirements, rest needs, and signs and symptoms to report to physician.
2. Client assesses daily for changes that are positive and negative in terms of progress.
3. Client administers medications correctly, and reports any untoward responses.
4. Client avoids stressful situations when possible.
5. Client adjusts sexual activities as needed.
6. Client avoids unrecognized treatments that may cause disappointment or injury.
7. Client maintains therapy regimens, laboratory testing schedule, and appointments with physician or other referrals.
8. Client participates in and accepts assistance from agencies and support groups as needed.
9. Client adapts to life-style changes in a realistic manner.

Fractured Hip; Hip or Knee Prosthesis or Replacement

Hip fractures include fractures of the head, neck, and trochanter parts of the femur. They usually result from osteoporosis or falls. The surgical procedure for hip/knee replacement includes the removal of the ball and socket of the hip joint and insertion of a prosthesis or the replacement of the surfaces of the tibia and femur with a prosthesis. Either procedure is done to correct damage caused by fracture, deformity, or rheumatoid or degenerative arthritis.

Home care is primarily concerned with the teaching of the medical and rehabilitative regimen to ensure optimal mobility.

Nursing diagnosis

Impaired physical mobility

Related factors: Musculoskeletal impairment

Defining characteristics: Inability to purposefully move within environment; reluctance to attempt movement; limited range of motion; fear of dislocating prosthesis

OUTCOMES

Short-term

Adequate activity and mobility, as evidenced by progressive ambulation and movement within imposed limitations (expected within 1 week)

Long-term

Optimal physical mobility and independence in activities of daily living (ADL) achieved within restrictions to maintain health and functioning without complications (expected within 1 month)

NURSING INTERVENTIONS/INSTRUCTIONS

1. Assess ability to participate in ADL, mobility status, and need for assistive aids for ambulation and self-care (see Musculoskeletal System Assessment, p. 29, for guidelines) (first visit and as needed).
2. Instruct client in transfer and pivoting techniques to get into car, bed, wheelchair, toilet, shower, or other places (first and second visits).
3. Instruct client in muscle-strengthening exercises to prepare for use of devices for ambulation and ADL; instruct client in use of walker, cane, or crutches as appropriate (each visit).
4. Instruct client in ROM exercises as permitted and instruct client to perform them on all functioning joints, including number of times and frequency (first visit and reinforce on second visit).
5. Instruct client in and encourage him or her to perform all personal care and to increase ambulation daily (each visit).
6. Instruct client in weight-bearing limitation on operative side (first visit).
7. Initiate referral to physical therapist, occupational therapist, and vocational therapist (any visit).
8. Refer home health aide to assist in ADL as needed.
9. Arrange for equipment in home, including hospital bed, wheelchair, walker, or other (first visit).

CLIENT AND FAMILY/CAREGIVER INTERVENTIONS

1. Client performs daily planned exercise regimen, including ROM exercises and ambulation using appropriate assistive aids.
2. Client progresses in independence in walking and in transfer techniques.
3. Client uses assistive aids for ADL, including raised toilet seat, long-handled tongs for reaching or picking up articles, and others, depending on needs associated with dressing, meal preparation, and bathing.
4. Client participates in physical therapy program.
5. Client carries out prescribed physical rehabilitation as instructed by therapist.

Nursing diagnosis

Risk for trauma

Related factors: Internal factors of surgical procedure affecting movement; external factors of unsafe environment

Defining characteristics: Weakness; reduced weight bearing; reduced movement of limb; lack of safety precautions; inability or refusal to use assistive aids

OUTCOMES

Short-term

Absence of falls or injury, as evidenced by ability to move without pain and weakness and by increased weight bearing using assistive aids (expected within 1 week)

Long-term

Ongoing absence of trauma, as evidenced by maintenance of optimal health and functioning, with length of extremity maintained without injury (expected within 1 month and ongoing)

NURSING INTERVENTIONS/INSTRUCTIONS

1. Assess for signs of prosthesis dislocation, such as shortening of or inability to move or bear weight on operative extremity and severe pain and spasms during movement, and instruct client to observe for these signs and symptoms (each visit).
2. Instruct client to maintain weight-bearing restrictions and to avoid hip flexion, elevation of knees, stooping, crossing legs, twisting of the limb, and positions during intercourse that cause hip to turn inward or rotation of the knee (first visit).
3. Instruct client to use assistive aids for ambulation and holding bars to assist with movement and provide stability (first visit).
4. Instruct client to turn only on side as instructed when in bed and to avoid lifting heavy objects (first visits).
5. Instruct client to provide clear pathways, to remove rugs, cords, furniture, or other objects, to avoid stairways, and to take plenty of time for all activities (first visit).
6. Instruct client to take rest periods and avoid activities when fatigued (first visit).

CLIENT AND FAMILY/CAREGIVER INTERVENTIONS

1. Client provides clear pathways, good lighting, and assistive aids to prevent falls.
2. Client avoids positions, turning, weight bearing, sitting, lifting, and stooping as instructed, to prevent dislocation.
3. Client avoids strain and fatigue as result of activity.
4. Client follows recommendations for positioning during sexual intercourse.
5. Client allows sufficient time for activities.
6. Client reports to physician any signs or symptoms indicating displacement.

Nursing diagnosis

Knowledge deficit

Related factors: Lack of information about postoperative care

Defining characteristics: Request for information about medical regimen and rehabilitation requirements

OUTCOMES

Short-term

Adequate knowledge, as evidenced by client's statement of signs and symptoms of complications to report and ability to perform postoperative wound care and administer medications correctly (expected within 1 week)

Long-term

Adequate knowledge, as evidenced by achievement of optimal health and return of functioning within prescribed limits (expected within 2 to 3 months)

NURSING INTERVENTIONS/INSTRUCTIONS

1. Assess life-style and ability to adapt, learning abilities, and family assistance and support (first visit).
2. Inform client of signs and symptoms of complications, including persistent or increased pain in extremity, numbness in extremity, bleeding, edema, redness, or pain at incision site, and

continued difficulty in bearing weight on extremity, and instruct client to report to physician (first visit).

3. Instruct client in administration of analgesics and antibiotics, including action, dose, frequency, route, and side effects (first visit).
4. Instruct client in sterile dressing changes and allow for return demonstration; instruct client to note drainage characteristics and report (first visit and reinforce on second visit).
5. Encourage client to participate in diversional activities according to interests (first visit).
6. Instruct client to report any changes in elimination pattern (constipation) for advice in taking stool softener or for changing fluid and nutritional intake (first visit).
7. Inform client of importance of compliance with physical and occupational rehabilitation program (any visit).

CLIENT AND FAMILY/CAREGIVER INTERVENTIONS

1. Client administers medications correctly as prescribed.
2. Client provides care to surgical site as needed, using sterile technique.
3. Client establishes and maintains bowel elimination pattern.
4. Client monitors for complications and reports to physician if present.
5. Client complies with rehabilitation program with satisfaction.
6. Client participates in diversional and stress-reducing activities.

Fractures; Cast Application

A fracture is a break in a bone caused by trauma (falls or accidents) or disease (osteoporosis with pathologic fracture). It is usually accompanied by contusion of the surrounding soft tissue. Fractures may be complete or incomplete, simple or compound, and may affect any bone in the body. A fracture is corrected by closed reduction or open reduction and immobilization of the part by casting, splinting, or traction.

Home care is primarily concerned with the teaching of care for the affected body part, ensuring immobilization and healing of the fracture, and preventing complications of the fracture.

Nursing diagnosis

Pain

Related factors: Physical injuring agents of bone fracture

Defining characteristics: Verbal descriptors of pain; guarding and protective behavior; alteration in muscle tone

OUTCOMES

Short-term

Minimal pain or absence of pain, as evidenced by client's statement that pain has been reduced or controlled and that measures to promote comfort are effective (expected within 3 days)

Long-term

Absence of pain, as evidenced by achievement of optimal comfort level and mobility for health and functioning in presence of casted body part (expected within 1 week or when cast removed)

NURSING INTERVENTIONS/INSTRUCTIONS

1. Assess, and instruct client and family to assess, type of fracture and associated pain, tight cast (insert finger between cast and skin), swelling, pallor or cyanosis, coolness of skin, loss of sensation, and decreased peripheral pulse in casted extremity; assess every 30 minutes for 24 hours and then every 3 to 4 hours (first visit).
2. Instruct client to handle involved extremity gently, with smooth movement, especially first 24 hours, and to elevate on pillow for comfort (first visit).
3. Instruct client in administration of analgesic, including dose, frequency, and relief to expect (first visit).
4. Instruct client to participate in diversional activities and relaxation exercises to reduce pain (music, reading, TV, imagery) (first visit).

5. Instruct client to change position every 2 hours to prevent pressure of cast to one area (first visit).

CLIENT AND FAMILY/CAREGIVER INTERVENTIONS

1. Client assesses pain and administers analgesic accordingly.
2. Client provides comfort measure to reduce pain.
3. Client utilizes diversional methods and interactions to relieve pain.

Nursing diagnosis

Risk for impaired skin integrity

Related factors: External factors of pressure of cast and physical immobilization

Defining characteristics: Redness, swelling, irritation of skin at cast edges or bony prominences; immobility of injury part

OUTCOMES

Short-term

Skin integrity preserved, as evidenced by intactness at pressure areas (expected within 2 to 3 days)

Long-term

Absence of skin damage, as evidenced by maintenance of optimal skin integrity and by return to normal functioning (expected ongoing)

NURSING INTERVENTIONS/INSTRUCTIONS

1. Assess skin at edges of cast, splint, or other device used to immobilize fractured bone; note redness, irritation, breaks, or pain, and instruct client to assess and report these signs and symptoms if they are present (first visit).
2. Petal edges of cast or device with soft adhesive, and inform client of rationale and of procedure to replace petaling (first visit).
3. Instruct client to avoid sticking things into cast to scratch itchy areas (first visit).
4. Encourage client to change positions frequently (first visit).

CLIENT AND FAMILY/CAREGIVER INTERVENTIONS

1. Client maintains skin integrity at areas prone to irritation.
2. Client protects skin from rough edges of cast or rubbing from device.
3. Client avoids skin damage caused by foreign objects in cast.

Nursing diagnosis

Impaired physical mobility

Related factors: Pain and discomfort; musculoskeletal impairment

Defining characteristics: Inability to purposefully move within physical environment; imposed restriction of movement by cast or splint; ability to use assistive aids and provide self-care

OUTCOMES

Short-term

Adequate activity and mobility within limitations of cast or splint, as evidenced by movement with use of assistive aids (expected within 2 to 3 days)

Long-term

Optimal physical mobility and independence in ADL achieved within restrictions to maintain health and functioning without complications (expected within 1 week or at time of cast removal)

NURSING INTERVENTIONS/INSTRUCTIONS

1. Assess mobility status with cast and ability to progress daily with or without assistive aids; assess for mobility with leg cast or for ADL with arm cast (see Musculoskeletal System Assessment, p. 29, for guidelines) (first and second visits).
2. Instruct client in use of walking cast, crutches, or arm sling as appropriate (first visit or when weight bearing is allowed).
3. Instruct client in transfer to bed, chair, car, and toilet and in use of aids for bathing, dressing, grooming, and personal hygiene activities as needed (first visit).
4. Instruct client to arrange furniture and clear pathways for ambulation and to place articles within easy reach and for convenience (first visit).

5. Instruct client in ROM exercises for uncasted parts and to move unaffected body parts frequently while progressing in ADL and other activities; include digits on casted extremity (first visit).
6. Initiate referral to physical therapist if needed (any visit).
7. Refer home health aide to assist in ADL as appropriate (first visit).

CLIENT AND FAMILY/CAREGIVER INTERVENTIONS

1. Client ambulates and participates in ADL at earliest possible time using assistive aids.
2. Client ambulates when weight bearing is allowed; applies sling properly; avoids activities that might damage cast.
3. Client provides and promotes activities that require use of all muscles and independence in ADL.
4. Client performs ROM and other strength-maintenance muscle exercises.
5. Client maintains clear, safe pathways and safe environment to prevent falls and injury and bumping or damage to cast.

Nursing diagnosis

Risk for peripheral neurovascular dysfunction

Related factors: Fracture; mechanical compression (cast)

Defining characteristics: Pallor; cyanotic color and coolness of skin at cast edges; decreased peripheral pulses; change in sensation or feeling proximal to cast edges; numbness or loss of sensation at cast site

OUTCOMES

Short-term

Neurovascular function preserved, as evidenced by digits or areas proximal to cast warm and pink and perception to touch present (expected within 2 to 3 days)

Long-term

Absence of neurovascular dysfunction in presence of cast, as evidenced by optimal color, temperature, sensation, and peripheral pulses until cast removed and fracture healed (expected for period of cast application[s])

NURSING INTERVENTIONS/INSTRUCTIONS

1. Assess skin at cast edges and on digits for color, presence of pain or numbness, peripheral pulses and capillary refill, and warmth or coolness, and instruct client to assess and report any changes to physician (first visit).
2. Instruct client in monitoring neurovascular status of casted part by noting swelling; taking peripheral pulses bilaterally and comparing them; placing pressure on digits to note capillary refill when pressure is released; and noting color of skin, which may be pink, red, pallid, or cyanotic, and temperature of skin, which may be cool or warm to touch; inform client of frequency (possibly twice daily) of assessment (first visit).
3. Position casted part for comfort, usually elevated; instruct client to avoid trauma or pressure to casted areas to prevent injury (each visit).

CLIENT AND FAMILY/CAREGIVER INTERVENTIONS

1. Client assesses neurovascular status of casted area at least daily.
2. Client provides positioning and comfort to casted area.
3. Client reports signs and symptoms of neurovascular complications of fracture and/or cast application.

Nursing diagnosis

Knowledge deficit

Related factors: Lack of information

Defining characteristics: Request for information about cast care and safety precautions to prevent falls or complications

OUTCOMES

Short-term

Adequate knowledge, as evidenced by client's statement of measures to care for cast and prevent complications of cast application (expected within 1 week)

Long-term

Adequate information, as evidenced by client's meeting requirements of modified life-style resulting from fracture and casted part to achieve optimal health and functioning as healing is completed (expected within 4 to 6 weeks or until cast removed)

NURSING INTERVENTIONS/INSTRUCTIONS

1. Assess client's life-style, ability to adapt to change and temporary disability, learning ability and interest, and family participation and support (first visit).
2. Inform client of cause and type of fracture and type and function of cast (first visit).
3. Instruct client to handle wet cast with palms of hands for at least 24 hours until cast is completely dry; use fan to dry cast by placing it 18 to 24 inches from the cast; expose all parts to air for drying, and avoid covering cast until dry (first visit).
4. Instruct client to wear comfortable, loose clothing to fit over cast (first visit).
5. Instruct client to maintain skin integrity (clean, dry, and free of irritants) and to assess for complications to report, including foul, musty odor from cast, evidence of staining that comes from wound under cast, elevated temperature, pallor or cyanotic color and cool skin, decreased peripheral pulse, change in sensation or feeling, and increasing pain (first visit).
6. Instruct client to decrease itching by using alcohol swabs or blowing cool air into cast with fan and to avoid use of powders or lotion under cast (first visit).
7. Instruct client to petal cast edges with soft tape or to pad edges to prevent irritation of skin (first visit).
8. Instruct client to cover cast with a plastic bag while bathing or taking a shower (first visit).
9. Instruct client to clean cast with a damp cloth if soiled (first visit).
10. Instruct client to protect cast from damage or breakage by avoiding weight bearing or activities until cast is completely dry (first visit).
11. If medications are prescribed, instruct client in administration, including dose, frequency, time, side effects, and food and drug interactions (first visit).

CLIENT AND FAMILY/CAREGIVER INTERVENTIONS

1. Client assesses for and reports signs and symptoms of complications of fracture and cast application, including circulatory, neurologic, or skin symptoms or presence of infectious process.
2. Client states purpose and importance of cast and immobilization of body part.
3. Client maintains dry, intact cast; cleans with damp cloth or shoe polish.
4. Client protects skin at edges of cast with petaling.
5. Client avoids inserting anything into cast or allowing cast to get wet.
6. Client administers medications correctly and safely.
7. Client secures rental or purchase of equipment and supplies.

Laminectomy/Spinal Fusion, Lumbar or Cervical

A laminectomy is the surgical removal of the posterior arch of a vertebra to treat a herniated nucleus pulposus (bulging disk), tumor, or bone fragment that creates pressure on the spinal nerve roots and causes chronic pain. The procedure is usually performed on a cervical or lumbar vertebra. The fusion of bone fragments from the iliac crest may be performed to provide stability for the spine if degenerative disease is present.

Home care is primarily concerned with the teaching aspects of postoperative care to promote healing and function, prevent complications, and achieve a successful outcome of the surgery.

Nursing diagnosis

Impaired physical mobility

Related factors: Pain and discomfort; neuromuscular and musculoskeletal impairment

Defining characteristics: Reluctance to attempt movement of legs or arms; limited range of motion; decreased muscle strength and control; difficulty in performing activities of daily living

OUTCOMES

Short-term

Adequate activity and mobility within prescribed limits, as evidenced by progressive ambulation within imposed limitations and movement within proposed restrictions (expected within 3 days)

Long-term

Return to optimal physical mobility and self-care activities within restrictions to maintain health and functioning without complications (expected within 2 to 3 weeks)

NURSING INTERVENTIONS/INSTRUCTIONS

1. Assess ability to participate in ADL, body alignment, ambulation limitations, and knowledge of prescribed restrictions (see Musculoskeletal System Assessment, p. 29, for guidelines) (first visit and as needed).
2. Instruct client to apply brace and collar before ambulation, to stabilize surgical site (first visit).
3. Instruct client in logrolling, ambulation, sitting, bending, and stooping using proper body mechanics (first visit and reinforce on second visit).
4. Instruct client to sit in straight-backed chair and seat for driving and to splint back when sitting or rising from chair (first visit).
5. Instruct client in range-of-motion and other exercises as permitted (first visit and reinforce on second visit).
6. Advise client to sleep on firm mattress with hips and knees flexed or in proper body alignment (first visit).
7. Instruct client in use of assistive aids for ADL within recommended restrictions (each visit).
8. Initiate referral to physical therapist (first visit).
9. Refer to home health aide to assist with ADL as needed (first visit).

CLIENT AND FAMILY/CAREGIVER INTERVENTIONS

1. Client performs progressive ambulation, ADL, and other activities allowed, using proper body mechanics.

2. Client participates in exercise regimen as instructed.
3. Client applies cervical collar, corset, and brace correctly, and wears as prescribed.
4. Client limits or avoids sexual activity, driving, and lifting as instructed.
5. Client takes rest periods as needed; stops activity if weak or tired or if painful response occurs.
6. Client changes mattress if necessary; utilizes aids in turning in bed or getting up.
7. Client participates in physical therapy program.
8. Client resumes work on a part-time basis, or considers the need for a change in occupation.

Nursing diagnosis

Knowledge deficit

Related factors: Lack of information about postoperative care

Defining characteristics: Request for information about postoperative activity restrictions, wound care, urinary and bowel elimination, medication regimen

OUTCOMES

Short-term

Adequate knowledge, as evidenced by client's statement of postoperative care requirements and performance of postoperative procedures (expected within 1 week)

Long-term

Adequate knowledge, as evidenced by compliance with postoperative medical regimen and meeting requirements to return to optimal health and functioning (expected within 4 to 6 weeks)

NURSING INTERVENTIONS/INSTRUCTIONS

1. Assess life-style, ability to adapt, learning ability and interest, and family participation and support (first visit).
2. Inform client of cause of vertebral abnormality and surgical procedure done to correct it (first visit).
3. Instruct client in administration of analgesics and muscle relaxants as ordered, including times, dose, frequency, side effects, and food and drug interactions (first and second visits).

4. Instruct client in wound care, including dressing change using sterile technique, and to report pain, redness, or swelling at site; allow for return demonstration of dressing change (first and second visits).
5. Instruct client to report leg or arm pain or numbness or weakness in leg or arm (first visit).
6. Inform client of bowel and bladder elimination changes and their causes and of use of stool softener, fluid intake, and exercises to assist in return to normal pattern (first visit).
7. Inform client of importance of compliance with activity and exercise regimen proposed and of avoiding activities that place stress on operative area (changing position, lifting, pushing, pulling, stooping) (first visit).
8. Instruct client in padding brace, cast, neck collar, or any other device to protect skin from rough edges or excessive tightness; check skin for changes caused by pressure when removing device (first visit).
9. Instruct client to comply with follow-up appointments with physician (first visit).

CLIENT AND FAMILY/CAREGIVER INTERVENTIONS

1. Client administers medications correctly as prescribed.
2. Client provides care to surgical site as needed, using sterile technique.
3. Client assesses skin under collar, brace, or other immobilizing device and provides skin care to prevent irritation and breakdown.
4. Client participates in prescribed activities safely and within restrictions imposed by surgery.
5. Client establishes and maintains bowel and urinary elimination pattern.
6. Client reports adverse effects of medications, treatments, and surgical intervention if appropriate.

Osteomyelitis

Osteomyelitis is an infection of the bone and may be acute or chronic. It may occur as a result of surgery or compound fractures, in which case the infectious agent is introduced directly into the bone, or the bloodstream may carry an infectious agent to the bone from infected soft tissue or joints. The infection may spread through the marrow, cortex, and periosteum. Causative agents include *Staphylococcus aureus* (most common), *Streptococcus* group A, *Escherichia coli, Pseudomonas,* and *Klebsiella.*

Home care is primarily concerned with symptomatic treatment and with teaching of the medication regimen and prevention of secondary infection or transmission of infection to others.

Nursing diagnosis

Pain

Related factors: Biologic injuring agents (infection)

Defining characteristics: Communication of pain descriptors; guarded or protective behavior toward painful part

OUTCOMES

Short-term

Pain minimized or controlled, as evidenced by client's statement that pain is relieved by initiation of measures to prevent discomfort; relaxed posture and expressions (expected within 3 days)

Long-term

Absence of pain and achievement of optimal functioning without pain (expected within 2 weeks)

NURSING INTERVENTIONS/INSTRUCTIONS

1. Assess, and instruct client to assess, pain and characteristics, as well as precipitating and alleviating factors, with an emphasis on early recognition of onset (first visit).
2. Assess pain for type, location over long bones with redness and edema, sudden onset, intensity, and duration (first visit).
3. Instruct client in administration of analgesics and antibiotics as ordered to control pain and reduce infectious process causing pain (first visit and reinforce on second visit).
4. Immobilize part with pillows and splints to prevent increased pain, and instruct client in need for bed rest and in methods to immobilize limb (first visit).

5. Instruct client in use of bed cradle and in supporting limb and handling gently when moving in bed, to prevent pressure or further injury to limb (first visit).
6. Maintain body alignment and correct positioning of limb (each visit).

CLIENT AND FAMILY/CAREGIVER INTERVENTIONS

1. Client maintains bed rest and position of comfort.
2. Client administers analgesic and monitors response in controlling pain.
3. Client performs measures to prevent pain and injury to limb.
4. Client maintains immobilization of part during acute phase.

Nursing diagnosis

Impaired physical mobility

Related factors: Pain and discomfort; intolerance to activity

Defining characteristics: Limited range of motion; imposed restrictions of movement by splint or traction; relunctance to attempt movement; decreased muscle strength

OUTCOMES

Short-term

Increasing tolerance to activity, as evidenced by increased endurance and participation in ADL within imposed restrictions (expected within 1 week)

Long-term

Optimal mobility, energy, endurance, and participation in activities, as evidenced by performance of ADL and progressive ambulation (expected within 1 month)

NURSING INTERVENTIONS/INSTRUCTIONS

1. Assess discomfort, weakness, muscle strength or atrophy, ROM in all joints, and presence of traction or splints (see Musculoskeletal System Assessment, p. 29, for guidelines) (first visit).
2. Perform ROM exercises within limitations set by physicians as healing allows, and instruct client to perform ROM and muscle exercises (first and second visits).

3. Progressively allow ambulation with use of assistive aids as needed when healing allows, and encourage client to comply daily as instructed while limiting activity (each visit).
4. Refer home health aide to assist in ADL until healing allows self-care (first visit).

CLIENT AND FAMILY/CAREGIVER INTERVENTIONS

1. Client performs ROM exercises, ADL, and ambulation daily, with increases as endurance and healing allow.
2. Client performs ADL with assistance and eventual independence.
3. Client applies and uses splint for ambulation.
4. Client prevents muscle wasting and contractures.
5. Client plans activities around rest periods.
6. Client uses assistive aids or device for ambulation if needed.

Nursing diagnosis

Risk for secondary infection

Related factors: Inadequate primary defenses (traumatized tissue)

Defining characteristics: Altered bone integrity with fracture or risk of fracture; spread of infectious agent; redness, swelling, drainage at entry site of catheter used for medication administration (right atrial); septicemia; meningitis

OUTCOMES

Short-term

Prevention of infection spread, as evidenced by normal range of temperature and vital signs and by absence of purulent drainage (expected within 1 week)

Long-term

Maintenance of infection-free state, as evidenced by the absence of septicemia, meningitis, or pathologic fracture (expected within 1 to 2 months)

NURSING INTERVENTIONS/INSTRUCTIONS

1. Assess temperature for elevation; note amount and characteristics of drainage if present (each visit).

2. Instruct client to avoid heat application to the area or exercises that would increase circulation to the part and stimulate the spread of infection (first visit).
3. Instruct client in antiinfective administration, including dose, frequency, method, route, food and drug interactions, and side effects, for oral administration and topical administration via dressing if applicable (first visit).
4. Instruct client in sterile dressing change (dry, wet) and in disposal of soiled dressings using universal precautions; allow for return demonstration (first visit).
5. Instruct client to avoid exposure to persons with infections or illnesses that might be transmitted to client (first visit).

CLIENT AND FAMILY/CAREGIVER INTERVENTIONS

1. Client administers antiinfective for 6 to 8 weeks as prescribed.
2. Client performs hand washing and sterile dressing changes.
3. Client takes temperature daily and reports to physician if chilled or drainage becomes purulent.
4. Client provides light clothing and linens in a comfortable, cool environment.
5. Client avoids exposure to persons with infections; prevents transmission of pathogens to client.
6. Client uses proper precautions in disposal of contaminated articles and supplies.

Nursing diagnosis

Knowledge deficit

Related factors: Lack of information about treatment measures

Defining characteristics: Request for information about medication regimen, nutrition, fluids, and activity requirements

OUTCOMES

Short-term

Adequate knowledge, as evidenced by client's statement of medical regimen requirements and adaptive life-style behaviors necessary to achieve optimal health (expected within 1 week)

Long-term

Adequate knowledge, as evidenced by compliance with medical regimen and meeting the requirements to achieve return to health and optimal functioning with absence of recurrent infection (expected within 1 to 2 months)

NURSING INTERVENTIONS/INSTRUCTIONS

1. Assess life-style; adapting abilities, learning interest, abilities, and readiness; and family participation and support (first visit).
2. Instruct client in high-protein and vitamin C diet inclusions to facilitate healing, and inform client of need for more than normal nutritional requirements; offer a list and sample menus that include preferences and meet the recommended standards for height and weight; instruct client to weigh weekly on same scale, at same time, and with similar clothing (first visit and second visit if needed).
3. Instruct client in administration of antiinfective, analgesic, and antipyretic, following guidelines and a schedule that are mutually planned (first visit).
4. Inform client of activity restriction and rationale (first visit).
5. Instruct client in daily requirements of fluid intake, especially if temperature is elevated (first visit).
6. Instruct client in skin protection and care if splints or traction is used and prolonged rest and immobilization are advised; instruct client in massage of bony prominences and in position changes and to report any reddened areas (first and second visits).
7. Discuss effect of disease process on self-concept and body image when long-term care is necessary and possible deformity occurs; allow client to express feelings and explore coping strategies (first visit).

CLIENT AND FAMILY/CAREGIVER INTERVENTIONS

1. Client administers medications correctly, and records any side effects.
2. Client complies with dietary and fluid requirements, and increases protein and vitamin C intake.
3. Client adapts to long-term immobilization and restriction in activity.
4. Client maintains intact skin, with protection to pressure points.

5. Client displays optimistic attitude for a recovery without deformity.

Osteoporosis

Osteoporosis is a condition characterized by reduced bone mass or density resulting from increased bone resorption. It is associated with liver or renal diseases, menopause, hyperthyroidism, hyperparathyroidism, and Cushing's syndrome. Reduced mobility and inadequate dietary calcium contribute to the disorder. Bone fracture and deformity are common results of long-term osteoporosis.

Home care is primarily concerned with the teaching of the medical regimen to prevent or control the progression of bone mass loss and subsequent fractures.

Nursing diagnosis

Risk for trauma

Related factors: Bone weakness from reduced bone mass

Defining characteristics: Falls, spontaneous fractures

OUTCOMES

Short-term

Minimal risk for trauma, as evidenced by client's compliance with safety measures to prevent falls and with treatment regimen (expected within 4 to 7 days)

Long-term

Absence of bone fracture, as evidenced by intact skeletal system and achievement of mobility and activities of daily living for optimal health and functioning (expected within 1 month and ongoing)

NURSING INTERVENTIONS/INSTRUCTIONS

1. Assess environment for safety hazards; assess client for weakness, past falls and fractures, and presence of back pain (first visit).
2. Instruct client to remove small rugs, obstructed pathways, and water on floors and to install hand grips, holding bars, and antislip equipment, to have adequate lighting and sturdy chairs, and to use low bed or footstool (first visit).
3. Instruct client to use cane, walker, or other method of support (first visit).
4. Instruct client in activity needs, daily walking and exercises, and other activities to maintain bone density (first visit and reinforce on second visit).
5. Inform client of and recommend therapist for weight-bearing exercises (first visit).

CLIENT AND FAMILY/CAREGIVER INTERVENTIONS

1. Client performs daily exercise regimen, including recommended frequency and number of times for each exercise.
2. Client joins activity group for exercises if appropriate.
3. Client wears corset to prevent vertebral collapse.
4. Client maintains mobility and activities of daily living without falls.
5. Client maintains a hazard-free environment to prevent trauma.
6. Client provides aids to maintain safe mobility and self-care.

Nursing diagnosis

Knowledge deficit

Related factors: Lack of information

Defining characteristics: Request for information about causes, treatment, and measures to prevent condition

OUTCOMES

Short-term

Adequate knowledge, as evidenced by client's verbalization of cause, medication regimen, and complications of the disease (expected within 3 days)

Long-term

Adequate knowledge, as evidenced by client's compliance with requirements for health and functioning and prevention of complications (expected within 2 weeks and ongoing)

NURSING INTERVENTIONS/INSTRUCTIONS

1. Assess client's life-style, ability to adapt, learning abilities and interest in health maintenance, and family participation and support (first visit).
2. Assess client's history to determine underlying cause of condition, including diabetes mellitus, cirrhosis of liver, kidney disease, hyperthyroidism, or hyperparathyroidism (first visit).
3. Instruct client in cause of disease, effects of bone loss, and risk for deformity or pathologic fracture (first visit).
4. Instruct client in prescribed medication regimen, including estrogen therapy and calcium and vitamin D supplements, with action, dose, frequency, time, side effects, and drug, food and alcohol interactions; calcium injection if prescribed (first visit and reinforce on second visit).
5. Inform client of foods containing calcium and vitamin D to include in diet if supplements are not prescribed (first visit).
6. Inform client of importance of follow-up x-ray studies and bone-density procedures if ordered (first visit).
7. Instruct client to report to physician bone pain or inability to move any part of the body (first visit).

CLIENT AND FAMILY/CAREGIVER INTERVENTIONS

1. Client verbalizes cause, treatment, and complications of the disease.
2. Client administers prescribed medications accurately as instructed.
3. Client includes foods high in calcium and vitamin D in dietary intake.
4. Client complies with requirement of 1000 mg/day of calcium and estrogen therapy if postmenopausal.
5. Client maintains appropriate follow-up appointments with physician and diagnostic laboratory.

Renal/urinary system

Kidney Transplantation

Kidney transplantation is the surgical placement of a donor kidney (from a cadaver or from a family member) into a matching–tissue type of recipient with end-stage renal disease. Recipients of a kidney transplant require immunosuppression to prevent rejection. The advisability of transplantation is dictated by the client's age and health problems, the availability of a donor kidney, and the client's preference for the procedure rather than relying on dialysis. Graft rejection may be acute or chronic, with the least acute response resulting from the most adequately matched donor and recipient.

Home care is primarily concerned with teaching the client about immunosuppressive therapy and monitoring for signs and symptoms of rejection

Nursing diagnosis

Anxiety

Related factors: Threat to or change in health status

Defining characteristics: Verbalization of fear of organ rejection and consequences; apprehension; uncertainty; focus on self

OUTCOMES

Short-term

Decreased anxiety, as evidenced by client's statement of increased interest in care, increased participation by client in care, and relaxed posture and facial expression (expected within 3 days)

Long-term

Optimal level of anxiety or control of anxiety, as evidenced by client's compliance with and acceptance of treatment and by positive treatment response (expected within 1 month)

NURSING INTERVENTIONS/INSTRUCTIONS

1. Assess client's mental and emotional status (see Psychosocial Assessment, p. 48, for guidelines) (first visit).
2. Provide an accepting environment, and allow for expression of fears and concerns about organ rejection (each visit).
3. Provide continuing information about progression to wellness; explain that one or more rejection episodes may occur within several months of transplant but they do not mean that kidney will be lost (each visit).
4. Initiate referral to counseling or support group if indicated (last visit).

CLIENT AND FAMILY/CAREGIVER INTERVENTIONS

1. Client seeks information that will reduce anxiety.
2. Client develops coping strategies for possibility of rejection.
3. Client maintains manageable level of anxiety.
4. Client consults with counselor or support group for control of anxiety.

Nursing diagnosis

Altered family processes

Related factors: Situational crisis from transplant surgery

Defining characteristics: Family system unable to meet needs of donor and recipient, both physical and emotional; inappropriate level and direction of energy; inability to accept or receive help; inability of family to adapt to situation

OUTCOMES

Short-term

Beginning progress toward family's acceptance of and adaptation to organ transplant, as evidenced by open communication, mutual support, and participation in care (expected within 1 week)

Long-term

Return of family to former positive interactions and support as client returns to wellness (expected within 1 to 2 months)

NURSING INTERVENTIONS/INSTRUCTIONS

1. Assess family interaction, dynamics, and supportive behaviors (see Family Assessment, p. 55, for guidelines) (first visit).

2. Include family members in teaching in a nonjudgmental environment; allow family members to ask questions (each visit).
3. Encourage openness among family members; inform them of importance of maintaining own health and social activities (first visit).
4. Suggest family counseling or support groups, rehabilitative services, or financial resources as needed (first visit).

CLIENT AND FAMILY/CAREGIVER INTERVENTIONS

1. Family verbalizes feelings and concerns.
2. Family identifies problems in family and ways to solve them together.
3. Family resolves life-style changes together.
4. Family seeks out and participates in support group activity.
5. Family participate in rehabilitation.
6. Client enters into family activities and contributes to family cohesiveness.

Nursing diagnosis

Knowledge deficit

Related factors: Lack of exposure to information about medical regimen

Defining characteristics: Request for information about immunosuppressive therapy, signs and symptoms of rejection to report, health-promotion behaviors

OUTCOMES

Short-term

Adequate knowledge, as evidenced by client's statement of treatment protocols, compliance with intensive medication regimen, and active participation in preventive health care (expected within 7 to 10 days)

Long-term

Adequate knowledge, as evidenced by client's meeting requirements for changed life-style and achievement of optimal level of health and functioning (expected within 4 to 6 weeks)

NURSING INTERVENTIONS/INSTRUCTIONS

1. Instruct client in progressive resumption of activity; emphasize avoidance of contact sports or any activity that might be traumatic to operative site (first visit).
2. Assess operative area for size, color, temperature, approximation of edges, and presence of drainage, and instruct client to notify physician of any changes in site (first visit).
3. Instruct client in administration of immunosuppressive agents, steroids, and antacids, including dose, frequency, multiple side effects, and possible interactions with OTC drugs, foods, and alcohol (first visit).
4. Assess client for side effects of drug therapy, including gastrointestinal irritation and bleeding, hepatotoxicity, cushingoid body changes, decreased wound healing, visual changes, and personality changes (each visit).
5. Instruct client in monitoring of weight, intake and output, and vital signs; demonstrate and have client return demonstration; instruct client to keep log on results (first visit and reinforce on second visit).
6. Inform client of possible signs and symptoms of organ rejection, including flulike symptoms, difficult urination, oliguria, weight gain, edema, increased blood pressure, and pain or tenderness over operative site; instruct client to report any of these signs to physician (first visit and reinforce each visit).
7. Instruct client to avoid active, live-virus immunizations and children with recent immunization (oral polio) (first visit).
8. Instruct client in proper collection of random, midstream, or 24-hour urine specimens (whichever is ordered), and stress importance of delivery to laboratory (first visit).
9. Inform client of importance of keeping physician appointments and laboratory testing for complete blood count, drug levels, electrolytes, renal function tests, urinalysis, and culture and sensitivities (first visit).
10. Instruct client to wear or carry identification and medical information, including surgery and date, medications, and physician's name and telephone number (first visit).
11. Initiate referral to nutritionist, dentist, and specialist physician as appropriate (first visit).

CLIENT AND FAMILY/CAREGIVER INTERVENTIONS

1. Client resumes activities within limitations and avoids trauma to site.
2. Client administers prescribed medications correctly and consistently and monitors for side effects to report.
3. Client monitors and records daily or weekly weight, vital signs, and intake and output.
4. Client lists signs and symptoms of graft rejection and reports to physician if they occur.
5. Client engages in multisystem regimen to avoid infection and reports any signs and symptoms of renal/urinary or respiratory infection.
6. Client maintains clean wound, with progressive healing stages.
7. Client maintains appointments with physicians and laboratory.
8. Client wears identifying medical information at all times.
9. Client consults with health professionals for regular health maintenance and advice.

Prostatic Hypertrophy/ Prostatectomy

Benign prostatic hypertrophy is the enlargement of the prostate gland, which is thought to be caused by an imbalance between the male and female sex hormones that occurs in men over the age of 50 years. The condition results in partial or complete obstruction of the urethra or incomplete emptying of the bladder. Prostatectomy, the partial or complete surgical removal of the prostate gland, can be done to relieve obstruction caused by compression on the urethra (suprapubic or transurethral) or to remove a malignant mass (perineal or retropubic). The surgical approach is dependent on age, size and location of the obstruction or mass, and severity of symptoms.

Home care is primarily concerned with the maintenance of urinary elimination before and after surgery, wound care after surgery, and the teaching of medical or surgical regimens and prevention of complications as applicable.

Nursing diagnosis

Urinary retention

Related factors: Blockage

Defining characteristics: Bladder distention; small, frequent voiding; absence of urinary output; dribbling; dysuria; residual urine; overflow incontinence; pain with bladder fullness and overdistention; small urinary stream; hesitancy in urinating

OUTCOMES

Short-term

Distress associated with urination minimized, as evidenced by client's statement of relief of retention with use of palliative measures (evidenced within 2 days)

Long-term

Urinary bladder distention and symptoms controlled, with optimal urinary elimination (expected within 1 to 2 weeks and ongoing)

NURSING INTERVENTIONS/INSTRUCTIONS

1. Assess renal/urinary and reproductive systems (see Renal/Urinary System Assessment, p. 32, and Reproductive System Assessment, p. 39, for guidelines), and note decreased size and force of urinary stream, difficulty in starting to urinate, urgency, frequency, dribbling, nocturia, hematuria, inability to completely empty bladder, and presence of overflow incontinence (first visit).
2. Assess for suprapubic distention by palpation and for possible complete retention with anuria and suprapubic pain (each visit).
3. Instruct client to note times and amounts of urinary elimination and to compare with times and amounts of fluid intake (first visit).
4. Instruct client to maintain hydration with intake of 8 to 10 glasses of water per day and to avoid alcohol and caffeine-containing beverages (first visit).
5. Instruct client to notify physician if client is unable to void

or if signs and symptoms of urinary elimination problems escalate (first visit).

6. Instruct client to avoid straining at bowel elimination; instruct client in administration of stool softener if needed (each visit).
7. Instruct client to take warm sitz baths to facilitate voiding and decrease distress (first visit).
8. Instruct client to empty bladder every 2 to 3 hours and not to delay voiding when urge is present (first visit).
9. Instruct client in administration of urinary antispasmodics and urinary analgesics as ordered, including dose, frequency, side effects, and food, drug and alcohol interactions (first visit).
10. Catheterize client using aseptic technique if ordered and when voiding has been absent for 6 to 8 hours (any visit).

CLIENT AND FAMILY/CAREGIVER INTERVENTIONS

1. Client records changes in urinary elimination patterns and signs and symptoms of distress in a diary.
2. Client notifies physician of failure of relief measures to control signs and symptoms.
3. Client avoids constipation and straining by administration of stool softener.
4. Client maintains fluid intake of 2 to 3 L/day; avoid fluids that increase diuresis.
5. Client empties bladder at designated times and when urge is present.
6. Client takes medications prescribed for specific complaints.

Nursing diagnosis

Risk for infection

Related factors: Inadequate primary defenses (stasis of urine, broken skin)

Defining characteristics: Invasive procedure (surgery); surgical wound with redness, edema, pain, purulent drainage; urinary retention; wound or urine culture positive for infectious organism; cloudy, foul-smelling urine

OUTCOMES

Short-term

Absence of infection, as evidenced by decreased urinary retention and by proper care of surgical site (expected within 3 to 4 days)

Long-term

Absence of infection, as evidenced by temperature and white blood count within normal ranges, surgical site clean and healing, urine clear, and urination without symptoms (expected within 4 to 6 weeks)

NURSING INTERVENTIONS/INSTRUCTIONS

1. Assess temperature, pulse, respiration, and blood pressure, and instruct client to report chills and fever over 100° F to physician (each visit).
2. Assess incisional drains and operative wounds as applicable for pain, color, temperature, swelling, drainage, and approximation of edges (each visit).
3. Perform sterile wound care and catheter or meatal care (each visit).
4. Instruct client in care of catheter, placement and emptying of drainage bag, and use of leg bag (first visit).
5. Instruct client to inform physician of changes in urine characteristics, including cloudiness and foul odor (first visit).
6. Monitor for hematuria and assess client's ability to empty bladder after catheter removed (each visit).
7. Instruct client to administer antibiotics and urinary antiseptics as ordered for treatment or prophylaxis (first visit).

CLIENT AND FAMILY/CAREGIVER INTERVENTIONS

1. Client monitors vital signs and temperature and reports changes.
2. Client reports changes in urine characteristics, hematuria, or changes in appearance of wound.
3. Client maintains closed drainage system for indwelling catheter.
4. Client performs wound and catheter care using sterile technique.
5. Client maintains adequate hydration.
6. Client administers antibiotics for full course and other medications for urinary bladder treatment.

Nursing diagnosis

Sexual dysfunction

Related factors: Altered body function

Defining characteristics: Impotence; decreased libido; erectile dysfunction following surgery; sterility

OUTCOMES

Short-term

Temporary dysfunction progressing to normal function, as evidenced by client's statement of understanding of surgical outcome and changes that can be expected in sexual functioning (expected within 1 week)

Long-term

Optimal sexual functioning within physiologic limitations resulting from surgical procedure (expected within 1 month)

NURSING INTERVENTIONS/INSTRUCTIONS

1. Provide a nonjudgmental, nonthreatening environment for client to have time and opportunity to ask questions or discuss sexual function according to comfort level (each visit).
2. Inform client of sexual implications of surgery and possibility of sterility or impotence (first visit).
3. Inform client of change in urine clarity after intercourse if transurethral procedure is done (first visit).
4. Inform client that sexual intercourse may resume 6 to 8 weeks after surgery, and provide information about alternate methods of gratification for partner (first visit).
5. Inform client about possible aids available to assist with penile erection if applicable (first visit).
6. Initiate referral for sexual counseling if indicated or requested (last visit).

CLIENT AND FAMILY/CAREGIVER INTERVENTIONS

1. Client expresses feelings and concerns about sexuality for resolution.
2. Client communicates needs and abilities to perform sexual intercourse and response of partner.

3. Client consults sex therapist with or without partner.
4. Client explores use of aids for impotence.

Nursing diagnosis

Anxiety

Related factors: Threat to health status; threat to change in role functioning

Defining characteristics: Urinary incontinence, blood in urine; change in role and relationships; altered body image if dribbling or incontinence is chronic or with use of retention catheter; urgency and inability to reach bathroom

OUTCOMES

Short-term

Decreased and manageable anxiety level, as evidenced by client's statements of knowledge of postoperative course and improved bladder control (expected within 3 days)

Long-term

Anxiety controlled, as evidenced by maintenance of improved urinary elimination pattern and by improved body image (expected within 1 month)

NURSING INTERVENTIONS/INSTRUCTIONS

1. Assess client's coping abilities and ability to adapt to changes in health status; assist in identification and utilization of positive and effective coping mechanisms and problem-solving skills (each visit).
2. Instruct client to avoid heavy lifting or carrying a heavy object or prolonged sitting or driving for 3 to 6 weeks (first visit).
3. Inform client that some blood may remain in urine for several weeks (first visit).
4. Instruct client to become acquainted with locations of bathrooms when away from home and to refrain from fluid intake before going out and at bedtime (first visit).
5. Inform client that postoperative dribbling and some incontinence are common and may be minimized by exercising; instruct client in perineal exercises (first visit).

6. Assist client to formulate an exercise schedule that is progressive in frequency and number of times (first visit).

CLIENT AND FAMILY/CAREGIVER INTERVENTIONS

1. Client utilizes positive coping strategies that reduce anxiety and improve body image.
2. Client avoids activities postoperatively that cause complications.
3. Client verbalizes normal postoperative course and expectations.
4. Client performs perineal exercises daily to strengthen sphincter tone.
5. Client reduces embarrassment of dribbling and incontinence by limiting fluids and wearing waterproof undergarment.
6. Client uses bathroom as frequently as needed, at least every 2 hours.

Renal Failure, Chronic (CRF)

Chronic renal failure is the progressive, gradual deterioration of kidney function, resulting in decreased glomerular filtration rate (GRF), renal blood flow, resorption ability, and function of the tubules. The condition is irreversible as it progresses toward uremia but may be controlled by dietary and fluid restrictions. As the kidneys lose the ability to maintain fluid and electrolyte balance, the client is provided with renal dialysis. Diseases that predispose a person to the development of CRF are immunologic (glomerulonephritis), infectious (pyelonephritis, tuberculosis), urinary obstructive (prostatic hypertrophy, renal calculi), metabolic (diabetes mellitus), congenital (polycystic disease), vascular (hypertension), or nephrotoxic (drugs). All organs of the body are affected by CRF.

Home care is primarily concerned with providing for activities of daily living as needed, administration of peritoneal dialysis if appropriate, and teaching the client about dietary and

fluid restrictions, compliance with hemodialysis, and prevention of complications of the disease.

Nursing diagnosis

Anxiety

Related factors: Threat of death; threat to or change in health status

Defining characteristics: Apprehension; uncertain outcome; increased helplessness and tension; possible future kidney dialysis or transplant; changes in life-style

OUTCOMES

Short-term

Decreased anxiety, as evidenced by client's statement of reduced fear and apprehension about change in health status and possible dialysis and transplant availability (expected within 3 days)

Long-term

Management or control of anxiety level, as evidenced by compliance with and acceptance of treatment regimen and change in life-style (expected within 1 to 2 months)

NURSING INTERVENTIONS/INSTRUCTIONS

1. Assess client's mental and emotional status regarding life-threatening illness (see Psychosocial Assessment, p. 48, for guidelines) (first visit).
2. Encourage expressions of fears, concerns, and questions regarding therapy and its effects in an accepting environment (each visit).
3. Assist client to identify needed changes in life-style and methods for making necessary changes (first visit and reinforce each visit).
4. Inform client of all activities, treatments, and tests and effects to expect (first visit).
5. Initiate referral to counseling or support group (any visit).

CLIENT AND FAMILY/CAREGIVER INTERVENTIONS

1. Client develops coping mechanisms for long-term treatment and possible outcome.

2. Client maintains manageable level of anxiety.
3. Client seeks information that will reduce anxiety.
4. Client expresses fears and concerns about necessary changes in life-style.
5. Client consults with counselor, clergy, or support group.

Nursing diagnosis

Fluid volume excess

Related factors: Compromised regulatory mechanism

Defining characteristics: Edema; weight gain; decreased urinary output; electrolyte imbalance (potassium, sodium, calcium, magnesium, phosphorus); increased blood pressure and pulse; decreased specific gravity; increased blood urea nitrogen and creatinine

OUTCOMES

Short-term

Balanced intake and output, as evidenced by decreasing edema, compliance with fluid and electrolyte restrictions, and stable weight and blood pressure (expected within 1 week)

Long-term

Adequate renal function, as evidenced by optimal intake and output ratio and by maintenance of renal status within limitations imposed by disease (expected within 1 to 2 months)

NURSING INTERVENTIONS/INSTRUCTIONS

1. Assess client's renal status (see Renal/Urinary System Assessment, p. 32, for guidelines); evaluate baseline weight, hydration, peripheral edema, vital signs, output trends, and urine characteristics (each visit).
2. Instruct client in techniques for taking blood pressure and weight and for monitoring edema and intake and output, and allow for return demonstration (first visit).
3. Instruct client in fluid restriction as prescribed: generally previous day's urinary output plus 500 to 800 ml over intake; include allotment and measurement of fluids, rationale for

therapy, and how to distribute fluids over 24 hours (first visit and reinforce on second and third visits).

4. Instruct client to restrict sodium intake by avoiding addition of table salt and eating of cold cuts, processed, canned, or convenience foods, and other foods high in sodium (first visit).
5. Instruct client to restrict potassium intake by avoiding citrus products, dried fruits, and bananas (first visit).
6. Instruct client to notify physician of increasing weight gain and edema, decreased urinary output, or increased blood pressure (first visit).
7. Instruct client, and reinforce instruction, in need for continual kidney dialysis, procedure for peritoneal dialysis in the home, and performance of procedure by client or family member if realistic and possible (first visit and ongoing visits).
8. Instruct client in administration of diuretics and antihypertensives, including dose, frequency, route, side effects, possible interferences with over-the-counter (OTC) drugs, and possible reactions with foods (first visit).

CLIENT AND FAMILY/CAREGIVER INTERVENTIONS

1. Client monitors and records blood pressure, weight, intake and output, and edema daily.
2. Client restricts fluid; uses ice chips, and spreads limited fluids over 24 hours; measures fluids at mealtime, snack time, and medication time.
3. Client restricts foods containing large amounts of sodium or potassium.
4. Client administers medications correctly and as instructed.
5. Client reports signs and symptoms of increasing failure or increased sodium or potassium levels.
6. Client participates in hemodialysis and performs peritoneal dialysis as appropriate in home.

Nursing diagnosis

Altered nutrition: less than body requirements

Related factors: Inability to ingest foods

Defining characteristics: Anorexia, dietary protein restriction, nausea, vomiting, hiccups

OUTCOMES

Short-term

Adequate nutrition, as evidenced by absence of anorexia and by ingestion of protein-restricted diet (expected within 1 week)

Long-term

Optimal nutrition, as evidenced by compliance with special dietary restrictions throughout illness, including achievement of caloric, electrolyte, and protein requirements (expected within 1 month)

NURSING INTERVENTIONS/INSTRUCTIONS

1. Assess nutritional status and eating patterns, including food preferences and cultural and religious adaptations; note presence of anorexia, nausea, vomiting, stomatitis, bad taste in mouth, or tissue wasting (each visit).
2. Instruct client in protein-restricted diet if client is not on dialysis; emphasize proteins with high biologic value (each visit).
3. Instruct client in adequate foods to increase caloric intake, derived primarily from carbohydrates and unsaturated fats; integrate information about fluid and electrolyte requirements or restrictions into instruction (each visit).
4. Instruct client in administration of vitamin supplements, phosphorus-binding agents, and calcium supplements (first visit).
5. Instruct client in oral hygiene, especially after meals; encourage client to brush teeth and use mouthwash, hard candy, or sour candy for breath control (first visit).
6. Instruct client to eat smaller, more frequent meals and to take antiemetics ½ hour before eating if nauseated (first visit).
7. Provide written instructions, sample menus, and recipes, and emphasize that compliance with dietary regimen will ease distressing symptoms of anorexia, nausea, vomiting, fatigue, and edema (each visit).

CLIENT AND FAMILY/CAREGIVER INTERVENTIONS

1. Client adjusts eating schedule to rest periods and to antiemetic administration.
2. Client performs mouth care frequently during day.
3. Client follows restrictions in diet (protein, sodium, potassium) using planned menus.

4. Client eats smaller, more frequent meals.
5. Client administers vitamin and mineral supplements and other medications as instructed.
6. Client maintains ideal weight as closely as possible.
7. Client reads labels on foods and avoids foods containing large amounts of sodium or potassium; notes caloric value of purchased foods.

Nursing diagnosis

Risk for impaired skin integrity

Related factors: External factors of immobility; internal factors of urea deposits and peripheral neuropathy

Defining characteristics: Pruritis; yellow pigmentation; scratching with breaks in skin; redness at pressure points; buildup of uremic frost on skin; dryness of skin; numbness in feet and legs

OUTCOMES

Short-term

Skin integrity intact, as evidenced by decreased pruritis and by compliance with skin care regimen (expected within 4 days)

Long-term

Skin integrity maintained, as evidenced by absence of skin disruption with skin in optimal condition (expected within 1 month and ongoing)

NURSING INTERVENTIONS/INSTRUCTIONS

1. Assess skin (see Integumentary System Assessment, p. 36, for guidelines), and note color, turgor, integrity, temperature, presence of scratch marks, and presence of uremic frost or pruritis (each visit).
2. Instruct client to bathe daily and to use a superfatted soap and emollients if itching is present (first visit).
3. Instruct client to maintain nails in short and clipped condition and to cut them straight across when trimming (first visit).
4. Instruct client to avoid scratching or rubbing skin (first visit).
5. Instruct client in perineal care after toileting (first visit).

6. Instruct client in use of antipruritics, oral and topical (first visit).
7. Instruct client in hand-washing technique.

CLIENT AND FAMILY/CAREGIVER INTERVENTIONS

1. Client bathes daily; uses lotion, moisturizer, emollients; pats skin and avoids rubbing.
2. Client performs perineal care after toileting.
3. Client avoids scratching; maintains nails in short, clean condition.
4. Client administers medications for pruritis as instructed.
5. Client reports skin breaks, rashes, or scratches to physician.

Nursing diagnosis

Risk for activity intolerance

Related factors: Deconditioned status, generalized weakness

Defining characteristics: Verbalization of fatigue and weakness; activity restrictions; inability to produce erythropoietin, causing anemia; defect in platelet function; faulty bone metabolism

OUTCOMES

Short-term

Adequate activity, as evidenced by participation in activities of daily living (ADL) within limitations (expected within 1 week)

Long-term

Mobility and self-care in ADL achieved for optimal level of functioning, within limitations imposed by illness (expected within 1 month)

NURSING INTERVENTIONS/INSTRUCTIONS

1. Assess client's level of participation in ADL, endurance, muscle strength, gait, peripheral neuropathy, and fatigue with activity (first visit).
2. Encourage independence in ADL; instruct client to prioritize and pace activities, to use aids to conserve energy, and to schedule rest periods between activities (first visit).

3. Instruct client in measures to take to protect feet and legs from trauma (first visit).
4. Initiate referral to physical and/or occupational therapy if indicated (any visit).
5. Refer home health aide to assist with ADL when appropriate.

CLIENT AND FAMILY/CAREGIVER INTERVENTIONS

1. Client schedules rest periods, and paces activities according to endurance and energy.
2. Client participates in ADL.
3. Client wears sturdy, well-fitted shoes and clean socks.
4. Client avoids injury caused by limited energy and fatigue.
5. Client equips environment with holding bars and aids for washing, dressing, grooming, toileting, and eating.

Nursing diagnosis

Altered thought processes

Related factors: Physiologic changes

Defining characteristics: Drowsiness, inability to concentrate, memory deficit, hallucinations, seizures, high level of nitrogenous wastes

OUTCOMES

Short-term

Minimal changes in thought processes, as evidenced by appropriate attitude, behavior, and communication (expected within 1 week)

Long-term

Thought processes maintained intact, as evidenced by optimal level of mental functioning within disease limitations (expected within 1 month and ongoing)

NURSING INTERVENTIONS/INSTRUCTIONS

1. Assess client's mental and orientation status, and compare findings with previous profiles (each visit).
2. Adapt communication style and instruction to client's needs and abilities (each visit).

3. Reinforce need for compliance with dietary restrictions and medication administration and dialysis to maintain thought processes (first visit and reinforce when needed).
4. Provide stimulating and diversional experiences, including reality-based experiences (each visit).

CLIENT AND FAMILY/CAREGIVER INTERVENTIONS

1. Client complies with medical regimen.
2. Client participates in reality-based activities, utilizing aids to reinforce orientation.
3. Client complies with dialysis protocol.
4. Client uses aids to assist with remembering medications, dietary, and fluid schedules.

Nursing diagnosis

Ineffective family coping: compromised

Related factors: Prolonged, progressive disease that exhausts supportive capacity of significant people

Defining characteristics: Less than satisfactory supportive behaviors and results; client's expression of concerns about response to health needs by others; expressed need by family for knowledge and understanding of client needs

OUTCOMES

Short-term

Improved coping by family, as evidenced by family's acknowledgement of disabling effects of disease and required life-style changes and by family's cooperation and participation in treatment regimen (expected within 1 week)

Long-term

Optimal level of participation and support of family members to facilitate client life-style and improvement in health status (expected within 1 to 2 months)

NURSING INTERVENTIONS/INSTRUCTIONS

1. Assess family interactions, coping abilities, strengths of individual members, level of participation and support, and re-

sources available and utilized by family (see Family Assessment, p. 55, for guidelines) (first visit).
2. Provide accurate information to family about treatment regimen and progress; allow time for questions and clarifications (each visit).
3. Encourage family to discuss strengths and options for change and to identify coping mechanisms used (each visit).
4. Include family members in teaching and planning of care (each visit).
5. Inform client of government and community agencies available for support and assistance (first visit).
6. Encourage family to contact counselor and to arrange for hospice care if appropriate (any visit).

CLIENT AND FAMILY/CAREGIVER INTERVENTIONS

1. Family verbalizes concerns and feelings about burden of caring for family member with long-term disorder.
2. Family seeks assistance if needed.
3. Family participates in planning and implementing care.
4. Family adapts to limitations of client and integrates them into family activity.
5. Family supports dialysis program.
6. Family continues family activities and open communication.

Nursing diagnosis

Anticipatory grieving

Related factors: Perceived potential loss of physiopsychosocial well-being

Defining characteristics: Altered sleep and communication patterns; sorrow; expression of distress at potential loss

OUTCOMES

Short-term

Progress in grieving, as evidenced by verbalization, attitude, and behavior changes manifested by stage in process (expected within days)

Long-term

Grief process resolving, as evidenced by resumption of life-style with or without changes as needed and by integration of grieving stage into life-style and activities (expected within 2 to 3 months and ongoing)

NURSING INTERVENTIONS/INSTRUCTIONS

1. Assess degree and stage of grief; include suicide potential (each visit).
2. Inform client of stages of grief and that client's behavior is acceptable for specific stage and that resolution will be final stage (first visit).
3. Allow expression of feelings about disabilities and potential loss and implications for the future (each visit).
4. Provide open communication and accepting environment for interactions (each visit).
5. Initiate referral for psychological or spiritual counseling (any visit).

CLIENT AND FAMILY/CAREGIVER INTERVENTIONS

1. Client progresses through grieving process to resolution.
2. Client seeks counseling as needed.

Nursing diagnosis

Knowledge deficit

Related factors: Lack of exposure to information about medical regimen

Defining characteristics: Request for information about dialysis and about care of abdominal site or arteriovenous fistula site

OUTCOMES

Short-term

Adequate knowledge, as evidenced by compliance with medication regimen, identification of signs and symptoms to report, and demonstration of shunt care or care of abdominal site for dialysis (expected within 1 week)

Long-term

Adequate knowledge, as evidenced by client's meeting requirements for a modified life-style without complications and maintaining optimal health and functioning within disease limitations (expected within 1 to 2 months)

NURSING INTERVENTIONS/INSTRUCTIONS

1. Instruct client in administration of prescribed drugs, including diuretics, exchange resins, sodium bicarbonate or citrate, antibiotics, and clofibrate; include dose, route, frequency, side effects, and fluid allotment (first visit).
2. Instruct client in measures for preventing constipation, including high-fiber diet and exercise (first visit).
3. Instruct client in measures to prevent infection, including hand washing, catheter care, avoiding persons with upper respiratory infections, and using sterile technique in shunt or peritoneal dialysis site care (first visit and reinforce on second visit).
4. Assess for cardiovascular changes (increased blood pressure, arrhythmias, visual changes), respiratory changes (decreased breath sounds, crackles, wheezes, chest pain, dyspnea, fever, restlessness), neurologic changes (lassitude, apathy, decreased mental acuity, paresthesias, muscle cramps, twitching, irritability, confusion), and hematologic changes (fatigue, pallor, easy bruising, petechiae, purpura, bleeding from any site) (each visit).
5. Assess for signs of hypocalcemia, including confusion, emotional lability, numbness, tingling or twitching of fingers or toes, Chvostek's sign or Trousseau's sign, muscle weakness, and stupor (each visit).
6. Instruct client to notify physician if symptoms increase in severity or any complications occur (first visit).
7. Instruct client in arteriovenous shunt or fistula care (first and second visits):
   - Avoid taking blood pressure or blood samples from affected arm.
   - Avoid carrying purse or heavy item over affected arm.
   - Avoid wearing tight clothing over affected arm.
   - Avoid tugging, pulling, or lying on affected arm.
8. Instruct client in dressing change at abdominal peritoneal site, and allow for return demonstration (first visit).

9. Instruct client to monitor patency of external shunt, including presence of bright red blood and a thrill or bruit on auscultation over site (first visit).
10. Instruct client to monitor patency of internal fistula, including checking pulsations at site (first visit).
11. Inform client of importance of compliance with total care regimen and of incorporation of regimen into daily activities (each visit).
12. Instruct client to follow up with physician and laboratory visits as scheduled; inform client of importance of dialysis schedule (each visit).
13. Instruct client to wear or carry identification information at all times, including condition and physician's name and telephone number (first visit).

CLIENT AND FAMILY/CAREGIVER INTERVENTIONS

1. Client complies with medication regimen.
2. Client manages constipation with diet and medication.
3. Client uses measures to prevent infection and other complications.
4. Client reports deteriorating condition or presence of signs and symptoms of complications associated with dialysis access site.
5. Client maintains patency of access site; takes measures to avoid injury to site.
6. Client maintains dialysis, physician, and laboratory appointments.
7. Client wears identification information for emergency care.
8. Client complies with total medical regimen and integrates into life-style.

Urinary Tract Infection (UTI)

Infection of the lower urinary tract (cystitis) is caused by gram-positive or gram-negative organisms that gain access to the bladder by sexual intercourse, urethral trauma, poor personal hygiene, or an indwelling catheter or by stasis of urine as a result of obstructive conditions, neurogenic bladder, or kidney disease. The condition is more common in women because of the proximity of the urethra to the vagina and anus. Cystitis may become chronic as microorganisms become resistant to therapy. Chronic cystitis is particularly common in elderly people who have indwelling catheters for long periods of time.

Home care is primarily concerned with the teaching of medication regimens to prevent or control recurrent bladder infections and possible spread to the kidneys.

Nursing diagnosis

Pain

Related factors: Biologic injuring agents (bacterial infection)

Defining characteristics: Communication of pain descriptors; urine culture positive for infectious organism; dysuria; cloudy and foul-smelling urine

OUTCOMES

Short-term

Minimal pain or decrease in pain, as evidenced by client's statement of compliance with urinary tract analgesic and antibiotic therapy (expected within 2 days)

Long-term

Absence of pain, as evidenced by completion of antibiotic regimen and increased comfort in lower abdomen and during urination (expected within 10 days)

NURSING INTERVENTIONS/INSTRUCTIONS

1. Assess client's pain, including site, duration, intensity, aggravating and alleviating factors, and characteristics associated with voiding (each visit).
2. Instruct client in administration of systemic antibiotics, urinary antiseptics, or urinary tract analgesics, including dose, frequency, side effects, and food, drug, and alcohol interactions; inform client that phenazopyridine may turn urine orange or orange-red and stain undergarments (first visit).

3. Instruct client in use of heating pad over suprapubic area or low back region and in use of sitz bath (first visit).

CLIENT AND FAMILY/CAREGIVER INTERVENTIONS

1. Client administers medications as instructed and for proper length of time.
2. Client applies heat for symptomatic relief.

Nursing diagnosis

Altered urinary elimination patterns

Related factors: Mechanical trauma of bladder infection

Defining characteristics: Dysuria; frequency; nocturia; urgency; urinary retention and stasis; small, frequent voidings

OUTCOMES

Short-term

Minimal urinary alteration, as evidenced by resumption of normal micturition pattern (expected within 2 days)

Long-term

Urinary elimination pattern within baseline and free from any abnormal changes (expected within 2 weeks)

NURSING INTERVENTIONS/INSTRUCTIONS

1. Perform renal and reproductive assessment (see Renal/Urinary System Assessment, p. 32, and Reproductive System Assessment, p. 39, for guidelines); note temperature and assess for history of UTI or renal problems, or presence of sexually transmitted diseases (first visit).
2. Instruct client to monitor pattern and frequency of voidings and characteristics of urine and to note pain or burning on urination, urgency, hesitancy, and force of flow (each visit).
3. Encourage client to consume up to 3000 ml of fluid per day if allowed (first visit).
4. Instruct client in acid-ash diet, including meat, fish, poultry, eggs, cheese, corn, cereals, cranberries, plums, and prunes; instruct client to avoid alcohol, caffeine, and pepper, since they aggravate symptoms (first visit).

CLIENT AND FAMILY/CAREGIVER INTERVENTIONS

1. Record all output and characteristics of urine, with symptomatology if present.
2. Drink 8 to 10 glasses of water or juice per day at regular intervals.
3. Include or avoid specific foods that affect condition.

Nursing diagnosis

Knowledge deficit

Related factors: Lack of exposure to information about infection

Defining characteristics: Request for information about medication administration and measures to prevent recurrence of infection

OUTCOMES

Short-term

Adequate knowledge, as evidenced by identification of and compliance with hygienic practices and medication regimen (expected within 3 days)

Long-term

Adequate knowledge, as evidenced by completion of medical regimen and hygienic measures to prevent recurrence (expected within 10 days)

NURSING INTERVENTIONS/INSTRUCTIONS

1. Instruct client in absolute necessity of taking full course of antibiotics even if symptoms disappear (first visit).
2. Instruct client in hygienic practices (first visit):
   - Wash with soap and water daily.
   - Void when urge is felt; do not delay, and void every 2 hours if possible.
   - Women should wipe from front to back.
   - Urinate after intercourse.
3. Instruct client to notify physician if symptoms persist or escalate or if flank pain or fever is present (first visit).
4. Suggest showers instead of tub baths (first visit).
5. Instruct female client to avoid use of feminine sprays and to wear cotton undergarments (first visit).

6. Advise client to have follow-up urine cultures if symptoms recur (last visit).

CLIENT AND FAMILY/CAREGIVER INTERVENTIONS

1. Client follows hygienic preventive procedures.
2. Client administers all medications as prescribed.
3. Client maintains consistency in daily care; avoids allowing irritating substances to come into contact with genital area.
4. Client collects midstream urine specimen and takes to laboratory if symptoms escalate or recur.

Integumentary system

Burns

Burns are injuries that destroy layers of the skin and, in some cases, underlying tissues. Burns are classified as partial thickness, which may be superficial (first degree) or deep (second degree) and which involve the dermis and epidermis, with potential for epithelial regeneration, and full thickness (third or fourth degree), which involve all skin layers, including nerve endings, as well as muscles, tendons, and bones, with scarring and loss of function, and which require skin grafting. With full thickness burns, all systems are affected: cardiovascular (impaired circulation and occluded blood supply), respiratory (edema and obstruction of the airway), renal (reduced blood flow to kidneys with ischemia), musculoskeletal (formation of scar tissue with contractures), neurologic (disorientation, withdrawal), gastrointestinal (stress ulcer), and endocrine (stress diabetes).

Home care is primarily concerned with the rehabilitation phase of burn care and includes teaching the client about the care and treatment of the healing wounds and supporting the client's compliance with the physical therapy regimen.

Nursing diagnosis

Pain

Related factors: Biologic injuring agents

Defining characteristics: Verbalization of pain descriptors; pain during physical therapy

OUTCOMES

Short-term

Pain minimized, as evidenced by performance of physical therapy with reduced pain (expected within 1 week)

Long-term

Absence of pain, as evidenced by ultimate restoration of function and by increased comfort during physical therapy (expected within 3 months or depending on extent of treatment)

NURSING INTERVENTIONS/INSTRUCTIONS

1. Assess pain severity during exercises and effect of pain on therapy in achieving function (first visit).
2. Assess itching of healing areas (first visit).
3. Administer analgesic and instruct client to take analgesic before therapy (first visit and when needed).

CLIENT AND FAMILY/CAREGIVER INTERVENTIONS

1. Client administers analgesic correctly.
2. Family supports client in physical therapy regimen.

Nursing diagnosis

Impaired skin integrity

Related factors: External factor of burn

Defining characteristics: Disruption of skin surface; destruction of skin layers; sensitivity of newly healed skin to slight pressure or trauma; itching and flaking during healing

OUTCOMES

Short-term

Preservation of skin integrity, as evidenced by healing with newly formed skin and nerve regeneration (expected within 1 week and ongoing)

Long-term

Absence of skin impairment, as evidenced by gradual return of function and new skin development (expected within 2 to 3 months, depending on extent of injury)

NURSING INTERVENTIONS/INSTRUCTIONS

1. Assess skin and grafted area for sensitivity to cold, heat, or touch; itching that occurs with healing; flaking; and formation of blisters with slight trauma (each visit).
2. Instruct client to apply topical antihistamine cream and palliative creams to itchy, dry, flaking skin on healed areas (first visit).
3. Instruct client to avoid direct sunlight and restrictive clothing (first visit).
4. Inform client of healing process, including discoloration and development of scar tissue with contours (first visit).
5. Instruct client in application of Jobst pressure garments for maintaining gentle pressure on the healed burn area and to wear 24 hours a day for possibly as long as 1 year (first visit).
6. Inform client that healing is usually complete within 6 weeks, with mature healing and return of suppleness and normal coloring within 6 to 12 months (first visit).
7. Instruct client in wound care and dressing changes using sterile technique (first and second visits).

CLIENT AND FAMILY/CAREGIVER INTERVENTIONS

1. Client protects healing skin from trauma and sensitivity reactions to cold, heat, sun, and excessive pressure or constriction.
2. Client applies topical medication to allay itching.
3. Client wears pressure garment continuously, as instructed.
4. Client performs dressing changes using sterile technique; notes and reports any drainage at wound edge or fluid under the graft.

Nursing diagnosis

Impaired physical mobility

Related factors: Pain and discomfort, musculoskeletal impairment, severe anxiety

Defining characteristics: Reluctance to attempt movement; limited range of motion; decreased muscle strength; muscle atrophy; contractures of major joints

OUTCOMES

Short-term

Adequate mobility, as evidenced by minimal discomfort during physical therapy and reduced risk for contracture formation of skin and underlying tissues (expected within 1 week)

Long-term

Adequate mobility and activity performance, as evidenced by skin healing and maturity, with the absence of contractures and client's acceptance of physical therapy as a part of daily living (expected within 2 to 3 months and ongoing)

NURSING INTERVENTIONS/INSTRUCTIONS

1. Assess client's ability for movement of all joints and muscles and ability to ambulate and perform activities of daily living (ADL) without assistance; note especially skin at neck area, axillae, antecubital spaces, fingers, groin, popliteal area, and ankles, as appropriate, for developing skin contractures and shortening of tendons and ligaments (each visit).
2. Perform and instruct client to perform active range-of-motion (ROM) exercises, muscle stretching, and ambulation progressively and concurrently with physical therapy (first visit and reinforce each visit).
3. Inform client of importance of continuous long-term physical therapy to achieve optimal function (first visit).
4. Refer to physical therapy and encourage client to comply with physical therapy program and to correlate with ADL and social and diversional activities (first and second visit).
5. Refer home health aide to assist with ADL as needed.

CLIENT AND FAMILY/CAREGIVER INTERVENTIONS

1. Client complies with daily rehabilitation program requirements and self-care activities, using assistive aids for eating, toileting, bathing, grooming, and dressing as needed.
2. Client performs joint and muscle exercises as instructed; takes analgesic before exercising.
3. Client notes and reports pain or resistance to exercising to therapist and possibly physician.

Nursing diagnosis

Body image disturbance

Related factors: Biophysical factor of effect of burns

Defining characteristics: Verbal and nonverbal response to change in body structure and function; negative feelings about body, scarring, deformity, disfigurement, discoloration, and contour of scarring; social isolation

OUTCOMES

Short-term

Improved adaptation to body image change, as evidenced by client's statement of feelings about changed appearance and limitations imposed by condition and need to change life-style until restoration of function is achieved (expected within 1 to 2 weeks)

Long-term

Optimal adaptation to body image change, as evidenced by client's statement of acceptance of appearance and by client's expression of ability to cope with life changes and meet needs for optimal health and functioning (expected within 2 to 3 months)

NURSING INTERVENTIONS/INSTRUCTIONS

1. Assess client's life-style, roles, and ability to adapt to and integrate long-term rehabilitation into treatment regimen (first visit).
2. Allow client to express feelings about appearance, loss of function, presence of any deformity or disfigurement, loss of control over life situations, and inability to meet role expectations (each visit).
3. Reassure client that feelings, anxiety, and expressions of concern are a normal part of adjustment to the changes in life-style that occur (first visit).
4. Encourage client to ask for help when needed, to identify strengths, and to suggest options for changing life-style, including ADL, social and occupational interactions, and recreation and leisure activities (any visit).
5. Assist client to identify coping mechanisms that have a positive effect on adjustment to body image changes (any visit).

6. Emphasize the positive aspects of rehabilitation and adjustment and what is achieved instead of what is not (each visit).
7. Assist client to identify clothing that will cover scarring or deformity as appropriate (first visit or as needed).
8. Refer client to counseling, occupational therapist, or social services as needed (any visit).
9. Refer to social worker for long-term planning and counseling (any visit).

CLIENT AND FAMILY/CAREGIVER INTERVENTIONS

1. Client verbalizes concern and feelings about appearance.
2. Client allows grieving over change in body image.
3. Client adapts to life-style change and frustrations of long-term treatment.
4. Client utilizes positive coping mechanisms with success.
5. Client adapts to change in appearance and limitations imposed by disability.
6. Client resumes close interpersonal relationships.
7. Client utilizes counseling and/or other services as needed.

Nursing diagnosis

Knowledge deficit

Related factors: Lack of information about long-term therapy

Defining characteristics: Request for information about risk of complications, nutritional needs, and long-term health maintenance

OUTCOMES

Short-term

Adequate knowledge, as evidenced by client's statement of basic needs for health promotion (expected within 1 week)

Long-term

Adequate knowledge, as evidenced by compliance with requirements to maintain optimal health and functioning (expected ongoing)

NURSING INTERVENTIONS/INSTRUCTIONS

1. Assess for daily basic needs based on progression toward wellness and past patterns (first visit).
2. Instruct client in need for scheduled rest periods, especially before or after physical therapy (first visit).
3. Instruct client in high-protein, high-calorie diet as appetite improves; refer client to dietitian if appropriate (first visit and reinforce on second visit).
4. Instruct client to assess for and report any redness, swelling, pain, or drainage at burn/healing site (first visit).
5. Inform client that cosmetic or reconstructive surgery may be needed if burn is extensive and tissue destruction is major; information should reinforce physician notification only (any visit).
6. Arrange visits from other burn victims for support if appropriate (any visit).

CLIENT AND FAMILY/CAREGIVER INTERVENTIONS

1. Assess and monitor would for infection and report to physician.
2. Provide suggested dietary inclusions and rest and sleep opportunities.
3. Promote morale and optimism during therapeutic regimen.
4. Express and fulfill daily basic needs for health maintenance.

Herpes Zoster

Herpes zoster is an acute, viral central nervous system infection that involves the dorsal root ganglia; it is characterized by painful skin eruptions in areas supplied by peripheral sensory nerves that arise in the affected ganglia.

Home care is primarily concerned with the relief of pain and discomfort and with teaching the client about medication administration and treatment of prolonged neuralgia.

Nursing diagnosis

Pain

Related factors: Biologic injuring agents

Defining characteristics: Communication of pain descriptors (severity, location, duration); guarding and protective behavior toward affected area(s); self-focusing; restlessness

OUTCOMES

Short-term

Increased comfort, as evidenced by client's statement that pain is decreased or absent (expected within 2 to 3 days)

Long-term

Absence of or minimal pain, with decreased incidence of recurrent episodes and achievement of optimal health and functioning without pain (1 to 2 months)

NURSING INTERVENTIONS/INSTRUCTIONS

1. Assess pain, burning, or neuralgia on side of trunk or other area; assess severity of pain before and during outbreak of vesicles (first visit).
2. Instruct client in administration of oral medications to reduce pain (analgesics), inflammation (steroids), and itching (antihistamines) (first visit).
3. Instruct client in application of topical medication to reduce itching and promote healing and comfort (calamine lotion, zinc oxide, benzoin, steroids) (first visit).
4. Apply wet, cool compresses or cool sprays, and instruct client in application (first visit).
5. Instruct client to take warm tub baths with Burow's solution and to avoid rubbing skin dry, extremes in temperature or pressure against painful area, and tight clothing around area (first visit).
6. Instruct client in diversional therapy, such as music, relaxation techniques, and guided imagery (each visit).
7. Instruct client to avoid lying on affected area (first visit).

CLIENT AND FAMILY/CAREGIVER INTERVENTIONS

1. Client administers medications correctly and effectively.

2. Client reports prolonged pain to physician.
3. Client maintains calm environment including diversion from pain.
4. Client avoids actions that cause or trigger pain, including rubbing, pressure or temperature extremes, and scratching.

Nursing diagnosis

Knowledge deficit

Related factors: Lack of information about disease

Defining characteristics: Expressed need for information about disease causes and treatment and prevention of complications

OUTCOMES

Short-term

Adequate knowledge, as evidenced by client's statement of cause, treatments, and prognosis for the disease (expected within 1 week)

Long-term

Adequate knowledge, as evidenced by client's meeting requirements to achieve optimal level of health by compliance with the treatment regimen (expected within 1 month)

NURSING INTERVENTIONS/INSTRUCTIONS

1. Assess client's life-style and ability to adapt, learning abilities and interests, readiness to learn, and family participation and support (first visit).
2. Inform client of cause, course, and unpredictability of the disease, and exacerbations in clear, honest language (first visit).
3. Instruct client in care of lesions and to prevent infection by avoiding scratching, touching, picking, or squeezing lesions (first visit).
4. Instruct client in hand washing and precautions to take (skin and protective isolation) if needed (first visit and thereafter).
5. Inform client of rest requirements and that inadequate rest may lengthen course of illness; instruct client to schedule rest periods and provide a stress-free, quiet environment (each visit).

6. Inform client of importance of nutrition and fluid requirements; instruct client to note and report weight loss (first visit).
7. Instruct client in antibiotic therapy to prevent or treat infection (first visit).

CLIENT AND FAMILY/CAREGIVER INTERVENTIONS

1. Client maintains measures to prevent infection and to meet fluid, nutrition, and rest requirements for healing lesions.
2. Client complies with medication regimen correctly.
3. Client provides restful, stress-free environment.
4. Client verbalizes cause of the disease, methods of transmission, and methods for control of disease manifestations and prevention of exacerbations or sequelae.
5. Client cares for lesions and takes steps to prevent infection.

Pressure Ulcers

Pressure ulcers (bedsores) are caused by the breakdown of the epidermal and underlying structures as a result of excessive pressure or shearing forces. Areas usually affected are the bony prominences. The risk for pressure ulcer is increased in those who are immobilized or malnourished or who have altered sensation or circulation or fecal or urinary incontinence.

Home care is primarily concerned with the care and teaching aspects of pressure ulcer prevention and control and with the healing of existing ulcers.

Nursing diagnosis

Impaired skin integrity

Related factors: External factors of pressure, shearing; internal factors of nutrition, circulation, level of consciousness, sensation

Defining characteristics: Redness, warmth at pressure area; disruption of skin, with pain, swelling, heat, induration, drainage, and tissue necrosis, depending on stage of pressure ulcer

OUTCOMES

Short-term

Reduction in skin impairment, as evidenced by absence of blanching, hyperemia, or disruption in skin over stress areas (expected within 2 weeks)

Long-term

Absence of skin impairment despite immobilization, negative nitrogen balance, incontinence, or impaired innervation or circulation (expected within 1 month and ongoing)

NURSING INTERVENTIONS/INSTRUCTIONS

1. Assess skin, creases, folds, and bony prominences, including color, temperature, tone, turgor, and integrity; note presence of edema, irritation, maceration, excoriation, induration, ulceration, drainage, or necrosis (each visit).
2. Locate and measure pressure ulcers, and document degree of breakdown (each visit).
3. Instruct client in hygienic measures, including personal and skin care, bathing and cleansing after toileting, and taking sponge bath in bed (first visit).
4. Instruct client in positioning in bed or sitting (first visit).
5. Instruct client in ROM exercises and in use of prophylactic and palliative measures, including pillows, heel and elbow guards, sheepskin, and air or fluid mattress and pads (each visit).
6. Apply protective topical agent and dressing as prescribed; irrigate pressure ulcer with sterile saline, and apply debriding agent as prescribed; instruct client in medication and dressing changes (each visit).
7. Massage bony prominences; avoid pulling or sliding client in bed if client is on bed rest (each visit).

CLIENT AND FAMILY/CAREGIVER INTERVENTIONS

1. Client maintains clean, dry skin; bathes daily with mild soap; rinses well and pats dry.
2. Client pads and protects heels, elbows, back of head, iliac crests, sacrococcygeal area; applies emollient to intact skin.
3. Client maintains clean bed, free of wrinkles and crumbs.
4. Client uses footboard and bed cradle as appropriate.

5. Client positions self hourly using overhead bar if able.
6. Family/caregiver positions every 2 hours; massages pressure areas; performs ROM exercises.
7. Client exposes pressure ulcer to air, light, and heat for prescribed intervals.
8. Caregiver avoids shearing forces when moving client; lifts and rolls instead of pulling or sliding.

Nursing diagnosis

Knowledge deficit

Related factors: Lack of information about care and prevention of pressure ulcer

Defining characteristics: Request for information about cleansing, dressing, heat application, and preventive measures to avoid new pressure ulcer formation or further breakdown of existing ulcer

OUTCOMES

Short-term

Adequate knowledge, as evidenced by client's statement about causes of skin breakdown and care to prevent or treat pressure ulcer (expected within 1 week)

Long-term

Adequate knowledge, as evidenced by client's compliance with medical regimen and meeting requirements for adaptation of activities of daily living to achieve optimal health and skin integrity (expected within 1 month)

NURSING INTERVENTIONS/INSTRUCTIONS

1. Assess client's nutrition and neurologic status for obesity or thinness, state of consciousness, paralysis, incontinence, immobility, and use of sedatives or tranquilizers (each visit).
2. Assess client's weight weekly and compare with actual and ideal weight (any visit).
3. Encourage and instruct client in high-calorie, high-protein diet with adequate fluid intake (2 L per day) as appropriate (first visit).

4. Institute bowel and bladder training program if indicated (each visit).
5. Instruct client in prescribed treatments for skin area and their frequency, such as massage, padding, heat application, cleansing and dressing area, and postition changes (first visit and reinforce on second visit).
6. Inform client of use and availability of cushions, egg crate or alternating pressure mattresses, or rice or bean bags to relieve pressure on skin (first visit).

CLIENT AND FAMILY/CAREGIVER INTERVENTIONS

1. Client maintains hydration and well-balanced meals that include protein and vitamin C; takes supplements as needed.
2. Client avoids medications that affect awareness and consciousness.
3. Caregiver offers toileting every 2 to 3 hours while client is awake; provides measures to prevent urine or bowel incontinence, or applies device to prevent exposure to the skin.
4. Client reports progressive skin breakdown that occurs in spite of preventive measures.
5. Client changes position and utilizes aids to reduce pressure on skin.

Psoriasis

Psoriasis is a noninflammatory chronic dermatologic condition in which many silvery, scaly-appearing red papules and plaques appear at bony prominences. The condition may affect any part of the body, including hands, feet, ears, nails, back, buttocks, and scalp. Recurrence may result from local trauma, environmental factors, withdrawal from systemic corticosteroids, emotional stress, or infection.

Home care is primarily concerned with the teaching aspects of treatments, resulting in comfort and prevention of exacerbation of the condition.

Nursing diagnosis

Impaired skin integrity

Related factors: Alterations in skin by dermatitis

Defining characteristics: Scales and plaques over any part of body; possible itching or scratching; disruption of skin surfaces

OUTCOMES

Short-term

Minimal skin impairment from eruptions, as evidenced by client's compliance with prescribed skin care and reduction of symptoms (expected within 1 week)

Long-term

Absence of skin impairment, as evidenced by adaptive life-style changes to minimize recurrences, continued compliance with prescribed skin regimen, and intact and lesion-free integument (expected within 4 to 6 weeks)

NURSING INTERVENTIONS/INSTRUCTIONS

1. Assess skin for color, integrity, and presence of papules, plaques, or pustules; include location, extent and distribution (see Integumentary System Assessment, p. 36, (each visit).
2. Relate skin manifestations to implications of prescribed drug use (each visit).
3. Instruct client in skin care and application of topical petrolatum-based emollients and combinations of topical corticosteroids, salicylic acid, crude coal tar, or anthralin preparations as prescribed (first visit and reinforce on second visit).
4. Instruct client in scalp care, including loosening and removal of scales, use of tar shampoo, and application of topical steroids (first visit).
5. Instruct client in medication administration (first visit).
6. Apply and instruct client in application of occlusive wraps, avoiding exposure of eye or other sensitive area to medications (first visit).
7. Inform client of methods to minimize staining of garments (first visit).

8. Administer and instruct in alternate therapies, such as light therapy alone or in conjunction with medication, photochemotherapy, and protection of sensitive areas (first visit).
9. Instruct client in practices regarding teratogenic drugs and effect of systemic antimetabolites or oral retinoids on hepatic, renal, and hematopoietic systems; monitor for toxicities (each visit).
10. Provide clear written instructions for all skin care and medication protocols (first visit and review on second visit).

CLIENT AND FAMILY/CAREGIVER INTERVENTIONS

1. Client takes tub baths instead of showers for 15 to 20 minutes daily and applies topical preparations to damp skin.
2. Client uses written protocol for scheduling time, type, and method of topical medications; administers as directed.
3. Client applies salicylic acid to affected areas on scalp at bedtime; sleeps with shower cap on.
4. Client loosens scales on scalp in morning, shampoos with tar preparation, and follows with topical steroid preparation.
5. Client uses salicylic acid on affected areas only; avoids use of plastic occlusive wrap with coal tar or anthralin application.
6. Client applies topical steroid with occlusive plastic dressing; modifies vinyl jogging suit for fuller body coverage.
7. Client applies anthralin with gloves to affected area only with a downward motion and wears old clothes; avoids contact with eyes or other sensitive areas.
8. Client avoids sunlight and artificial light for 24 hours following photochemotherapy; wears full protective ultraviolet filtering glasses.
9. Client follows planned schedule and family planning practices before, during, and following therapies using retinoids and methotrexate.
10. Client consults with physician when needed for clarification and assistance in therapies.

Nursing diagnosis

Knowledge deficit

Related factors: Lack of information about disorder

Defining characteristics: Request for information about skin disruptions, cause, treatments, and prevention of exacerbations

OUTCOMES

Short-term

Adequate knowledge, as evidenced by client's identification of measures to take to minimize recurrence and to comply with skin care and medication protocols (expected within 3 days)

Long-term

Adequate knowledge, as evidenced by client's meeting requirements for changes in life-style and medical regimen to achieve optimal level of health and functioning (expected within 2 weeks)

NURSING INTERVENTIONS/INSTRUCTIONS

1. Inform family members and/or caretakers that condition is not contagious (first visit).
2. Inform client of cause of condition and that although it is chronic, it does not affect overall health and that control of condition is possible in most cases (first visit).
3. Instruct client in general measures to reduce recurrence (first visit).
4. Identify support systems, and refer client to psychological counseling if indicated for coping, effects on body image and self-concept, and feelings of loss, grief, or isolation (any visit).
5. Refer client to social services for assistance with occupation changes (first visit).
6. Refer client to National Psoriasis Foundation for information and support (first visit).

CLIENT AND FAMILY/CAREGIVER INTERVENTIONS

1. Client verbalizes chronicity and limitations imposed by condition.
2. Client actively employs general measures to reduce relapses or recurrences: avoids skin injury or irritation; avoids overexposure to sunlight; manages emotional stress constructively; and avoids infections.
3. Consult with appropriate agencies or individuals for assistance, information, and support.

Reproductive system

Mastectomy

Mastectomy, or the surgical removal of a breast, is usually done to treat breast malignancy. A radical mastectomy is the removal of an entire breast, including the pectoral muscles, the lymph nodes of the axilla, and the pectoral fascia; a modified radical mastectomy does not include the pectoral muscles and pectoral fascia; a simple mastectomy is the surgical removal of an entire breast. Mastectomy may be followed by the surgical reconstruction of the breast (mammoplasty).

Home care is primarily concerned with functional maintenance of the operative side and with the psychological consequences of such a loss.

Nursing diagnosis

Body image disturbance

Related factors: Loss of body part; psychosocial effect on self-concept, sexuality

Defining characteristics: Verbalization of actual change in structure of body part, missing breast, disfigurement, significance of part in regard to sexual function and desirability, negative feelings about body, change in social involvement

OUTCOMES

Short-term

Progressive improvement in body image and adaptation to changes in function and structure, as evidenced by client's ventilating feelings, expressing concerns, and considering prosthetic purchase, reconstructive surgery, and sexual activity alterations (expected within 1 to 2 weeks)

Long-term

Optimal acceptance of changes in body structure, with positive self-concept and body image (expected within 1 to 2 months)

NURSING INTERVENTIONS/INSTRUCTIONS

1. Assess client's mental and emotional status and ability to adapt and cope (see Psychosocial Assessment, p. 48, for guidelines) (first visit).
2. Accept feelings of mutilation, grief, depression, and anxiety as result of surgery (each visit).
3. Allow time and opportunity for client to ventilate feelings, express concerns, and ask questions. Note nonverbal as well as verbal cues for assistance to communicate feelings (each visit).
4. Explore client perception of effect of breast loss on self-concept, self-image, and sexuality (first and second visits).
5. Give specific and accurate information about sexual activity (third or fourth visit):
   - Fear of exposure, rejection, or pain is common.
   - Sexual activity may be resumed in 4 to 6 weeks with physician approval.
   - Initial use of breast prosthesis during sexual activity may be a transitory buffer.
   - Instruction in sensate focusing can increase awareness of other sensitive and erotic zones.
6. Discuss availability of a proper prosthesis; include types of prostheses, emotional readiness for fitting, clothing to be worn when shopping for prosthesis, and cost (first visit).
7. Initiate referral to counseling if appropriate (fourth or fifth visit).
8. Refer to occupational therapy as needed.

CLIENT AND FAMILY/CAREGIVER INTERVENTIONS

1. Client verbalizes feelings and concerns; asks questions if needed.
2. Client participates in personal care and grooming; selects clothing that enhances body image without revealing prosthesis.
3. Client initiates purchase of a breast prosthesis.
4. Client considers sexual options, with gradual resumption of activity and satisfaction.

5. Client considers reconstructive breast surgery; speaks with others who have had this surgery.

Nursing diagnosis

Fluid volume excess

Related factors: Compromised regulatory mechanisms

Defining characteristics: Lymphedema in arm on operative side; fear or refusal to exercise arm and shoulder

OUTCOMES

Short-term

Minimal or absence of fluid accumulation in operative arm, as evidenced by arm circumference at baseline measurements and client's compliance with postoperative mastectomy exercises (expected within 1 to 2 weeks)

Long-term

Adequate lymph drainage with absence of arm swelling, optimal fluid balance, and full range of motion in arm on operative side (expected within 1 to 2 months)

NURSING INTERVENTIONS/INSTRUCTIONS

1. Assess operative site, chest wall, posture, bilateral upper arm circumference (6 cm above elbow), and complaints of arm heaviness (each visit).
2. Assess ability of client to demonstrate hospital exercise regimen for baseline; note instructions given at discharge (first visit).
3. Encourage self-care in activities of daily living (bathing, grooming, dressing, washing and brushing hair) (first and second visits).
4. Demonstrate and establish an activity and exercise regimen as ordered (first visit).
   Avoid strenuous activity and heavy lifting or carrying until sutures are removed and incision is healed.
   Begin resumption of light tasks at home and work as tolerated.
   Exercise regularly, three or four times a day; stop when pulling or pain occurs, and resume when discomfort ceases.

Practice fist clenching, shoulder rotation, hand climbing up and down wall, hand swinging, and abduction exercises of arm.

Rest affected arm above heart level; elevate arm during sleep.

5. Initiate referral to a structured postmastectomy exercise program such as that offered by a physical therapist or YWCA's Encore.

CLIENT AND FAMILY/CAREGIVER INTERVENTIONS

1. Client participates in self-care, including activities that involve raising the arms over the head.
2. Client performs exercises three or four times per day; takes analgesic before exercise if needed; stops and rests between exercises when needed.
3. Client resumes household, occupational, and recreational tasks and activities.
4. Client participates in community-sponsored programs for rehabilitation or physical therapy.
5. Client uses pneumatic sleeve or elastic arm stocking to relieve edema.

Nursing diagnosis

Knowledge deficit

Related factors: Lack of knowledge about disease and postoperative care

Defining characteristics: Request for information on and instruction in postoperative care regimen and chemotherapy regimen

OUTCOMES

Short-term

Adequate knowledge, as evidenced by client's statements about disease, treatment expectation and progression, and measures to prevent injury or infection (expected within 1 week)

Long-term

Adequate knowledge, as evidenced by compliance with treatment regimens, resulting in optimal health and return to optimal functioning (expected within 1 month).

NURSING INTERVENTIONS/INSTRUCTIONS

1. Assess life-style, ability to adapt, learning abilities, and family participation and support (first visit).
2. Assess operative site for size, color, temperature, approximation of edges of incision, presence of drainage, and need for dressing change (each visit).
3. Instruct client to notify physician of changes in incisional area or temperature elevation (first visit).
4. Assess changes in vital signs, posture, gait, balance, and use of operative side (each visit).
5. Instruct client in administration of analgesics, including dose, frequency, side effects, and food, drug, and alcohol interactions; differentiate between operative and phantom breast pain, numbness and pins-and-needles sensation in area, and advise that these will eventually disappear (first visit).
6. Instruct client in measures to prevent or minimize injury or infection, to protect arm from exposure and bumping, and to have all blood pressure checks, injections, and blood withdrawals done on unaffected arm (first visit and reinforce on second visit).
7. Avoid any burns, cuts, nicks, scratches, or insect bites or stings of affected arm on operative side (first visit).
8. Instruct client to wear clothing over arm that is protective, loose, and nonrestrictive and to avoid carrying purse or parcels with arm on affected side (first visit).
9. Instruct client to always cleanse all skin breaks and apply antiseptic and to notify physician if arm becomes red, hot, or swollen (first visit).
10. Discuss and provide written information about prescribed adjuvant therapy, such as chemotherapy or radiation, and inform client of protocols regarding these treatments and when to appear at clinic or agency for therapy (each visit).
11. Demonstrate and instruct client in breast self-examination (BSE) for remaining breast and to perform examination each month after menstrual period or if menopausal (third or fourth visit).
12. Instruct client to keep physician appointments and to have yearly mammogram, and ultrasound if needed, on remaining breast (fourth visit).
13. Initiate referral to support groups such as Reach for Recov-

ery, I Can Cope, or psychological counseling if appropriate (first visit).

CLIENT AND FAMILY/CAREGIVER INTERVENTIONS

1. Client monitors wound healing and notifies physician of changes at site or fever.
2. Client administers analgesic for pain and verbalizes pain descriptors and causes.
3. Client prevents any injury to arm on operative side; protects and supports arm as needed.
4. Client reads and interprets written information on adjuvant therapies and asks questions to clarify information and modify behaviors.
5. Client performs monthly BSE correctly and has yearly mammogram.
6. Client keeps appointments with physician and for therapies and tests.
7. Client participates in support group and/or counseling focusing on breast diseases and surgery.

Eye, ear, nose, and throat

Auditory/Visual Impairment

Auditory impairment is the inability to hear adequately as a result of the aging process (presbycusis) or other physical or psychological condition. Visual impairment is the inability to see adequately as a result of the aging process (presbyopia) or other physical or psychological condition. Each type of loss imposes life-style changes upon an individual that require the use of an aid (hearing aid or glasses) to compensate for the impairment.

Home care is primarily concerned with teaching of the use and care of sensory aids and with prevention of injury as a result of the deficit.

Nursing diagnosis

Altered sensory perception (auditory, visual)

Related factors: Chronic illness; aging; neurologic disease or deficit; altered status of sense organ; psychologic stress

Defining characteristics: Hypoxia; electrolyte imbalance; use of drugs that affect the central nervous system (stimulants or depressants, mind altering); anxiety (narrowed perceptual fields); visual and auditory distortions; change in usual response to stimuli; expressed impairment in auditory and/or visual perception

OUTCOMES

Short-term

Adequate sensory perception, as evidenced by client's awareness of need for life-style changes to compensate for auditory or visual loss (expected within 3 to 7 days)

Long-term

Optimal sensory perception, as evidenced by incorporation of lifestyle changes into activities of daily living and other activities to achieve health and functioning within identified limitations (expected within 1 month)

NURSING INTERVENTIONS/INSTRUCTIONS

1. Assess sensory abilities, limitations in activities of daily living imposed by sensory loss, and need for supplementary aids (see Eye, Ear, Nose, and Throat Assessment, p. 45 for guidelines) (first visit).
2. Interact with client in well-lit, quiet room free from external distractions, and allow time to process communication and respond (each visit).
3. Use as many sensory modalities as the client is comfortable with (each visit).
4. When communicating with a hearing-impaired individual (each visit):

   Avoid covering mouth or chewing gum when speaking.

   Face client.

   Speak slowly and clearly; avoid shouting; a lower-pitched voice may help.

   Repeat instruction or conversation if client does not respond or responds inappropriately.

   Be sure hearing aid is turned on if present or that hearing aid is used.
5. When communicating with a visually impaired individual (each visit):

   Announce arrival and departure.

   Use touch only if indicating that you will do so and if client does not object.

   Include client in all conversation, and speak in moderate tone.

   Sit directly in front of client, in a well-lit room.

   Be sure glasses or contact lenses are used.
6. Encourage use of assistive aids or devices, such as large-print reading material or Braille, large-numbered telephone dials, amplified telephone box, and closed-caption or narrative TV (first visit).
7. Instruct client about importance of annual examination for eye or ear disorders or deficits (first visit).

8. Instruct client in administration of eyedrops, ointments, eardrops, or other prescribed treatments (first visit).
9. Support referral to community resources for assistance and information (first visit).

CLIENT AND FAMILY/CAREGIVER INTERVENTIONS

1. Family members and/or caregiver use communication skills that are meaningful for client with a particular sensory deficit.
2. Client uses supplementary and assistive aids.
3. Client consults physician about changes in perception and for yearly or more frequent examinations.
4. Client seeks out community resources that assist hearing or visually impaired individuals and families.

Nursing diagnosis

Risk for trauma

Related factors: Poor vision or hearing; lack of safety precautions and education

Defining characteristics: Request for information on preventing falls or other injury; reluctance to engage in activities (self-care and social)

OUTCOMES

Short-term

Absence of injury, as evidenced by compliance with safety precautions and use of assistive aids (expected within 2 days)

Long-term

Maintenance of optimal health and functioning without injury (expected within 2 weeks and thereafter)

NURSING INTERVENTIONS/INSTRUCTIONS

1. Assist client in identifying limitations and safety hazards in the environment (first visit).
2. Assess ability of client to solve problems and to resolve these threats to safety (first visit).
3. Instruct client and family to provide and maintain clear path-

ways, remove throw rugs and clutter, and maintain intact cords and electrical appliances (first visit).

4. Instruct family to provide constant, adequate, well-distributed, glare-free light in all rooms and to place night-light in bathroom (first visit).
5. Instruct client to take time when adjusting to changes in light intensity, especially when climbing stairs (first visit).
6. Emphasize importance of using aids at all times (first visit).
7. Supply client with a list of available supplemental aids for telephone, reading material, doorbell, and others specific to client (first visit).
8. Instruct family and client to retain furniture placement and familiarity of environment and to provide rails or objects to hold on to when moving about (first visit).

CLIENT AND FAMILY/CAREGIVER INTERVENTIONS

1. Client identifies hazards and eliminates or modifies them.
2. Client allows time for all activities; seeks assistance when needed.
3. Client uses assistive and supplemental aids.
4. Client maintains familiar environment; obtains assistance from trained pet for hearing or vision if appropriate.

Cataract Removal and Lens Implantation

Cataract removal is the surgical removal of a lens that has become cloudy or opaque, causing visual impairment. Cataract development may be caused by senile degeneration, congenital trauma, disease (diabetes mellitus), or drug therapy (corticosteroids). The method of removing a cataract depends on a client's particular type of cataract and particular eye, and the time for removal is determined by the extent of impairment experienced (reading, driving, participation in activities). A cataract may be removed by intracapsular extraction, in which the entire lens is removed, including the capsule that surrounds it, by touching the lens with a cold probe that freezes the lens and then removes it from the eye.

Another method is extracapsular extraction, in which the back portion of the capsule is left behind to help secure an intraocular lens implant and hold the vitreous fluid in proper position inside the eye. A third method is extracapsular extraction in which the cataract is broken into small particles by ultrasound and then suctioned out of the eye. A hard or soft lens may be implanted to replace the lens that has been removed. An alternative to the intraocular lens implant is the use of cataract glasses or contact lenses.

Home care is primarily concerned with the teaching of medication regimens (eyedrops and ointment) and measures to prevent complications of infection, glaucoma, retinal detachment, or corneal damage.

Nursing diagnosis

Altered sensory perception (visual)

Related factors: Altered status of sense organ

Defining characteristics: Bandaged eye; reduced visual acuity in nonoperative eye; change in visual acuity until operative eye stabilizes

OUTCOMES

Short-term

Improved visual acuity in operative eye, as evidenced by client's statements that vision is improving to baseline expectation and by compliance with postoperative eye medication regimen (expected within 3 days)

Long-term

Return of visual acuity and stabilization, as evidenced by return to 20/20 or 20/30 vision (expected within 4 weeks)

NURSING INTERVENTIONS/INSTRUCTIONS

1. Announce your presence when entering room while client's eye is covered; use normal tone of voice (each visit).
2. Advise client that someone should be in attendance while anesthesia is metabolized and eye is covered (first visit).

3. Inform client of activities that require assistance and determine if referral for home health aide is needed (first visit).
4. Inform client of postoperative visits to physician on first, second, and seventh postoperative days for examination of operative eye and possible suture removal (first visit).
5. Inform client of visual progression (first visit):
   - Dark glasses may be suggested to reduce glare.
   - New prescription for lens in glasses on operative eye may be secured.
   - Diplopia may result after unilateral correction.
   - Use of interim glasses will result in clear central vision only, and head must be turned to bring peripheral objects into central vision.
   - Depth perception will be affected if one eye covered or implant not performed.
   - Contact lenses may be used in some instances and require fewer adaptations.
   - If lens is not implanted, permanent lenses in glasses will be prescribed 4 to 12 weeks postoperatively.
   - Gradual adaptation and full adjustment occur for optimal vision.

CLIENT AND FAMILY/CAREGIVER INTERVENTIONS

1. Client participates in activities of daily living (ADL) and other activities (driving, reading, TV) within 1 week of surgery with physician recommendation.
2. Client wears corrective lenses as prescribed.
3. Client notifies physician if vision changes or decreases.
4. Client complies with postoperative physician visits until discharged.

Nursing diagnosis

Knowledge deficit

Related factors: Lack of exposure to information about postoperative care

Defining characteristics: Request for information about medication regimen to prevent infection, prevent increased intraocular pressure, and reduce inflammation and about protection of eye from trauma

OUTCOMES

Short-term

Adequate knowledge, as evidenced by client's stating responsibilities to be carried out postoperatively to prevent complications (expected within 2 to 3 days)

Long-term

Adequate knowledge, as evidenced by absence of infection, glaucoma, or trauma of operative eye and by compliance with treatment regimen (expected within 4 weeks)

NURSING INTERVENTIONS/INSTRUCTIONS

1. Inspect eye after dressing removed; note color, and check for edema and presence of purulent drainage (each visit).
2. Assess for return of vision and increased acuity (each visit).
3. Assess for headache or pain and severity; instruct client to notify physician if pain sharp and sudden and not relieved (first visit).
4. Instruct client in eye care (cleansing from inner to outer area), hand washing, and administration of eyedrops and eye ointment (steroids, antibiotics, mydriatics), and include dose, technique, frequency, side effects, and implications for activity (first visit).
5. Instruct client to protect eye with shield during sleep for 1 week after physician removes initial dressing and shield (first visit).
6. Instruct client to avoid lifting, stooping, straining, bending, rubbing or bumping eye, or sneezing; instruct client to use stool softener and/or cough suppressant if needed (first visit).
7. Instruct client in positioning during sleep: rest on back or on nonoperative side; avoid lying flat; use small pillow or raise head of bed with foam-rubber wedge (first visit).
8. Instruct client to ambulate carefully to avoid bumping or jostling (first visit).
9. Instruct client to use eye medications until entire amount is administered or to follow physician's instructions for length of therapy (first visit).

CLIENT AND FAMILY/CAREGIVER INTERVENTIONS

1. Client performs medical asepsis procedures before eye care and medication administration.
2. Client uses warm compress to remove discharge from operative eye.
3. Client protects eye with shield, glasses, or both.
4. Client avoids activities that will cause injury or increase intraocular pressure.
5. Client participates in ADL with assistance if needed or independently.
6. Client instills eyedrops or applies eye ointment correctly and safely, as instructed and prescribed.
7. Client rests and sleeps in optimal position without placing pressure on eye.
8. Client reports any sudden pain or change in vision to physician immediately.

Psychiatric care plans

Alcohol/Drug Abuse

Alcohol or drug abuse is a progressive disorder that affects all body systems. It can precipitate cirrhosis of the liver, esophageal varicies, coma, and death. Several theories describe the alcoholic or drug abuser as having a fixed outlook, retarded emotional development, poor impulse control, chronic low self-esteem, and low frustration tolerance and as being highly dependent. Serious family dysfunction can contribute to alcohol or drug abuse.

Home care primarily focuses on the teaching of a medication regimen and on life-style changes

Nursing diagnosis

Altered thought process

Related factors: Physiologic changes; impaired judgment

Defining characteristics: Inaccurate interpretation of environment; distractibility; egocentricity; hypervigilance or hypovigilance

OUTCOMES

Short-term

Adequate thought process, as evidenced by client's identifying correctly activities happening in his or her environment and by client's being oriented to surroundings after prompting by health care worker (expected in 3 days)

Long-term

Adequate thought processes, as evidenced by client verbalizing that alcohol or drugs have caused alteration in thought (expected in 2 months)

NURSING INTERVENTIONS/INSTRUCTIONS

1. Assess for memory deficits (long, short) by asking questions about the past and the present (first visit).
2. Provide an unhurried, patient, reassuring approach to the client that is both positive and empathetic (each visit).
3. Assist in helping the client to order recent events according to time sequence. Provide support for correct answers (each visit).
4. Explore with the client his or her perception of self; reinforce reality when appropriate (each visit).
5. Plan and implement a consistent approach to the client's care (each visit).
6. Repeat for the client instructions or information; ask the client to restate information in his or her own words (each visit).
7. Use patterns of recall (each visit).
8. Limit sensory input and choices to decrease distractions and frustrations (each visit).
9. Ask the client to make realistic commitments, and hold the client accountable for fulfillment of commitments (any visit).

CLIENT AND FAMILY/CAREGIVER INTERVENTIONS

1. Family maintains calm, caring attitude during treatment; stays with client.
2. Client attempts to prevent or discourage stressful situations.
3. Client develops and uses effective coping skills that decrease anxiety.

Nursing diagnosis

Ineffective individual coping

Related factors: Personal vulnerability; difficulty handling new situations; previous ineffective or inadequate coping skills; inadequate coping skills, with substitution of alcohol, anxiety, fear

Defining characteristics: Verbalization of inability to cope or inability to ask for help; inability to meet role expectations; inability to meet basic needs; inability to solve problems; alteration in societal participation; destructive behavior toward self or others; inappropriate use of defense mechanisms; change in usual communication patterns; verbal manipulation

OUTCOMES

Short-term

Effective individual coping, as evidenced by client's attending support group (such as Alcoholics Anonymous) and verbalizing relationship of alcohol or drug abuse to difficulty in present life situation (expected within 7 days)

Long-term

Effective individual coping, as evidenced by client's making necessary life-style changes (expected within 2 months)

NURSING INTERVENTIONS/INSTRUCTIONS

1. Assess for psychosomatic symptoms; sleep, eating, bowel problems (each visit).
2. Assess support system, how the system functions, and if it is adequate (first visit).
3. Establish rapport, show acceptance of the person, and establish a positive relationship with him or her (each visit).
4. Reduce the number of decisions that the client must make, including the need to solve problems (first visit).
5. Allow client sufficient time to make decisions; start with decisions that have only two options (first and second visits).
6. Discuss alternative ways of coping; allow these new coping techniques to be tried in a safe, nondestructive environment (each visit).
7. Use positive rather than negative reinforcement during the testing of new coping mechanisms (each visit).
8. Allow client time to verbalize feelings of denial, anger, guilt, or grief regarding crisis situation (each visit).
9. Acknowledge the validity of fear and other feelings (each visit).
10. Encourage client to talk about the changes the crisis will cause (each visit).
11. Listen and clarify the client's perception of the crisis situation (each visit).
12. Assist client to sort out the facts concerning the crisis (any visit).
13. Assist client in seeking and accepting help, and provide referral to psychiatrist or psychologist if needed (each visit).

14. Identify defense mechanisms used and whether they are being used positively or negatively. Reinforce positive coping mechanisms that have been successfully used in the past but that are not being used now (any visit).

CLIENT AND FAMILY/CAREGIVER INTERVENTIONS

1. Client includes the family in sorting out information regarding the crisis.
2. Client discusses with the family the need to avoid judgments regarding the client's behavior.
3. Client refers family to Al-Anon or other support group.

Nursing diagnosis

Knowledge deficit

Related factors: Lack of recall; misinterpretation of information; cognitive limitation; lack of interest in learning

Defining characteristics: Verbalization of the problem; inappropriate or exaggerated behavior (e.g., hysterical, hostile, agitated, apathetic); inaccurate follow-through of instructions; inaccurate performance on test

OUTCOMES

Short-term

Adequate knowledge, as evidenced by client's explaining needed life-style changes and medication regimen and by client's ability to verbalize the effects of substance abuse and its effects on therapies (expected within 5 days)

Long-term

Adequate knowledge, as evidenced by client's demonstrating change in life-style, following through with medication regimen and rehabilitation, and verbalizing the advantages of abstaining from alcohol or drug abuse (expected within 1 month)

NURSING INTERVENTIONS/INSTRUCTIONS

1. Assess client's strengths and weaknesses through interviewing, and determine previous interests or areas of success (first visit).

2. Assess client's knowledge regarding Antabuse therapy: action, side effects, and response if patient drinks while on Antabuse (first visit).
3. Assess client's developmental level, educational level, vocabulary level, and past decisions regarding health practices (first visit).
4. Assess information client has about life-style change that is needed by asking specific questions (first visit).
5. Discuss what needs to be taught and who needs to be taught, including family members who may be responsible for health care (first and second visits).
6. Provide positive feedback for participation and adequate information (each visit).
7. Demonstrate techniques using several sessions; increase difficulty at each session; require return demonstration after each session.
8. Evaluate teaching plan (any visit).

CLIENT AND FAMILY/CAREGIVER INTERVENTIONS

1. Family determines progress with the client and revises schedules on the basis of observed progress.
2. Family uses available resources for health maintenance and delivery, with client's input.
3. Client institutes appropriate referrals and use of support systems through community agencies.

Depression

Depression is an affective disorder characterized by an altered mood with symptoms of poor self-esteem, sadness, guilt, hopelessness, emptiness, and despondency. Views about the cause of depression include environmental, societal, genetic, and biomedical theories.

Home care is primarily concerned with the teaching of medication regimens and life-style changes that may be needed, providing a safe environment (frequently after hospitalization), and maintenance of daily well-being.

Nursing diagnosis

Hopelessness

Related factors: Prolonged activity restriction, creating isolation; failing or deteriorating physiologic condition; long-term stress; abandonment; lost belief in transcendent values (i.e., God)

Defining characteristics: Passivity, decreased verbalization; decreased affect; verbal cues (despondent content); turning away from speaker; closing eyes; decreased appetite; increased sleep; lack of initiative; decreased response to stimuli

OUTCOMES

Short-term

Decreased hopelessness, as evidenced by decreased negative verbalization and increased eye contact with health care provider (expected within 3 days)

Long-term

Decreased hopelessness, as evidenced by increased involvement in care and activities (expected within 1 month)

NURSING INTERVENTIONS/INSTRUCTIONS

1. Assess for isolation (physical, emotional, spiritual), chronic stress, and poor physical health (first visit).
2. Assess for defense mechanisms used: denial, isolation, regression (first visit).
3. Assess for nonverbal and verbal indicators of hopelessness; poor eye contact, slumped posture, flat affect, monotone speech, retarded speech (first visit).
4. Discuss how life used to be and activities performed when client was happy (first visit).
5. Allow client to take as much responsibility as possible in own care (each visit).
6. Assist client to set realistic goals in areas of life that he or she can control (first and second visits).
7. Discuss how life has changed and what would make life satisfying again (any visit).
8. Provide referral to appropriate groups, depending on client's condition (any visit).

CLIENT AND FAMILY/CAREGIVER INTERVENTIONS

1. Client includes family in planning, including referrals to outside agencies for help.
2. Client attempts to prevent or discourage stressful situations.
3. Client develops and uses effective coping skills that decrease depression.

Nursing diagnosis

Ineffective individual coping

Related factors: Personal vulnerability; difficulty in handling new situations; previous ineffective or inadequate coping skills; inadequate coping skills, with substitution of alcohol, anxiety, fear

Defining characteristics: Verbalization of inability to cope or inability to ask for help; inability to meet role expectations; inability to meet basic needs; inability to solve problems; alteration in societal participation; destructive behavior toward self or others; inappropriate use of defense mechanisms; change in usual communication patterns; verbal manipulation

OUTCOMES

Short-term

Effective individual coping, as evidenced by client's statement of life-style changes that relieve depression (expected within 5 days)

Long-term

Effective individual coping as evidenced by client's achievement of necessary life-style changes and by client's understanding of relationship between feelings and antecedent event (expected within 1 month)

NURSING INTERVENTIONS/INSTRUCTIONS

1. Assess for psychosomatic symptoms: sleep problems, eating problems, bowel problems (first visit).
2. Assess support system and how the system functions (first visit).

3. Encourage and assist client to identify feelings and relationship between feelings and event or stressor when event is known (each visit).
4. Establish rapport, show acceptance of the person, and establish a positive, concerned relationship with him or her (each visit).
5. Reduce the number of decisions that the patient must make, including the need to solve problems (first and second visits).
6. Allow client sufficient time to make decisions; start with decisions that have only two options (first and second visits).
7. Discuss alternative ways of coping; allow these new coping techniques to be tried in a safe, nondestructive environment (any visit).
8. Use positive rather than negative reinforcement during the testing of new coping mechanisms (each visit).
9. Allow client time to verbalize feelings of denial, anger, guilt, or grief regarding crisis situation (each visit).
10. Acknowledge the validity of fear, hostility, and anxiety (any visit).
11. Encourage the client to talk about the changes the situation has caused (any visit).
12. Listen to and clarify the client's perception of the situation (any visit).
13. Assist the client to sort out the facts concerning the situation (any visit).
14. Identify defense mechanisms used, and determine whether they are being used positively or negatively. Reinforce positive coping mechanisms that have been successfully used in the past but that are not currently being used (any visit).
15. Avoid giving false reassurance (each visit).
16. Assist the client to recognize early symptoms of depression and ways to alleviate them (first visit).

CLIENT AND FAMILY/CAREGIVER INTERVENTIONS

1. Client seeks and accepts help and utilizes referral to day care, crisis center, psychiatrist, or psychologist, if needed.
2. Client sorts out and analyzes information from the family regarding the crisis.
3. Family avoids judgments regarding the client's behavior.

Nursing diagnosis

Impaired social interaction

Related factors: Knowledge and/or skill deficit about ways to enhance mutuality; communication barriers; absence of available significant others or peers; limited physical mobility; therapeutic isolation; sociocultural dissonance; environmental barriers; altered thought processes

Defining characteristics: Verbalized or observed discomfort in social situation; verbalized or observed inability to receive or communicate a satisfying sense of belonging, caring, interest, or shared history; observed use of unsuccessful social interaction behaviors; dysfunctional interaction with peers, family, and/or others; family report of change of style or pattern of interaction

OUTCOMES

Short-term

Adequate socialization, as evidenced by client's communicating with significant others and requesting other people to interact with him or her (expected within 1 week)

Long-term

Adequate socialization, as evidenced by client's expressing interests that are appropriate to developmental age or stage, use of eye contact while interacting, and absence of hostility in voice and behavior (expected within 1 month)

NURSING INTERVENTIONS/INSTRUCTIONS

1. Assess for limited social contacts, preoccupation with own thoughts and feelings, and number of social contacts per week (first visit).
2. Assess for positive feelings that occur from contact with others (first visit).
3. Discuss being alone, amount of time needed, and how client feels during this time (any visit).
4. Acknowledge feelings of loneliness, and discuss feelings of rejection, hostility, and insecurity (any visit).
5. Identify cultural norms, and discuss how isolation occurs when social norms are not followed (any visit).

6. Identify behaviors that are not considered socially acceptable to dominant culture; acknowledge and reinforce acceptable behaviors (any visit).
7. Discuss frequent testing of relationships and how testing may lead to social isolation (any visit).
8. Encourage verbal communication, eye contact, and involvement in community functions (any visit).

CLIENT AND FAMILY/CAREGIVER INTERVENTIONS

1. Client attempts to prevent or discourage interactions with negative individuals.
2. Client develops and uses effective coping skills that decrease isolation.

Nursing diagnosis

Knowledge deficit

Related factors: Lack of exposure to information; lack of recall; misinterpretation of information; cognitive limitation; lack of interest in learning; unfamiliarity with information resources

Defining characteristics: Verbalization of the problem; inappropriate or exaggerated behavior (e.g., hysterical, hostile, agitated, apathetic); inaccurate follow-through of instructions; inaccurate performance on test

OUTCOMES

Short-term

Adequate knowledge, as evidenced by client's ability to explain reasons for depression (expected within 3 days)

Long-term

Adequate knowledge, as evidenced by client's ability to demonstrate needed life-style changes, participate in treatment programs, and identify resources (expected within 1 month)

NURSING INTERVENTIONS/INSTRUCTIONS

1. Assess strengths and weaknesses through interviewing, and determine previous interest areas of success (first visit).
2. Assess developmental level, educational level, vocabulary

level, age, and past discussion regarding health practices (first visit).
3. Assess extent of client's information about depression by asking specific questions (first visit).
4. Provide information about drug therapy, potential side effects, precautions, and benefits, and emphasize that client is not to stop drug suddenly (first visit).
5. Refer client to support agencies and resources (any visit).
6. Discuss progress with the client, and revise schedules based on observed progress (any visit).
7. Provide written instructions as well as verbal instructions (each visit).

CLIENT AND FAMILY/CAREGIVER INTERVENTIONS

1. Client administers drug therapy correctly and consistently and notes progress to report or need for change in therapy.
2. Client uses available resources for health maintenance and delivery.

Physical/Emotional Abuse

Physical abuse is considered to be a destructive act or injury inflicted by a caregiver. Emotional abuse includes threats and acts of degradation that are damaging to a person's self-worth.

Home care is primarily concerned with the teaching aspects of symptoms of abuse and with adequate prevention, evaluation, and reporting of abuse.

Nursing diagnosis

Risk for trauma

Related factors: Interactive conditions between individual and environment that pose a risk to the defensive and adaptive resources of the individual

Defining characteristics: Internal environment: weakness; poor vision; balancing difficulties; lack of safety or drug education; lack of proper precautions; cognitive or emotional difficulties. External environment; people or provider.

OUTCOMES

Short-term

Absence of trauma, as evidenced by client's statement that trauma has not occurred (expected within 1 week)

Long-term

Absence of trauma, as evidenced by absence of falls, injuries, or death from abuse (expected within 2 months)

NURSING INTERVENTIONS/INSTRUCTIONS

1. Assess client, situation, and environment for potentially abusive situation (first visit).
2. Identify and remove actual dangers in the environment (see Defining Characteristics) (each visit).

CLIENT AND FAMILY/CAREGIVER INTERVENTIONS

1. Client increases awareness of the possibility of abuse by family and caregivers.
2. Family provides for respite care of client to relieve caregiver.

Nursing diagnosis

Altered family processes

Related factors: Situational transition or crisis; developmental transition or crisis

Defining characteristics: Family system unable to meet physical needs of its members; family system unable to meet emotional needs of its members; family system unable to meet spiritual needs of its members; inability to express or accept wide range of feelings; inability to express or accept feelings of members; family unable to meet security needs of its members; inability of family members to relate to each other for mutual growth and maturation; family uninvolved in community activities; inability to accept or receive help appropriately; rigidity in function and roles; family not demonstrating respect for individuality and autonomy of its members; family unable to adapt to change or deal with traumatic experience constructively; family failing to accomplish current or past developmental tasks; unhealthy family decision-making process; failure to send and receive clear messages; inappropriate boundary maintenance; inappropriate or poorly communicated family rules, rituals, symbols; unexamined family myths; inappropriate level and direction of energy

OUTCOMES

Short-term

Family allows for individual differences of its members (expected within 1 week)

Long-term

Family allows for all individuals to be involved in the decision-making process; all family members state that basic needs (physical, emotional, spiritual) are being met within the family (expected within 3 months)

NURSING INTERVENTIONS/INSTRUCTIONS

1. Assess decision-making or problem-solving techniques used in the family (who influences the decisions in the family, who makes the final decision, all persons involved in the process) (first visit).
2. Assess the developmental stage of the family and of each member (are there developmental lags in any one of the members) (first visit).
3. Assess for coalitions in the family (who takes whose side during arguments), triangling, and scapegoating (first visit).
4. Assess the realistic view of the crisis (first visit).
5. Assess the availability of support systems outside the family (any visit).
6. Identify ineffective coping mechanisms used; acknowledge and encourage positive coping mechanisms (each visit).
7. Discuss ambivalence, hostility, guilt, and anxiety and how these emotions affect the family; discuss verbalizing these feelings and emotions (each visit).
8. Assist the family to identify the major stressors in the family (each visit).
9. Allow client and family to verbalize about situational or maturational crises that are occurring within the family; determine whether family crises are occurring at the same time as individual crises (each visit).
10. Discuss the concept of tolerance and how a nonjudg-

mental attitude leads to feelings of security in the family (first visit).

11. Identify the family's need for further professional help, and refer the family to appropriate agencies (any visit).

CLIENT AND FAMILY/CAREGIVER INTERVENTIONS

1. Family is involved in decision making related to the client.
2. Family members avoid severe stressors in the family and develop more appropriate coping mechanisms.

Nursing diagnosis

Impaired home maintenance management

Related factors: Disease or injury of family member; insufficient family organization or planning; insufficient finances; unfamiliarity with neighborhood resources; impaired cognitive or emotional functioning; lack of knowledge; lack of role modeling; inadequate support systems

Defining characteristics: Household members express difficulty in maintaining their home in a comfortable fashion; household requests assistance with home maintenance; household members describe outstanding debts or financial crises; disorderly surroundings; unwashed or unavailable cooking equipment, clothes, or linens; accumulation of dirt, food wastes, or hygienic wastes; offensive odors; inappropriate household temperature; overtaxed family members (e.g., exhausted, anxious); lack of necessary equipment or aids; presence of vermin or rodents; repeated hygienic disorders; infestations, or infections

OUTCOMES

Short-term

Absence of dirt, food wastes, or hygienic waste; absence of offensive odors; washed or available cooking equipment, clothing, linens; absence of hygienic disorders, infestations, infections; absence of vermin (expected within 1 week)

Long-term

Household members state ease in maintaining home in comfortable fashion (expected within 3 months)

NURSING INTERVENTIONS/INSTRUCTIONS

1. Assess mental status, including orientation, affect, and level of consciousness (first visit).
2. Assess mobility (ambulation, equipment needed) (first visit).
3. Assess self-care abilities (hygiene, dressing, eating) (first visit).
4. Assess housekeeping skills (first visit).
5. Assess ability to organize housekeeping activities (first visit).
6. Provide referral for outside help or preparation of meals if needed (any visit).
7. Discuss making an organizational plan to be followed daily; include all family members (first visit).
8. Discuss rotation of household chores (first visit).
9. Discuss preparation of meals for 2 days or the entire week (any visit).

CLIENT AND FAMILY/CAREGIVER INTERVENTIONS

1. Family reorganizes family chores.
2. Client utilizes family and persons in the community who may help with home maintenance.

Nursing diagnosis

Knowledge deficit

Related factors: Lack of exposure to information; lack of recall; misinterpretation of information; cognitive limitation; lack of interest in learning; unfamiliarity with information resources

Defining characteristics: Verbalization of the problem; inappropriate or exaggerated behavior (e.g., hysterical, hostile, agitated, apathetic); inaccurate follow-through of instructions; inaccurate performance on test

OUTCOMES

Short-term

Adequate knowledge, as evidenced by client's ability to verbalize definition of signs and symptoms of abusive behavior (expected within 3 days)

Long-term

Adequate knowledge, as evidenced by client's ability to report abuse (expected in 2 weeks)

NURSING INTERVENTIONS/INSTRUCTIONS

1. Assess strengths and weaknesses of relationship between caregiver and client (first visit).
2. Assess information known about abuse; ask specific questions (first visit).
3. Discuss what needs to be taught (first visit).
4. Discuss abuse, symptoms, and prevention (any visit).

CLIENT AND FAMILY/CAREGIVER INTERVENTIONS

1. Caregiver uses available resources for prevention of abuse; uses client's input.
2. Client institutes appropriate use of support systems and referrals to community agencies.

Special care plans

Chemotherapy and External Radiation Therapy

Chemotherapy and radiation therapy are treatment modalities that are used to cure, control, or palliate cancer. Radiation therapy may be administered alone or in combination with surgery or chemotherapy. Chemotherapy protocols include alkylating agents, antimetabolites, antitumor antibiotics, plant alkaloids, nitrosoureas, corticosteroids, hormones, and unclassified miscellaneous and investigational drugs. These agents are given in combination for prescribed periods of time and frequency, depending on the malignancy being treated. They may be administered by oral, intramuscular, intravenous, intrathecal, intraarterial, intracavity, subcutaneous, topical, intraperitoneal, or perfusion routes, depending on tumor site.

Home care is primarily concerned with administration of chemotherapy, teaching of the physical and emotional effects and resulting care and needs during administration of chemotherapy and/or radiation therapy, and assessment and treatment of side effects.

Nursing diagnosis

Ineffective individual coping

Related factors: Multiple life changes; inadequate coping methods

Defining characteristics: Verbalization of inability to cope or ask for help; inability to solve problems; chronic worry and anxiety; inappropriate use of defense mechanisms

OUTCOMES

Short-term

Improved coping, as evidenced by client's statement of understanding of need for adaptations in life-style and positive coping strategies (expected within 1 week)

Long-term

Optimal coping, as evidenced by client's participation in and adaptation to altered life-style and by client's compliance with medical regimen to maintain optimal health and functioning (expected within 1 to 2 months)

NURSING INTERVENTIONS/INSTRUCTIONS

1. Assess for developmental level and dependency needs, mental status, behavioral and emotional changes, use of defense mechanisms and their effectiveness, and ability to solve problems (first visit).
2. Establish a trusting relationship and facilitate an open discussion to explore options and develop skills in coping and problem solving (each visit).
3. Help client to identify coping skills that work, and encourage positive feeling about success of any adaptation or changes (each visit).
4. Include client in all planning and formulation of realistic goals; assist if requested to do so (each visit).
5. Provide accepting, nonjudgmental attitude and environment when teaching and discussing needs and changes to be made in life-style (each visit).
6. Encourage expressions of fears, concerns, and questions regarding therapy and effects (each visit).
7. Initiate social services and counseling referrals (any visit).

CLIENT AND FAMILY/CAREGIVER INTERVENTIONS

1. Client develops coping strategies for long-term treatment and possible outcome.
2. Client shares feelings, fears, concerns with caregiver, family.
3. Client plans and participates in own care and health promotion.

4. Client sets goals and strategies for coping with life-style changes.
5. Client participates in support group with those who have similar conditions.
6. Client utilizes social services, counseling, and clergy as needed.

Nursing diagnosis

Altered nutrition: less than body requirements

Related factors: Inability to ingest and absorb nutrients because of biologic factors (chemotherapy and/or radiation therapy)

Defining characteristics: Anorexia; lack of interest in food; weakness; fatigue; weight loss; inadequate nutritional intake; stomatitis; vomiting; altered taste perception; mucositis of bowel

OUTCOMES

Short-term

Adequate nutrition, as evidenced by intake of prescribed dietary regimen and stabilization of weight without anorexia, nausea, and vomiting (expected within 1 to 2 weeks)

Long-term

Adequate nutritional status, as evidenced by intake of required nutrients for optimal health and functioning during and after therapy (expected within 1 month and ongoing)

NURSING INTERVENTIONS/INSTRUCTIONS

1. Assess nutritional status, including food preferences, cultural and religious restrictions, caloric requirements, and effect of different medications on food intake (first visit).
2. Calculate ideal weight for size, sex, frame, and height; instruct client in measuring weight weekly (first visit).
3. Assess for diarrhea, nausea, vomiting, anorexia, weight loss, fatigue, malaise, and reactions to meals (each visit).
4. Instruct client to schedule rest periods after meals and to have 6 to 8 hours of sleep per night (first visit).

5. Inform client of measures to facilitate eating, including eliminating odors; relaxed atmosphere; quiet environment; eating smaller, more frequent attractively prepared meals; taking antiemetics ½ hour before meals (first visit).
6. Inform client of newer antiemetics and success in controlling nausea and vomiting, and instruct in administration (first visit).
7. Instruct client to maintain a food diary for one week that includes type and amount of food consumed and method of preparation (first and second visits).
8. Instruct and include client in food selections for a high-protein, high-carbohydrate, high-calorie diet and to avoid hot, spicy foods; incorporate assessment data and food diary into menu planning (first and second visits).
9. Provide information for calorie and vitamin supplements (first visit).
10. Suggest oral hygiene before each meal (first visit).
11. If client's appetite is poor, suggest eating more frequent meals in smaller amounts and increasing amounts slowly as tolerated (first visit).
12. Initiate referral to nutritionist if needed (any visit).
13. Refer home health aide to assist with feeding and meal preparation as needed.

CLIENT AND FAMILY/CAREGIVER INTERVENTIONS

1. Client maintains or gains weight as determined.
2. Client participates in planning and ingestion of well-balanced diet with restrictions as determined.
3. Client promotes pleasant environment, preferred food preparation, and dietary pattern that enhances intake.
4. Client weighs weekly using same scale, at same time of day, wearing same amount of clothing and records in a log.
5. Client maintains a 7-day food diary listing types and amounts of all foods eaten.
6. Client eats a high-protein, high-carbohydrate, high-calorie diet; to assist with meal preparation, secures a cookbook for cancer clients.
7. Client uses high-calorie supplements as needed.
8. Client takes daily vitamins.
9. Client administers antiemetic 30 minutes before meals.

Nursing diagnosis

Diarrhea

Related factors: Inflammation or irritation of bowel; malabsorption of bowel (chemotherapy and/or radiation therapy)

Defining characteristics: Abdominal pain; cramping; increased frequency; loose, liquid stools; urgency; mucus in stool; increased frequency of bowel sounds; mucositis

OUTCOMES

Short-term

Return of baseline bowel pattern, as evidenced by decrease in the frequency of bowel eliminations and by stool characteristics within baseline parameters (expected within 1 week)

Long-term

Minimal or absence of diarrheal bowel eliminations, as evidenced by soft formed stools eliminated according to baseline pattern (expected within 2 weeks)

NURSING INTERVENTIONS/INSTRUCTIONS

1. Assess bowel elimination patterns and stool characteristics (see Gastrointestinal System Assessment, p. 20, for guidelines) (first visit).
2. Instruct client to maintain a record of bowel movements, including number and when they occur and characteristics such as color, amount, consistency, odor, and presence of mucus, blood, or pus (first visit).
3. Monitor medication administration, and instruct in intake and output, antidiarrheals, and anticholinergics, monitor intake and output ratio with increased fluid intake (each visit).
4. Instruct client to notify physician if diarrhea becomes more severe or frequent, if bleeding is noted, or if fatigue or weakness is noted (first visit).

CLIENT AND FAMILY/CAREGIVER INTERVENTIONS

1. Client administers antidiarrheal correctly as needed.
2. Client reports diarrhea that is not controlled or reveals blood, pus, or mucus.

3. Client adjusts diet and avoids foods irritating to bowel.
4. Client monitors fluid intake and output and increases fluid intake up to 3000 ml/day as needed.

Nursing diagnosis

Altered oral mucous membrane

Related factors: Medication (chemotherapeutic agents)

Defining characteristics: Stomatitis, oral lesions or ulcers, oral pain or discomfort

OUTCOMES

Short-term

Minimal changes in oral mucous membrane, as evidenced by decreased inflammation and oral pain and by intact mucous membrane (expected within 4 to 7 days)

Long-term

Oral mucous membrane maintained intact, as evidenced by absence of stomatitis and associated signs and symptoms (expected within 1 to 2 weeks and ongoing during therapy)

NURSING INTERVENTIONS/INSTRUCTIONS

1. Assess oral cavity for redness, pain, ulcerations, dysphagia, and dryness (each visit).
2. Instruct client to provide mouth care after meals, to rinse mouth with saline, hydrogen peroxide or sodium bicarbonate solution, or viscous lidocaine every 2 hours or as needed and to avoid commercial mouthwashes or alcohol (first visit).
3. Instruct client to avoid mouth breathing, smoking, and hot and spicy or irritating foods (first visit).
4. Instruct client to avoid using a hard toothbrush and to remove dentures except for meals (first visit).
5. Instruct client to apply petroleum jelly or cocoa butter to lips and artificial saliva preparation to oral cavity; instruct client to use topical anesthetic and fungal antibiotic if prescribed (first visit).
6. Instruct client to take cool beverages, popsicles, and ice cream to soothe oral cavity (first visit).

CLIENT AND FAMILY/CAREGIVER INTERVENTIONS

1. Client assesses oral cavity for stomatitis and reports condition that deteriorates in spite of treatments.
2. Client performs oral care using soft brush, unwaxed floss, soft-tipped applicator, and mouthwash consisting of acceptable solution.
4. Client applies topical preparations for dryness.
5. Client avoids commercial products for mouth care and irritants to oral cavity, such as hot, spicy foods, alcohol, and tobacco, and ingests cool fluids and bland, smooth foods.

Nursing diagnosis

Impaired skin integrity

Related factors: Internal factor of medication (chemotherapy); external factor of radiation

Defining characteristics: Disruption of skin surfaces; dryness; pruritis; blistering, allergic rashes; hyperpigmentation; irritation and excoriation of perianal area from diarrhea

OUTCOMES

Short-term

Skin intact, as evidenced by absence of irritation, dryness, rash, or breaks (expected within 1 week)

Long-term

Skin integrity maintained, as evidenced by absence of skin disruption and by skin protection to achieve optimal condition during treatments (expected ongoing during treatments)

NURSING INTERVENTIONS/INSTRUCTIONS

1. Assess for skin condition at irradiation site, itching, irritation at perianal area; assess skin for dryness, pruritis, rashes; review skin care protocol for clients receiving chemotherapy and/or radiation therapy (each visit).
2. Instruct client to cleanse skin with mild soap and warm water and pat dry; avoid using soap, lotions, or deodorants or washing or removing marks of any kind placed on skin at irradiation site (first visit).

3. Instruct client to avoid any massage, scratching, adhesive tape, pressure, or sun exposure to skin, to wear soft, loose clothing, and to use a sun screen for a year following treatment (first and second visits).
4. Instruct client to expose irradiation site to the air and to apply only prescribed preparations to skin twice a day, such as A & D Ointment for dryness, cornstarch to absorb moisture, and hydrocortisone cream to reduce inflammation (first visit).
5. Instruct client to cleanse and dry perianal area after each bowel elimination and to apply A & D Ointment or karaya gel to area (first visit).
6. Instruct client to assess for skin breakdown and to report any open areas to physician (first visit).

CLIENT AND FAMILY/CAREGIVER INTERVENTIONS

1. Client performs measures to protect skin integrity during chemotherapy and/or radiation therapy.
2. Client provides safe cleansing and protection to skin.
3. Client avoids exposure of skin to harmful pressure, rubbing, or irritants.
4. Client applies ointments to prevent or treat dryness, itching, or irritation of skin.
5. Client preserves markings placed on skin by x-ray personnel.
6. Client reports skin breakdown to physician.

Nursing diagnosis

Altered protection

Related factors: Abnormal blood profile (chemotherapy and/or radiation)

Defining characteristics: Leukopenia from bone marrow depression; thrombocytopenia from bone marrow depression; anemia from bone marrow depression; proneness to bleeding, infection, fatigue, weakness

OUTCOMES

Short-term

Control of bleeding or infection tendency, as evidenced by absence of bleeding or infection at any site (expected within 1 week)

Long-term

Absence of bleeding or infectious process, with blood profile within acceptable parameters during therapy (expected for duration of therapy)

NURSING INTERVENTIONS/INSTRUCTIONS

1. Assess for bleeding, including petechiae, ecchymoses, oozing or frank bleeding from any orifice or skin site, or blood in stool or urine; assess joints for pain and swelling; assess for increased weakness and fatigue (each visit).
2. Assess for fever; chills; decreased breath sounds, dyspnea with or without exertion; cough; chest pain; cloudy, foul-smelling urine; and frequency, burning, and urgency in urinary elimination (each visit).
3. Assess, as available, levels of white blood cells, red blood cells, hematocrit, hemoglobin, and platelets, and urine or sputum culture results, and compare to levels at which bleeding or infection is probable (any visit).
4. Instruct client to avoid any trauma to skin and to take measures to prevent falls or other injury in home environment (first visit).
5. Instruct client to avoid exposure to others with infections or illnesses that might be transmitted (first visit).
6. Instruct client in hand-washing technique, to wear mask if needed, and to avoid sharing utensils or articles such as linens or clothing (first visit).
7. Instruct client to avoid use of safety razor, hard toothbrushing, blowing nose hard, or straining at defecation (first visit).
8. Inform client of importance of having laboratory tests done as scheduled to determine bone marrow function and possible effects (first visit).
9. Instruct client to report any persistent symptoms to physician (each visit).

CLIENT AND FAMILY/CAREGIVER INTERVENTIONS

1. Client takes and records temperature, respirations, and pulse as needed.
2. Client adapts activities of daily living (ADL) and other activities to physical tolerance and rests when feeling fatigued.
3. Client assesses daily for bleeding or infectious process and reports any findings to physician.

4. Client avoids trauma to skin or mucous membranes resulting from straining or using harsh implements.
5. Client administers stool softeners and vitamin K as prescribed; avoids aspirin or aspirin products.
6. Client avoids exposure to persons with infections, crowded places, and use of or exposure to contaminated articles.
7. Client provides protective isolation measures based on laboratory results.
8. Client reports for all appointments for laboratory tests and physician follow-up.
9. Client secures and transports blood, urine, and sputum specimens to laboratory.

Nursing diagnosis

Body image disturbance

Related factors: Biophysical effect of chemotherapy and/or radiation

Defining characteristics: Alopecia; negative feeling about body; physical changes caused by therapy or surgery

OUTCOMES

Short-term

Improved body image, as evidenced by client's statement of reason for change and measures to take to disguise the change (expected within 2 to 3 days)

Long-term

Enhanced body image, as evidenced by client's verbalization of more positive feelings about appearance and the temporary state of the changes caused by chemotherapy and/or radiation (expected within 2 to 4 weeks and duration of therapy)

NURSING INTERVENTIONS/INSTRUCTIONS

1. Before therapy, inform client of potential for hair loss and instruct client to prepare with purchase of a wig or to use a scarf, turban, or large hat (first visit).
2. Allow client to express, in an accepting and nonjudgmental environment, feelings about hair loss, weight loss, nail changes, skin discoloration, and surgical scarring (each visit).

3. Instruct client to use a mild shampoo and to avoid use of curlers, dryers, hair spray, hot iron, or harsh brushing of hair (first visit).
4. Inform client that hair will grow back after treatment regimen but may be coarser and a slightly different color (first visit).
5. Inform of clothing with high necks, loose fit, long sleeves, or leg covering (slacks) to select to cover exposed surgical areas or prostheses (first visit).

CLIENT AND FAMILY/CAREGIVER INTERVENTIONS

1. Client secures wig, hairpiece, scarf, or other clothing to deal with concerns such as hair loss, thinness, skin discoloration, scarring, or prosthesis.
2. Client uses makeup to cover discoloration of skin.
3. Client expresses feelings about appearance and coping skills to maintain life-style and improved body image.
4. Client avoids actions that injure hair, skin, or nails.

Nursing diagnosis

Knowledge deficit

Related factors: Lack of information about therapy

Defining characteristics: Expressed need for information about chemotherapy and/or radiation therapy and effects and about health maintenance needs

OUTCOMES

Short-term

Adequate knowledge, as evidenced by client's statement of therapy regimen and of its temporary effect on health status (expected within 2 to 3 days)

Long-term

Adequate knowledge, as evidenced by client's compliance with medical protocol and actions to maintain optimal health and functioning during therapy (expected for duration of therapy)

NURSING INTERVENTIONS/INSTRUCTIONS

1. Assess client's life-style, ability to adapt, and learning ability and interest, family participation and support, and availability

of community agencies that offer information and support (first visit).

2. Assess client's knowledge of reason for therapy and what effects can be expected (first visit).
3. Instruct client in administration of each chemotherapeutic drug, including what action the drug has on the malignant cells, route of administration, dose, frequency, and combination protocols, with length of time given, side effects, and treatments given to prevent or control them; provide client with a written protocol and check-off sheet to take to physician for administration of chemotherapy (first and second visits).
4. Instruct client in radiation site, effect of radiation, frequency of treatment, length of therapy, and protection of irradiated area (first visit).
5. Inform client that fatigue and other effects of therapy begin during first week and gradually disappear 2 to 4 weeks after therapy ends (first visit).
6. Inform client of medications administered to counteract toxic effects of therapy and those given to treat complications of therapy (first visit).
7. Assist client to plan for fluid, nutritional, activity, rest, and sleep requirements and to modify them according to effects of therapy (each visit).
8. Instruct client to notify physician of any severe side effects and to keep all follow-up appointments for medications, treatments, and laboratory tests (first visit).
9. Initiate referral to community agencies and social and economic services to assist with transportation, meals, homemaking, shopping, economic problems, medical equipment and supplies, information, and psychological support (any visit).

CLIENT AND FAMILY/CAREGIVER INTERVENTIONS

1. Client meets fluid, dietary, exercise, and sleep requirements on the basis of assessment and abilities.
2. Client verbalizes chemotherapy and/or radiation protocol and measures to take to promote desired effect.
3. Client maintains positive attitude regarding effect and result of treatment.
4. Client administers medications as instructed to treat side effects of therapy.
5. Client reports uncontrolled side effects to physician.

6. Client keeps all appointments during therapy.
7. Client contacts American Cancer Society or other agencies as appropriate to needs.

Hospice Care

Hospice care is a concept of holistic care that provides compassion, concern, support, and skilled care for the terminally ill client. It includes physical, psychologic, social, and spiritual care by a medically supervised interdisciplinary team of professionals and volunteers. Hospice care in the home is based on client and family need and may be part time, intermittent, scheduled on a regular basis, or provided on a 24-hour on-call basis. Support for grieving before and after the death of the client is included in the care plan for client and family.

Home care is primarily concerned with the control of symptoms and promotion of comfort through palliative care.

Nursing diagnosis

Chronic pain

Related factors: Chronic physical disability; progressive invasion of malignant tumor

Defining characteristics: Altered ability to continue previous activities; long-term pain that becomes progressively more severe; tumor metastasis and pressure as mass becomes larger

OUTCOMES

Short-term

Pain decreased, as evidenced by client's statement that severity has been reduced with appropriate analgesic therapy (expected within 1 week)

Long-term

Pain absent or controlled with continuous or intermittent analgesic therapy administered intramuscularly, intravenously, or subcutaneously and based on need (expected for duration of terminal state)

NURSING INTERVENTIONS/INSTRUCTIONS

1. Assess status of pain and client's ability to tolerate pain (each visit).
2. Administer intravenously or intramuscularly analgesic of choice that will achieve pain control, or instruct client in subcutaneous self-administration with a pump device (first and second visits).
3. Provide a quiet, restful environment, and reduce stimuli to a minimum (first visit).
4. Instruct client to place self in position of comfort and to change positions gently and carefully to prevent additional pain (first visit).
5. Instruct client in guided imagery or relaxation techniques and provide music if these actions are appropriate (any visit).

CLIENT AND FAMILY/CAREGIVER INTERVENTIONS

1. Client or caregiver administers analgesic therapy as needed to relieve or control pain.
2. Caregiver maintains quiet, well-ventilated, temperature-controlled, and restful environment.
3. Client avoids any stressful or anxiety-provoking situations.
4. Caregiver provides music or other desirable diversions as appropriate.

Nursing diagnosis

Ineffective family coping: compromised

Related factors: Situational crisis of dying family member

Defining characteristics: Significant persons preoccupied with personal reactions of fear, grief, guilt, and anxiety regarding client's condition

OUTCOMES

Short-term

Improved coping, as evidenced by client's and family's acknowledgment of terminal state of illness and ability to grieve and support palliative treatment of family member (expected within 1 week)

Long-term

Optimal coping abilities and support of family members to facilitate client's comfort and care (expected during hospice experience)

NURSING INTERVENTIONS/INSTRUCTIONS

1. Assess family interactions, ability to cope, strengths and inner resources, ability to support family member who is terminally ill, and presence of or need for an advance directive in compliance with the Patient Self-Determination Act (each visit).
2. Inform family that care and concern extend to all family members according to their needs (first visit).
3. Provide accurate information to family about treatment and goal of hospice care and about what can and cannot be changed; allow for questions and clarifications (each visit).
4. Provide client with written information about right to know what treatment is planned and right to decide in advance what treatment is wanted or not wanted under special or serious conditions, in order to control medical treatment decisions. Inform client of right to execute advance directives through a living will or a durable power of attorney for health care according to state laws (first visit).
5. Encourage family to discuss strengths and options for use of coping skills that are helpful (each visit).
6. Include family members in as much care of client as they feel ready and able to perform; allow family to plan client's needs around family routines if possible (each visit).
7. Allow for family members to grieve in an accepting and nonjudgmental environment; assist family to identify grieving behaviors (each visit).
8. Inform family of government and community agencies and referral to interdisciplinary caregivers as needed and as available for hospice care (any visit).
9. Encourage family to accept social services, counseling from clergy, and psychotherapy as needed (first visit).

CLIENT AND FAMILY/CAREGIVER INTERVENTIONS

1. Client completes an advance directive stating choice for health care or names someone to make these choices if unable to make decisions about medical treatment.
2. Family members support and perform care if possible.

3. Family members verbalize concerns and feelings about client's condition during terminal stage of illness.
4. Family members cope with the imminent loss of a loved one.
5. Family members participate in planning and assisting with care.
6. Family members seek assistance from other professionals as needed.
7. Family members progress through grieving process.
8. Family prepares for death of family member.
9. Family maintains an open, honest approach and communication among family members and client.

Nursing diagnosis

Fatigue

Related factors: Overwhelming psychologic or emotional demands; state of physical discomfort

Defining characteristics: Weakness; inability to maintain and perform usual routines and activities of daily living

OUTCOMES

Short-term

Minimal fatigue, as evidenced by client's obtaining needed assistance in personal care (expected within 1 to 2 weeks)

Long-term

Optimal level of energy maintained and fatigue level minimized during terminal phase of illness (expected during length of hospice care)

NURSING INTERVENTIONS/INSTRUCTIONS

1. Provide assistance or complete care, including bathing, grooming, personal hygiene, toileting or urinary and bowel elimination care, feeding and drinking as appropriate, and gown changing (each visit).
2. Provide position changes, skin care, and aids to prevent pressure on susceptible areas (each visit).
3. Provide clean linens, massage with lotion, glycerin to lips, and mouth care with rinses or glycerin swabs (each visit).

4. Perform range-of-motion exercises for all joints, and maintain body alignment without compromising comfort (each visit).
5. Provide necessary assistance and care for all body processes as needed, support all body parts, and provide for every physical need without causing additional fatigue to client (each visit).
6. Anticipate needs of client and family, and pace activities according to energy level of client and family (each visit).
7. Utilize touch to exhibit caring (each visit).
8. Provide all interventions on a continuous basis.

CLIENT AND FAMILY/CAREGIVER INTERVENTIONS

1. Client accepts total physical care and support of all failing systems on a continuous basis.
2. Family promotes quality of life with comfort and support to client.
3. Family conserves client's energy and preserves client's emotional and physical status.
4. Family and caregiver comply with legal and ethical issues regarding terminal care (witholding basic needs, nonresuscitation).

Neoplasms (Malignant)

Malignant neoplasms, or cancer, is a term used to identify disease processes characterized by unregulated cell changes that are capable of metastasis, or spread to other organs of the body. Cancer is classified according to the type of tissue involved: lymphomas originate in the lymphatic or infection-preventing system organs; leukemias originate in the blood-forming organs; sarcomas originate in connective tissue, bone, or muscle; and carcinomas originate in the epithelial cells of organs. Metastasis occurs via the vascular system or the lymphatic system or by implantation from the primary site of the tumor. In addition to the classification of cancer by anatomic site or tissue of origin, the cells are graded by appearance and differentiation, from grade I through grade IV, and the extent of the disease is described by staging, from stage 0 through stage IV. Typing, grading, and staging are used as a basis to determine treatment modalities, whose goal may be cure, control, or palliation of the disease. There are at least 200 diseases in this group, and this care plan for clients with malignant conditions is presented to assist with the problems common to all or most of these clients who receive care in the home. Since treatment for this condition consists of surgical intervention, chemotherapy, and/or radiation therapy, the Postoperative and Chemotherapy and External Radiation Therapy care plans should be used in conjunction with this one for a comprehensive approach to care of the client with cancer.

Home care is primarily concerned with the teaching and caring aspects of the client's physical and emotional needs and with implementation of the medical protocol to preserve and maintain optimal physical health and function.

Nursing diagnosis

Anxiety

Related factors: Threat of death; threat to or change in health status

Defining characteristics: Apprehension; uncertain outcome; increased tension and helplessness; fearfulness; poor prognosis; possible early death; changes in life-style and temperament; powerlessness; depression; withdrawal

OUTCOMES

Short-term

Decreased anxiety, as evidenced by client's statement of reduced fear, worry, and apprehension regarding change in health status and possible poor prognosis (expected within 1 to 3 weeks)

Long-term

Management or control of anxiety level, as evidenced by adaptation to change in life-style and by compliance with and acceptance of treatment regimen to achieve desired goal of medical protocol (expected within 1 to 2 months and ongoing)

NURSING INTERVENTIONS/INSTRUCTIONS

1. Assess client's mental and emotional status regarding life-threatening illness (see Psychosocial Assessment, p. 48, for guidelines) (first visit).
2. In an accepting environment, encourage expressions of fears and concerns and questions regarding therapy and its effects (each visit).
3. Assist client to identify needed changes in life-style and methods to make necessary changes (first visit and reinforce each visit).
4. Inform client of all activities, treatments and tests, and effects to expect; reinforce information about the disease and client condition given by the physician (each visit).
5. Allow client to direct own care and make own choices when possible regarding treatment regimen and plan of care (each visit).
6. Initiate referral to counseling, support group, and agencies that may assist with social services and economic and health care needs (first visit).
7. Instruct client in relaxation exercises, music therapy, or imagery, or introduce other techniques to reduce anxiety (first and second visits).

CLIENT AND FAMILY/CAREGIVER INTERVENTIONS

1. Client develops coping methods for long-term treatment and possible outcome.
2. Client maintains manageable level of anxiety.
3. Client seeks information that will reduce anxiety.
4. Client expresses fears and concerns about necessary changes in life-style.
5. Client contacts and consults with support services available.

Nursing diagnosis

Anticipatory grieving

Related factors: Perceived potential loss of physiopsychosocial well-being

Defining characteristics: Expression of distress at potential loss; anger; guilt; denial of potential loss; sorrow; choked feelings; changes in sleep, eating, and activity patterns

OUTCOMES

Short-term

Progress in grieving, as evidenced by attitude and behavior changes manifested by stage in process (expected within days)

Long-term

Grief process resolving, as evidenced by resumption of life-style with or without changes as needed and by integration of grieving stage into life-style and activities (expected within 2 to 3 months and ongoing)

NURSING INTERVENTIONS/INSTRUCTIONS

1. Assess degree and stage of grief (each visit).
2. Inform client of stages of grieving process and that behavior is acceptable for specific stage, that progress goes back and forth, and that acceptance will be final stage (first visit).
3. Allow expression of feelings and perception of effects of therapy, potential loss, and death in a nonjudgmental environment (each visit).
4. Initiate referral for psychological and spiritual counseling as appropriate (any visit).

CLIENT AND FAMILY/CAREGIVER INTERVENTIONS

1. Client progresses through grief process to acceptance.
2. Client seeks counseling as needed.
3. Client verbalizes stages and behaviors during grief process.

Nursing diagnosis

Knowledge deficit

Related factors: Lack of information about disease

Defining characteristics: Expressed need for information, at understandable level, about cancer, treatment modalities, and limitations imposed by the disease

OUTCOMES

Short-term

Adequate knowledge, as evidenced by client's statement of disease process and type of cancer, diagnostic and classification methods, proposed treatment, and expected results (expected within 1 week)

Long-term

Adequate knowledge, as evidenced by client's understanding of and compliance with treatment protocol to achieve optimal physical and functional status within identified therapeutic goal (expected within 2 to 3 months and ongoing, depending on disease progression)

NURSING INTERVENTIONS/INSTRUCTIONS

1. Assess client's life-style, ability to adapt, learning ability and interest, family participation and support, and need for reinforcement of information given by physician (first visit).
2. Inform client of disease process, possible causes, reasons for signs and symptoms, and changes in body appearance and function (first visit).
3. Inform client of importance of maintaining all follow-up care and appointments with physician, laboratory testing, and scheduled chemotherapy and/or radiation therapy during treatment protocol (first visit and reinforce second visit).
4. Provide client with accurate information about the benefits of proven therapies and fallacies of unproven methods of cancer treatment, which might include chemicals or drugs, dietary supplements, and occult or mechanical devices or techniques (first visit).
5. Outline treatment protocol, length of therapy, expected discomforts and results, and side effects in honest, understandable terms (each visit).
6. Inform client of any limitations or restrictions to follow during therapy, including performance of activities of daily living within energy tolerance, avoiding sun exposure and alcohol intake, and arranging for leaving work or loss of work during therapy.
7. Inform client of common problem of fear associated with the disease and methods of coping with and reducing it after

diagnosis and during the initial phases of treatment (first visit).

8. Inform client of and refer to hospice care if appropriate, and explain the availability of this care in the future if appropriate (any visit).
9. Refer client to American Cancer Society for information, support groups, and equipment or supplies as needed (any visit).
10. In a realistic manner, inform client of importance of a hopeful attitude about the disease and the progress that has been made in curing the disease (any visit).

CLIENT AND FAMILY/CAREGIVER INTERVENTIONS

1. Client verbalizes information about the disease and important factors that contribute to its effect on the body.
2. Client verbalizes needed changes in life-style to accommodate treatment regimen.
3. Client establishes and maintains hope.
4. Client adapts to presence of cancer and complies with scheduled follow-up appointments.
5. Client avoids unproven therapies and methods of controlling disease.
6. Client contacts and utilizes community agencies for information and support.
7. Client participates in goal setting and decisions regarding care.

Postoperative Care Following Inpatient or Outpatient Surgery

Postoperative care involves the physical and emotional care of a client following surgery and discharge from the hospital or care of a client after surgery done in an outpatient surgical unit and discharge to home on the day of surgery. Outpatient surgery usually involves minor procedures that are done with administration of local anesthetics and/or short-acting inhalation anesthetics.

Home care is concerned with the teaching of safety management and preservation of health and function following

outpatient surgery and with maintenance and reinforcement of the hospital discharge teaching for follow-up care at home.

Nursing diagnosis

Risk for infection

Related factors: Inadequate primary defenses; invasive procedure

Defining characteristics: Surgical wound (broken skin) with redness, swelling, pain, drainage; respiratory changes (stasis of secretions) with decreased breath sounds, shortness of breath; urinary changes (stasis of body fluids) with cloudy, foul-smelling urine with or without indwelling catheter

OUTCOMES

Short-term

Reduced risk of infectious process following surgery, as evidenced by client's compliance with postoperative measures to prevent bacterial contamination (expected within 1 to 2 weeks)

Long-term

Absence of infectious process, as evidenced by wound healing without complication and by absence of postoperative complications, with return of optimal health and functional status (expected within 1 to 2 months)

NURSING INTERVENTIONS/INSTRUCTIONS

1. Assess, and instruct client to assess, wound site(s) for edge approximation and healing; drainage device for characteristics and amount of wound drainage; changes in color, temperature, or drainage; presence of swelling at surgical site; and increased pain (each visit).
2. Assess urine for characteristic changes and for catheter patency if one is in place; assess for respiratory changes in rate, depth, and ease and for changes in sputum to yellow or other color (each visit).
3. Instruct client in hand-washing technique and to perform before direct care, before meals, and after using bathroom (first visit).
4. Instruct client in continued use of incentive spirometry, coughing and deep breathing exercises, and assist client to plan daily schedule for times and frequency (first visit).

5. Instruct client in wound care and dressing change using sterile technique; how to care for and dress wound drains and device; how to remove dressing and application of smaller dressing; reporting pain, redness, or swelling at site; allow for return demonstration (first visit and reinforce on second visit).
6. Instruct client in need to void every 2 hours and to report any change in color or odor; teach client how to care for catheter and prevent entry of bacteria into the bladder (first visit).
7. Instruct client to monitor temperature and note chilling or elevation to over 100° F and to report to physician (first visit).
8. Instruct client in administration of antibiotic therapy to prevent or treat infection, whether oral or topical (ointment, drops), including route, dose, time, frequency, side effects, and drug and food interactions, and to instruct client to complete entire prescription (first visit).
9. Instruct client to avoid exposure to people with upper respiratory infections or who are ill (first visit).

CLIENT AND FAMILY/CAREGIVER INTERVENTIONS

1. Client administers antibiotic therapy correctly and as prescribed.
2. Client provides care to surgical site as needed, using sterile technique.
3. Client monitors temperature and condition of site(s).
4. Client assesses respiratory and urinary function and reports signs and symptoms of infection.
5. Client utilizes hand-washing technique when appropriate.
6. Client avoids exposure to persons with infections or touching wound site.

Nursing diagnosis

Self-care deficit (bathing/hygiene, dressing/grooming, toileting)

Related factors: Pain; discomfort with movement; intolerance to activity

Defining characteristics: Decreased strength and endurance; inability to perform or complete ADL independently; reluctance to attempt movement and activity; fear of injury to incision

OUTCOMES

Short-term

Improvement in self-care performance, as evidenced by progressive participation in ADL and increased activity within prescribed limitations (expected within 1 to 2 weeks)

Long-term

Independence in ADL, as evidenced by client's meeting requirements for self-care within limitations or restrictions for optimal postoperative health and function and return to work (expected within 2 months, depending on surgical procedure)

NURSING INTERVENTIONS/INSTRUCTIONS

1. Assess client's ability to perform ADL, fatigue level, pain on movement or during activity, and need for special procedures or treatments before, during, or after ADL (see Functional Assessment, p. 51, for guidelines) (each visit).
2. Instruct client to assist with ADL as needed without compromising client independence or progressive self-care (first visit).
3. Allow client to develop own plan of progressive care and goals to achieve during convalescence and to revise plan as needed (each visit).
4. Instruct client to accept assistance when needed until weakness and fatigue diminish (first visit).
5. Instruct client to avoid strenuous activity or activities (first visit).
6. Instruct client in use of energy-saving devices and techniques for ADL (first visit).
7. Instruct client in administration of analgesics for pain on the basis of assessment before activities (first visit).
8. Instruct client to rest after activity, pace activities, and set limits if needed (first visit).
9. Refer home health aide to assist in ADL as needed.

CLIENT AND FAMILY/CAREGIVER INTERVENTIONS

1. Client schedules rest and activity on the basis of individual needs and condition.
2. Client participates in ADL within set limits, with goals for daily or weekly progress toward independence.
3. Client assists with any activity requiring support; asks for as-

sistance when needed until independence achieved.

4. Client uses energy-saving devices or aids in ADL.
5. Client administers analgesics when needed, based on assessment, to allow for optimal activity and ADL performance.

Nursing diagnosis

Knowledge deficit

Related factors: Lack of information about follow-up postoperative care

Defining characteristics: Expressed need for information about postoperative activity restrictions, nutrition and fluid needs, bowel and urinary elimination, and prevention of complications

OUTCOMES

Short-term

Adequate knowledge, as evidenced by client's statement of postoperative medical regimen requirements and performance of postoperative procedures and treatments (expected within 1 to 2 weeks)

Long-term

Adequate knowledge, as evidenced by client's compliance with postoperative care regimen to achieve return to optimal health and functioning (expected within 4 to 6 weeks)

NURSING INTERVENTIONS/INSTRUCTIONS

1. Assess client's life-style, ability to adapt, learning ability and interest, and family participation and support (first visit).
2. Assess knowledge of surgical procedures, reason for surgical intervention for correction of problem, and where procedure performed (hospital or outpatient unit), and provide information needed or reinforce information already received if necessary (first visit).
3. Instruct client in medication administration as ordered, including times, dose, frequency, side effects, and food and drug interactions (first and second visits).
4. Inform client of bowel and bladder elimination changes and causes and about use of stool softener, fluid intake, and ex-

ercising to assist in return to normal pattern (first visit).

5. Inform client of importance of compliance with activity and exercise regimen proposed, and instruct client to avoid activities that place stress on operative area (changing position, lifting, pushing, pulling, stooping) and to avoid heavy lifting, carrying, or straining (first visit).
6. Instruct client in incision care and in protecting it during bathing with a plastic cover taped to skin on the sides in shape of a picture frame (first visit).
7. Instruct client in appropriate amount of daily fluids, up to 3 L per day, and inclusion of protein and vitamin C in dietary planning; offer food lists and sample menus, and assist client to coordinate with food and fluid preferences (first and second visits).
8. Inform client of time to resume work schedule and activities to avoid (any visit).
9. Instruct client to report incisional pain, increased drainage, elevated temperature, or any discomfort or changes in other body areas (first visit).
10. Instruct client to comply with follow-up schedule to see physician as advised after surgery or hospital discharge (first visit).

CLIENT AND FAMILY/CAREGIVER INTERVENTIONS

1. Client administers all medications accurately; uses check-off sheet as a reminder and to avoid errors.
2. Client establishes and maintains bowel and urinary elimination patterns.
3. Client reports adverse effects of medications, treatments, and surgical intervention if appropriate.
4. Client participates in approved activities and avoids those that place stress on incisional area.
5. Client provides and ingests fluids and nutrients to facilitate health.
6. Client maintains a written daily plan for compliance with postoperative requirements.
7. Client returns to work or seeks occupational rehabilitation or retraining if appropriate.

Appendixes

Basic Life Support for the Adult Victim*

1. ADULT ONE-RESCUER CPR

1. • Establish unresponsiveness.
   • Activate the EMS system.
2. • Open airway (head tilt–chin lift or jaw thrust).
   • Check breathing (look, listen, feel).
3. • Give 2 slow breaths (1½ to 2 seconds per breath), watch chest rise, allow for exhalation between breaths.
4. • Check carotid pulse.
   • If breathing is absent but pulse is present, provide rescue breathing (1 breath every 5 seconds, about 12 breaths per minute).
5. • If no pulse, give cycles of 15 chest compressions (rate, 80 to 100 compressions per minute) followed by 2 slow breaths.
6. • After 4 cycles of 15:2 (about 1 minute), check pulse.
   • If no pulse, continue 15:2 cycle, beginning with chest compressions.

2. ADULT TWO-RESCUER CPR

1. • Establish unresponsiveness.
   • EMS system has been activated.

Rescuer 1

2. • Open airway (head tilt–chin lift or jaw thrust).
   • Check breathing (look, listen, feel).
3. • Give 2 slow breaths (1½ to 2 seconds per breath), watch chest rise, allow for exhalation between breaths.
4. • Check carotid pulse.

---

*Reprinted with permission from American Heart Association: Basic life support for the adult victim, Currents 1993, p 6.

Rescuer 2

5. • If no pulse, give cycles of 5 chest compressions (rate, 80 to 100 compressions per minute) followed by 1 slow breath by Rescuer 1.
6. • After 1 minute of rescue support, check pulse.
   • If no pulse, continue 5:1 cycles.

3. ADULT FOREIGN BODY AIRWAY OBSTRUCTION—CONSCIOUS

1. • Ask "Are you choking?"
2. • Give abdominal thrusts (chest thrusts for pregnant or obese victim).
3. • Repeat thrusts until effective or victim becomes unconscious.

If victim becomes unconscious—

4. • Activate the EMS system.
5. • Perform a tongue-jaw lift followed by a finger sweep to remove the object.
6. • Open airway and try to ventilate; if still obstructed, reposition head and try to ventilate again.
7. • Give up to 5 abdominal thrusts.
8. • Repeat steps 5 through 7 until effective.

4. ADULT FOREIGN BODY AIRWAY OBSTRUCTION—UNCONSCIOUS

1. • Establish unresponsiveness.
   • Activate the EMS system.
2. • Open airway and try to ventilate; if still obstructed, reposition the head and try to ventilate again.
3. • Perform up to 5 abdominal thrusts.
4. • Perform a tongue-jaw lift followed by a finger sweep to remove the object.
5. • Repeat steps 2 through 4 until effective.

Documentation and Insurance Payment Guidelines

BASIC CONSIDERATIONS

1. Homebound status documented weekly with specific notations of physical, mental, or emotional limitations or restrictions that prevent leaving home except for therapy, physician, or laboratory appointments (usually determined by insurance plan). Examples include bed- or wheelchair-bound, severe pain, shortness of breath with slight exertion, indwelling catheter, dizziness, weakness, poor balance, or unsteady gait as result of surgery or illness, fractures or disabilities that prevent ambulation without assistance or use of aids, draining wounds or dressing changes, partial or complete paralysis, mental confusion, and extreme anxiety or paranoia.
2. Documentation of home care is included in the criteria for agencies seeking to meet state certification and licensure requirements.
3. Documentation is the basis for Medicare, Medicaid, and third-party payors, and the information recorded determines the billing statements for services to receive payment for continued or specific number of care visits, depending on need. Some payors require a copy of the nurses' notes with billing to receive reimbursement. It is advisable for agencies to request what services or types of care can be included in billing and maintain ongoing communication with the payment source(s) regarding documentation requirements during home care.
4. Documentation allows for continuity of planned care by providing a method of communication to others involved in a variety of care procedures and treatments by interdisciplinary professionals.
5. Documentation and maintenance of an accurate record is considered a legal document and ensures that profession-

al standards have been followed in the delivery of home care.

6. Documentation and maintenance of an accurate record provides data for research and audits for payment review.
7. Documentation can include the written narrative, flow sheets for checks and notes related to frequent monitoring of highly technical equipment, and frequent assessments of vital physiologic functions and complete care plans.
8. Documentation must be factual, objective, succinct, descriptive, and relevant; omit items or words that do not relate or contribute to essential information.
9. In home care, clients and family members are taught assessment procedures and use of flow sheets or graphs to note daily monitoring information within established parameters.

GENERAL DOCUMENTATION REQUIREMENTS FOR ALL CARE PLANS

1. Date and signature of nurse preparing the care plan
2. Assessment data and client status in major areas affected
3. Changes in client's health status
4. Client and family response and adaptation to illness
5. Care plan with inclusion of all accepted components
6. Nursing activities, including all assessments and teaching
7. Need for further assessment, instruction, referrals
8. Plan and timing for next visit
9. Readiness and plan for discharge from home visits
10. Dates and signatures of all professional and nonprofessional personnel performing care, and evaluation when and where appropriate
11. Copy of the plan available for the client and family

ESSENTIAL DOCUMENTATION COMPONENTS

1. Health history and physical assessment with emphasis on system(s) related to the client's medical diagnosis (listing all medical diagnoses but documenting the most acute one as the principal diagnosis)
2. Qualified medical diagnoses when possible by including words such as newly diagnosed, unstable, uncontrolled, or acute exacerbation

3. Identified nursing diagnoses with dates for each problem on the care plan
4. Client-focused (what client is to achieve), measurable (specific success achievement), realistic (definitely achievable) goals or outcomes (short- and long-term in collaboration with the client) and achievement dates documented (designated time) at least weekly, with the nursing interventions that achieve the specific outcomes, the frequency performed, and personnel responsible for the activities
5. Specific, descriptive choices or alternate nursing interventions or actions to solve problems and implement goals that lead to increased capacity for self-care and that reduce functional limitations; developed by the nurse, interdisciplinary professionals, adjunct personnel, client, and family members
6. Evaluation of goal fulfillment at designated time intervals (days, weeks, or months) by changes in the client's condition or need to reassess and modify the care plan based on these findings
7. Exact services being provided that require skilled professional nursing care, indication of other care needed
8. Time frames in which care will be provided (number of times per week), depending on condition and insurance parameters, plans for more frequent visits at the beginning of home care
9. Inclusion in each notation of why the visit was needed, using specific information from assessment to affirm medical necessity and specific care given
10. All care (specific and general) that relates to the medical diagnoses and physician orders; physician signature should appear on the document according to agency and insurance requirements
11. Unstable states or technology-dependent client that require skilled nursing care and response to changes in treatments or care; confirm that skilled care matches the diagnoses and physician orders
12. Treatments, exercise, and other rehabilitation regimens to restore function lost because of illness and described by the medical diagnosis; any obstacles (mental capabilities, language barrier) that need to be overcome to achieve optimal health
13. All teaching to client and family to develop ability to perform care and procedures, including disease-related information, assessments, strategies, demonstrations, record keeping; note

poor comprehension and lack of capability by client and need for reteaching

14. Referrals to professional therapists, community resources
15. Supervision visits (every 2 to 4 weeks, depending on insurance requirements) noting evaluation of licensed vocational nurse (LVN), home health aide (HHA), client and family response to care, need for care plan revision or restatement of existing plan
16. Discharge plan and instructions, summary to physician, case closing date; discharge must be considered if nursing interventions are not needed for up to 3 weeks and no problems exist or recur for which insurance benefits would apply

UNACCEPTABLE WORD USAGE AND STATEMENTS

1. Use of chronic for acute exacerbation
2. Use of monitor for assess or evaluate if condition has stabilized
3. Use of reinforce or repeat instruction instead of reinstruct
4. Use of discussed instead of instructed
5. Use of check or observe instead of assess
6. Use of words such as stabilized or reviewed instead of responding to treatment
7. Use of provide emotional support instead of making a referral
8. Use of prevent if instruction has already been given
9. Use of improvement, indicating that care is no longer needed (respiration rate, depth, and ease improved), instead of need for care with specific assessment data (respirations remaining at 28/minute with exertional dyspnea present)
10. Use of subjective general statement (general weakness) instead of objective statement (ambulates only 10 feet without fatigue, dizziness, dyspnea)
11. Lack of progress when progress should be seen instead of inability to participate in therapy because of mental or physical disabilities
12. Repetitive teaching unless client has limited intelligence or increased anxiety, use of specific care and skills performed (instructed to draw insulin into a syringe using sterile technique)
13. Private sitter or companion
14. Trips that client takes

15. Medications reviewed
16. Maintenance care
17. Unstable states instead of noting specific interventions and changes in treatment (medications, pulmonary physiotherapy, catheter change, sterile irrigations, wound care)

*INSURANCE PAYMENT GUIDELINES**

1. Usually all clients over 65 years of age disabled for 2 years or more or on renal dialysis receive Medicare benefits for health care. They also may have supplemental private health insurance (Medi-Gap) that covers expenses not paid for by Medicare or belong to a health maintenance organization (HMO) that accepts Medicare benefits without additional private coverage; these plans vary and benefits are policy specific.
2. Medicaid is a government assistance plan that differs from state to state. Coverage is reserved for a segment of the population whose economic status complies with the payment standards set by government regulations (usually 50% federal and 50% state funded).
3. CHAMPUS insurance benefits and coverage are reserved for government employees eligible to receive these payments via past or present employment or service to the government.
4. Private health insurance can be individually owned and paid for or part of a group policy sponsored and paid for completely or in part by the client's employer. The coverage also can include varied options for deductibles, prescription drugs, vision and dental health, HMOs, preferred provider organizations (PPO), and others.
5. Private long-term facility care insurance can include home care benefits following a hospitalization or long-term facility stay or private home care exclusively as a single policy or as a rider to a long-term nursing home policy.
6. Private combination health care insurance plans may cover long-term facility care, alternate or assistive facility care, and home care that includes case management planning.

---

*Requirements and benefits for government and private insurance plans change periodically, and guidelines should be compared with and validated as to what is and what is not covered at a given time.

7. Major areas of coverage usually include assessment, teaching, and performing complex hands-on care and procedures, with hours or number of visits allowed depending on acuity and type of skilled care needed; skilled care and lack of someone to perform personal care is needed before an HHA is assigned and will be paid.
8. Medicare, Medicaid, and some third-party payors require documentation of homebound status and skilled care need with specific, detailed functional limitations, dates of onset, and appropriate descriptive adjectives included in the medical diagnoses, a medical plan of care, and medical orders for home care.
9. The frequency of paid visits depends on the diagnosis, acuteness of the illness, homebound status, client or caregiver ability to learn, presence of a caregiver to teach, stability of client's condition, multiple medical diagnoses, and finally insurance criteria. Parameters may or may not be given as a basis for the number of visits that would be acceptable. Usually one begins with a higher frequency of visits, tapers down if possible, and schedules for 2 or 3 times per week. Daily visits can be allowed only during an acute phase or teaching; however, proper documentation will allow coverage for daily or twice daily visits.
10. Private home care insurance usually provides a designated amount of money available for daily care for a specified number of years based on the amount selected by the client. Criteria for payment commonly includes medical necessity and need for care in at least two or three of the five activities of daily living (ADL).
11. Nursing history, assessments, and care plan documentations that include all the specific requirements identified in the Essential Documentation Components must be present.

EXAMPLES OF ACTIVITIES USUALLY COVERED

1. New diagnosis of diabetes requiring insulin administration, glucose monitoring, foot care, and dietary regimen
2. New intestinal or urinary diversion surgical care
3. Unstable hypertension or other cardiac conditions requiring medication, dietary changes
4. Intramuscular, intravenous injections or infusion therapy
5. Renal dialysis

6. Nasogastric, gastrostomy feedings and care
7. Tracheostomy care and tube change, assisted ventilation
8. Wound care and dressing changes
9. Foley catheter changes, disimpaction
10. Medication regimen related to disease, one medication per visit
11. Disease pathology and signs and symptoms
12. Any assessment and teaching function

EXAMPLES OF ACTIVITIES NOT USUALLY COVERED (UNLESS NOT ABLE TO BE PERFORMED BY CLIENT OR CAREGIVER)

1. Vital signs (VS), intake and output (I&O)
2. Stable client who continues to be monitored
3. Repetition and reinforcement of instruction (medications, treatments)
4. Any preventive care, especially if previously taught (pressure ulcers)
5. Emotional support
6. Positioning in bed, active or passive range-of-motion (ROM) exercises
7. Medication injections if not medically necessary
8. Procedures performed by person not considered to be skilled

EXAMPLES OF PROBLEM AREAS FOR COVERAGE

1. Frequent physician contacts with no new orders
2. Chronic diagnosis with no change in treatment plan by physician
3. Too few or too many visits
4. Medical necessity for procedure
5. Procedures not corresponding with diagnoses
6. Rehabilitative claims of more than 3 months unless properly documented
7. Repeated instruction
8. Custodial care
9. Not homebound (varies in different areas)
10. Unskilled or intermittent care
11. Daily visits for more than 3 weeks unless estimated time of healing and necessity of teaching are documented

Text continued on p. 411.

Laboratory Values*

Test	Value Range	SI Range
BLOOD		
Acetone	Negative	Negative
Acid phosphatase	0.13-0.63 U/L at 37° C	2.2-10.5 U/L at 37° C
Albumin	3.2-5.6 g/dl (method related)	32-56 g/L
Aldolase	3-8 U/dl at 37° C	22-59 mU/L at 37° C
Alkaline phosphatase	20-130 IU/L at 37° C	20-130 U/L at 37° C
Ammonia	12-48 μg/dl (method related)	7-28 μmol/L
Amylase	16-120 Somogyi units/dl	30-220 U/L
Arterial blood gases		
pH	7.38-7.44	7.38-7.44
P_{CO_2}	35-40mm Hg	4.7-5.3 kPa
P_{O_2}	95-100 mm Hg	12.7-13.3 kPa
Bilirubin		
Total	0.1-1.2 mg/dl	2-21 μmol/L
Direct (conjugated)	<0.3 mg/dl	<5μmol/L
Indirect (unconjugated)	0.1-1.0 mg/dl	2-17 μmol/L
Calcium		
Total	9.2-11.0 mg/dl	2.30-2.74 mmol/L
Ionized	4.0-4.8 mg/dl	1.00-1.20 mmol/L
Chloride	95-103 mEq/L	95-103 mmol/L
Cholesterol	150-250 mg/dl (age, diet related)	3.88-6.47 mmol/L
Complete blood count		
Hematocrit	40%-54% (male)	0.40-0.54
	38%-47% (female)	0.38-0.47
Hemoglobin	13.5-18.0 g/dl (male)	135-180 g/L
	12.0-16.0 g/dl (female)	120-160 g/L
Red cell count	$4.6\text{-}6.2 \times 10^6/\mu l$ (male)	$4.6\text{-}6.2 \times 10^{12}/L$

*Modified from Henry JB: *Clinical diagnosis and management by laboratory methods*, ed 18, Philadelphia, 1991, WB Saunders.

Continued

Laboratory Values—cont'd

Test	Value Range	SI Range
BLOOD—cont'd		
	4.2-5.4 × 10^6/μl (female)	4.2-5.4 × 10^{12}/L
White cell count	4.5-11.0 × 10^3/μl	4.5-11.0 × 10^9/L
Creatine kinase		
Male	55-170 U/L at 37° C	55-170 U/L at 37° C
Female	30-135 U/L at 37° C	30-135 U/L at 37° C
Creatinine	0.6-1.2 mg/dl	53-106 μmol/L
Erythrocyte sedimentation rate	<15 mm/hr (male)	
	<20-30 mm/hr (male over 50)	
	<20 mm/hr (female)	
	<30-42 mm/hr (female over 50)	
Fatty acids	9.0-15.0 mmol/L (total)	9.0-15.0 mmol/L
	300-480 μEq/L (free)	300-480 μmol/L
Folate	>2.3 ng/ml (RIA method)	>5 nmol/L
Glucose	70-110 mg/dl (fasting)	
Immunoglobulins		
IgG	800-1801 mg/dl	8.0-18.0 g/L
IgA	113-563 mg/dl	1.1-5.6 g/L
IgM	54-222 mg/dl	0.5-2.2 g/L
IgD	0.5-3.0 mg/dl	5.0-30.0 mg/L
IgE	0.01-0.04 mg/dl	0.1-0.4 mg/L
Iron	60-150 μg/dl (total)	10.7-26.9 μmol/L
Lactate dehydrogenase	30%-60% of total	0.30-0.60 fraction of total
Lipase	14-280 mU/ml	14-280 U/L
Magnesium	1.3-2.1 mEq/L	0.65-105 mmol/L
Partial thromboplastin time (activated)	25-35 sec (reagent dependent)	

Laboratory Values—cont'd

Test	Value Range	SI Range
BLOOD—cont'd		
Phosphorus	2.3-4.7 mg/dl	0.74-1.52 mmol/L
Platelet count	150,000-450,000/μl	150-400 × 10^9/L
Potassium	3.8-5.0 mEq/L	3.8-5.09 mmol/L
Proteins		
Total	6.0-7.8 g/dl	60-78 g/L
Albumin	3.2-4.5 g/dl	32-45 g/L
Globulin	2.3-3.5 g/dl	23-35 g/L
Prothrombin time	10-13 sec (reagent dependent)	
Reticulocyte count	25,000-75,000 cells/μl	25-75 × 10^9/L
Sodium	136-142 mEq/L	136-142 mmol/L
Thyroid tests		
Thyroxine	5.5-12.5 μg/dl (total)	71-161 nmol/L
	0.9-2.3 ng/dl (free)	12-30 pmol/L
Triiodothyronine	80-200 ng/dl	1.23-3 nmol/L
	25%-38% (resin uptake)	0.25-0.38 uptake fraction
Transferases		
Aspartate aminotransferase	8-33 U/L at 37° C	8-33 U/L at 37° C
Alanine aminotransferase	4-36 U/L at 37° C	4-36 U/L at 37° C
Gamma glutamyl	5-40 U/L at 37° C	5-40 U/L at 37° C
Triglycerides	10-190 mg/dl	0.11-2.15 mmol/L
Urea nitrogen	8-23 mg/dl	2.9-8.2 mmol/L
Uric acid	4.0-8.5 mg/dl (male)	0.24-0.51 mmol/L
	2.7-7.3 mg/dl (female)	0.16-0.43 mmol/L
THERAPEUTIC DRUG LEVELS		
Digoxin	0.5-2 ng/ml	0.5-2 nmol/L
Phenytoin	10-20 μg/ml	40-79 μmol/L
Salicylate	100-200 μg/ml	1.09-1.45 mmol/L
Theophylline	10-20 μg/ml	44-111 μmol/L

Continued

Laboratory Values—cont'd

Test	Value Range	SI Range
URINE		
Acetone	Negative	Negative
Albumin	Negative (random)	Negative
	15-150 mg/24hr	0.015-0.150 nmol/24 hr
Bilirubin	Negative (random)	Negative
Catecholamines	<14 μg/dl (random)	<828 nmol/L
	<100 μg/dl/24 hr	<591 nmol/24 hr
Creatinine	20-26 mg/kg/24 hr (male)	177-230 μmol/kg/24 hr
	14-22 mg/kg/24 hr (female)	124-195 μmol/kg/24 hr
Glucose	Negative (random)	Negative
	130 mg/24 hr	0.72 mmol/24 hr
Osmolality	500-800 mOsm/kg water	500-800 mmol/kg
Specific gravity	1.016-1.022	1.016-1.022
Uric acid	250-750 mg/24 hr	1.5-4.5 mmol/24 hr
Uribilinogen	0.05-2.5 mg/24hr	0.1-4.2 μmol/24 hr
Vanillylmandelic acid	1.5-7.5 mg/24 hr	7.6-37.9 μmol/24 hr
FECES		
Bile	Negative (random)	Negative
Fat	<5 g/24 hr (total)	<5 g/24 hr
Occult blood	Negative	Negative
Trypsin	2+ to 4+	2+ to 4+
Urobilinogen	Positive (random)	Positive
	40-200 mg/24 hr	68-339 μmol/24 hr

Medication Administration and Teaching Guidelines

Medication administration to clients in the home by the caregiver or self-administration is the focus of these guidelines. Major responsibilities of the home care nurse are teaching the client and/or family to perform this procedure correctly and assessing the effects. Some of the more complex administration methods and routes require adequate or more extensive instruction and practice time to ensure safe compliance with a medication regimen. Medications administered in the home are prescribed by the physician or other prescriber and include those given orally, sublingually, topically, intramuscularly, subcutaneously, intrathecally, intravenously, by inhalation, and by feeding tube and are scheduled for regular administration or in response to requests when needed. The following information provides helpful tips as well as actual procedures and teaching performed by the nurse for the client and/or family to ensure safe administration and effective results from drug therapy:

TIPS FOR TEACHING SAFE ADMINISTRATION

1. Assess for age, weight, drug allergies.
2. Teach about compatibility with foods, other medications.
3. Note medications taken, both prescribed and over-the-counter.
4. Assess past dependency or risk for present dependency on drugs.
5. Instruct regarding use of alcohol, caffeine-containing beverages, herbal products, tobacco.
6. Provide information about each drug and special recommendations for administration.
7. Determine daily routines and best times for medication administration.
8. Assess ability to swallow medications, use of alternate forms or routes.
9. Assess client's cognitive, intellectual capacity, developmental level, and understanding of drug administration.

10. Give thorough instructions that include the drug name, reason for use, dose, frequency, route, form, length of time, measurement device to use, expected effects, adverse side effects to report or what actions to take.
11. Encourage return demonstrations until client feels comfortable with the procedure (usually more appropriate for injections).
12. Offer or maintain a written procedure and time schedule for administration of medications, check sheet, reminder compartmental devices and daily replenishment.
13. Inform that if drug is forgotten, wait until next dosage time unless dose can be taken within 1 hour after scheduled time (depends on frequency of dosage).
14. Note expiration dates and store in a cool, dry, locked cabinet with lid tightly fixed on the original container and labeled with the written instructions; refrigerate if medicine is to be kept at a lower temperature.
15. Ensure that devices used in medication administration are accompanied by inserts with instructions for use or pamphlet with manufacturer's directions for use, care, and type of administration set to use.

ORAL MEDICATIONS

1. Check medication label for the name, amount, and time before, during, and after administration to ensure accuracy; compare with drug container or checklist.
2. Administer according to special instructions such as before or after meals, at bedtime, number of times per day, with or without food, use of a straw, under the tongue, or in the cheek.
3. Select device to give the medication based on form and ability to swallow and prepare medications:
   - Measuring spoon, calibrated cup for liquid form, paper medicine cup
   - Pill crusher to crush tablets and water, juice, or soft food for mixing
4. Place tablet toward the back of the mouth and offer a glass of water to swallow.
5. Note side effects and instruct client to stop the medication and report to the physician immediately.

TOPICAL MEDICATIONS (TRANSCUTANEOUS, SUPPOSITORY, OINTMENT)

Gloves and sterile technique are used to perform all topical procedures when exposure to body fluid or breaks in skin are anticipated or present.

1. Check medication as for oral administration.
2. Expose area to be treated, position and drape if needed, remove dressings.
3. Uncap ointment and squeeze small amount and discard, apply to affected area with a sponge or applicator.
4. Cleanse skin and apply patch to administer via transcutanous route for prescribed time.
5. Insert correct dosage suppository, removed from wrapper, into the rectum past the internal sphincter with a cot-protected finger that has been moistened with water; hold buttocks together for about 5 minutes to prevent expulsion if needed.

EYE, EAR, NOSE MEDICATIONS

Nose administration:

1. Cleanse around nose and remove any accumulated secretion from the nares with a warm damp cloth, leave in place if crusted secretions are present until soft enough to be wiped away, draw up medication into the nose dropper.
2. Place in a supine position and gently tilt head backwards to rest on a small pillow or over side of the bed.
3. Place the correct number of drops into each side of the nose and retain head in tilted position for a minute; avoid allowing tip of dropper to touch nose.
4. Wipe excess from nose and allow to resume normal position.

Ear Administration:

1. Warm bottle of medication in a pan of water and check to assess warmth to avoid cold or hot drops, draw up medication into the ear dropper.
2. Cleanse outside of ears to remove any drainage with a tissue or cotton-tipped applicator, avoid touching the external ear canal.

3. Place on side to expose ear to receive medication and then on the other side to receive the medication.
4. Pull the outer ear upward and backward to straighten canal, place correct number of drops in each ear toward the side of the canal; avoid allowing tip of dropper to touch ears.
5. Maintain position of the head for a minute following the drops in each ear and wipe away excess from the outer ear if needed.
6. Place a cotton ball in each ear to prevent medication from leaking, change with each administration of drops to ears.

Eye Administration:

1. Cleanse around eyes with a warm damp cloth to remove any secretions, leave in place if crusted material is present until soft enough to be wiped away, draw medication up into the eyedropper.
2. Position in supine position with head slightly tilted backward and to the side of the eye to receive the medication.
3. Request the client to look up, gently pull the lower lid downward and place the correct number of drops into the lower lid using the other hand; avoid allowing the tip of the dropper to touch any part of the eye or skin.
4. Request client to close eyes tightly and open again to disperse the fluid, wipe any excess medication from around the eye with tissue.
5. For eye ointment follow same procedure and squeeze the ointment across the inner aspect of the lower lid from the canthus to the outer aspect of the eye.

INHALATION MEDICATIONS

Handheld small-volume nebulizer (SVN) administration:

1. Prepare nebulizer by attaching tubing and plugging into electric outlet with machine on OFF.
2. Assemble nebulizer chamber by attaching mouthpiece to the piece that is connected to the cap of the chamber containing prescribed medication dose (measured and poured or premeasured unit dose and poured).
3. Place cap on chamber by turning clockwise and attach the tubing from the nebulizer (compressor) to the chamber.
4. Check that all connections are tight, turn machine to ON, and note mist coming from the mouthpiece.

5. Place the mouthpiece into the mouth with lips around it and inform client to breathe through mouth.
6. Allow to breathe slowly and deeply, turn off machine to rest if fatigued and continue when able, until all solution is gone.
7. Turn machine OFF, disassemble chamber and cleanse with mild detergent, rinse with warm water, and air dry on paper towel.

Handheld metered-dose inhaler (MDI) administration:

1. Insert metal canister tightly into the holder and shake well to mix medication with the propellant.
2. Remove cap, request to exhale fully, place the inhaler in an upright position and hold mouthpiece up to mouth, or in the mouth resting on lower teeth with lips around it.
3. Request to press on top of canister with finger and inhale slowly and deeply, then hold breath for 5 to 10 seconds or as long as possible.
4. Release finger and remove from mouth, wait for 30 seconds, and repeat the procedure for a second dose.
5. Repeat the procedure if a second medication is to follow by inhalation.
6. Perform at frequency prescribed, remove canister, rinse holder daily, and allow to dry on paper towel.
7. Instruct to rinse mouth following inhalation of corticosteroid medication.

ENTERAL TUBE MEDICATIONS

Indwelling tubes include nasogastric (NG) and gastrostomy types. They are placed in position for short- or long-term feedings when the oral route is not possible. Medications administered via these small-bore feeding tubes are in liquid form or crushed tablet(s) mixed in a small amount of liquid (10 ml) and administered by the gravity method as follows:

1. Unclamp tube and check for placement in stomach and amount of residual, and discontinue or delay any feeding for 15 minutes prior to medication administration.
2. Place the prescribed dose in the barrel of a syringe, unclamp the tube end, and connect the barrel to the tubing.
3. Hold barrel 6 inches above insertion site and allow the liquid to flow into the tube by gravity; when the syringe barrel is almost

empty, add 30 ml water and allow to flow and clear the tubing to ensure that all the medication has reached the stomach.

4. Check patency of tubing for clogging if crushed or viscous medications are administered.

INTRAMUSCULAR (IM) AND SUBCUTANEOUS (SC) MEDICATIONS

Medication preparation:

1. Open proper-sized packaged syringe and needle, assemble if needed.
2. Cleanse top of vial with alcohol swab or remove top of ampule.
3. Remove cap from needle, draw in amount of air equal to amount of medication needed, place needle into top of vial, inject air into the vial, and withdraw the amount of medication needed; or place needle into the ampule and withdraw amount of medication needed.
4. Remove the needle from the vial or ampule, remove any air bubbles, and replace the cap loosely for easy removal when ready to administer the injection.

Medication administration:

1. Place client in sitting or lying position with proposed site exposed.
2. Cleanse the site with an alcohol swab in a circular motion from center outward and allow to air dry.
3. Remove cap from needle, hold the skin firmly at the appropriate site, and insert the needle at a 90-degree angle (intramuscular) or 45-degree angle with bevel of point facing upward (subcutaneous).
4. Pull the plunger to check for blood, remove and change needle if blood appears, or inject contents of syringe if blood does not appear.
5. Quickly and smoothly withdraw syringe and gently swab area with a tissue; apply an adhesive strip.
6. Dispose of syringe and needle, without recapping or breaking needle, in a waterproof, punctureproof, unbreakable container (covered coffee can) for proper disposal of hazardous materials.

SYRINGE PUMP SUBCUTANEOUS MEDICATIONS

A syringe pump contains a battery-powered motor that pushes fluid through the syringe in measured amounts and intervals for infusion of medication. It is usually used for insulin administration when multiple injections are necessary to receive insulin therapy. Gloves and sterile technique are used to perform syringe pump procedures.

1. Fill syringe, with the infusion tubing attached, with the prescribed type and amount of insulin (usually a 24-hour supply of fast-acting insulin) and place in the pump correctly; close the cover while leaving the tubing clamped and exposed on the outside of the pump.
2. Attach needle to the tubing, unclamp, and prime; insert into the prepared abdominal site subcutanously at a 30- to 60-degree angle, secure in place on the abdomen with a transparent dressing over the needle and tubing to prevent dislodgement, and allow for site assessment.
3. Set the program pump for continuous dose injections or manually for dose intervals with amounts (as prior to meals) that are balanced with activities and dietary regimens.
4. Place pump in carrying case and attach to belt or place in pocket.
5. Perform pump alarm checks, alternate the injection sites, change tubing and needle every 48 hours, and change batteries as needed.
6. Instruct client to perform blood glucose and urine testing and report altered levels that indicate need for modification of insulin dosage or dietary regimen. (See Diabetes Mellitus.)

MEDIFUSE SYRINGE PUMP INTRAVENOUS (IV) MEDICATIONS

A Medifuse syringe is a portable, disposable, nonelectric mechanical system for a continuous delivery of medications. It is an infusion device that contains a mechanism that applies the force needed to push the medication through a syringe that holds 10 to 35 ml. Small predictable amounts of 0.25 ml or less in a set infusion time and rate can be delivered. The infusion device system contains the infusion holder, the syringe to hold the medication, the administration set-up (tubing), and a belt. It is used to deliver analgesics, antibiotics, or chemotherapeutic agents intravenously at a preset volume, time, and rate. Gloves and sterile technique are used to perform any Medifuse procedures.

1. Prepare the syringe containing the appropriate amount and dose of medication (can be prepared by a pharmacist), connect to the administration set, expel air, and cover end of tubing.
2. Position the syringe in the holder in the infuser device and set the time and rate ordered (set is color coded for time).
3. Attach to access site and start infusion; flow will cease when correct amount of medication has been administered without allowing a backflow of blood.
4. Carry device in a case attached to a belt and hang over shoulder or place in a pocket.
5. Remove when completed, provide site care, and dispose of syringe.

HOMEPUMP INTRAVENOUS MEDICATIONS

A Homepump is a single-use, disposable, small (3 inches in height), lightweight (2 oz if empty) infusion pump available in various sizes to administer antibiotics and chemotherapy IV in home care. It is an infusion pump that controls the flow rate by the pressure of an elastometric membrane and microbore cannula. It is a one-piece closed system that can deliver 50 to 200 ml/hr of antibiotics in single doses and 2 to 5 ml/hr of chemotherapeutic doses. It consists of a pump device with a port cap, a container, tubing and a clamp, filter, adapter, cap, and carrying pouch. Gloves and sterile technique are used when performing Homepump procedures.

1. Select the proper-sized pump, close the clamp, and place the proper dose of medication at room temperature through the top port with a syringe into the multilayer membrane.
2. Remove the cap of the pump set-up at the distal end to release air from the line, then reclamp and attach the Luer adapter to the IV access site.
3. Unclamp pump set-up and begin the infusion.
4. Place in a carrying bag or pocket to permit mobility.
5. At conclusion of medication administration, disconnect the pump and set-up and dispose of the entire device because it cannot be reused.
6. Provide site care and apply dressing.

VERIFUSE INFUSION PUMP FOR INTRAVENOUS MEDICATIONS OR FLUIDS

A Verifuse infusion pump is capable of multiple-therapy delivery of medications by continuous, intermittent, or continuous with bolus, and tapering capabilities for delivery of total parenteral nutrition (TPN). It is a single-channel peristaltic pump that can be powered by battery or AC electric power. It includes the small, lightweight pump device, remote bolus control, programing software, administration set-up with filter and multiple injection ports, a universal spike, TPN kit, battery pack, AC power adapter, and carrying case.

1. Have the client protocol or prescription parameters entered into the computer to convert the data into a bar code by the software.
2. Print bar is printed onto a label for the medication container or entered by the nurse (bar code simplifies programing of an infusion, prevents client tampering, improper programing, and prolonged instruction).
3. Spike administration set tubing into the solution container, clamp and thread through the pump, unclamp and prime the tubing, reclamp and attach to the IV access.
4. Scan bar code, press VERIFY, and check for the correct protocol on the pump's display screen.
5. Unclamp tubing, press START, and initiate infusion to deliver as little as 0.1 ml/hr or a total of 0.1 ml with a maximum rate of 300 ml/hr with the capability to deliver a total of 6000 ml.
6. Place case carrying the device in pocket or within reach during infusion.
7. Press STOP to discontinue intermittent or bolus infusion, disconnect from IV site, remove set-up for proper disposal.
8. Attach Homebase to the side of the pump for remote programming of the pump or to check infusion status by telephone via a built-in modem to a computer for viewing by the pharmacist (allows for Homebase to receive a new protocol and send pump status for evaluation and client compliance that can reduce home visits to monitor IV therapy).

PATIENT-CONTROLLED ANALGESIA (PCA)

This is a method of self-administered drugs that uses a programmable infusion pump for IV and SC routes to allow for intermittent doses at preset time intervals. The analgesic can be administered by initial bolus and then continuous infusion. Time between doses is known as the lockout interval and should be length of time needed for the onset of drug action. Infusion of medication is initiated by pushing a button when pain is experienced.

EPIDURAL OR INTRATHECAL MEDICATIONS

Medication administration via these routes is usually reserved for terminal care. A catheter is inserted into the epidural or intrathecal space for intermittent or continuous infusion of analgesia to provide consistent drug levels and a long-lasting effect by the direct action on receptors in the spinal cord.

INFUSION PUMPS FOR INTRAVENOUS MEDICATIONS OR FLUIDS

A variety of ambulatory, small, portable microcomputer-controlled peristaltic infusion pumps are available to deliver prescribed amounts of medications, fluids, or TPN via central venous lines (right atrial catheter, port catheter). The infusion pump controller is used when a sustained slow flow rate is desired. Another available infusion pump delivers fluids at a high flow rate. Both of these stationary types of pumps have safety alarms that go off when air gets in the line, the line becomes occluded, or when the infusion has been completed. In general, ambulatory and stationary pumps are selected according to the type of infusion fluid, amount and rate of infusion, and route of administration.

They are selected for use depending on their capability of delivering continuous (with or without bolus) and intermittent infusion of analgesics, antibiotics, chemotherapeutics, TPN, and hydration fluids. Depending on the model, they can deliver 1 to 400 ml/hr for 1 minute to 100 hours and deliver two independent programs with one device for bolus, intermittent, or continuous infusion. The ambulatory devices operate via internal or external battery power. The device and solution container(s) can be placed in a carrying case and hung over the shoulder or kept in the open for viewing. Various brands of delivery systems are available for home intravenous therapy (Pancreatec, Cormeds, IVAC, IMED).

HEPARIN LOCK INTRAVENOUS MEDICATIONS

A catheter is inserted into a vein and maintained over time to eliminate the need for multiple peripheral venipunctures to administer IV medication in the home. The primary care involves maintaining and monitoring tube for patency and insertion site for infection and safe medication administration. Gloves and sterile technique are used when performing heparin lock procedures.

Site assessment and protection:

1. Note redness, edema, pain, and drainage at the site daily.
2. Change sterile gauze dressing over the heparin lock, tape in place with capped end exposed; gently wash around the insertion site while avoiding the tube when needed, cover the tube and area with plastic when bathing to protect from wetness.
3. Change catheter periodically according to policy or if problem develops.

Patency and use of heparin lock:

1. Prepare heparin and medication in separate syringes as outlined in IM and SC injections.
2. Flush catheter with a specified amount of heparin solution at prescribed frequency and following all medication administration.
3. Cleanse heparin lock hub or cap with antiseptic, insert needle of syringe with the medication into the hub or cap center and inject the contents slowly over 3 to 4 minutes.
4. Remove the needle from the heparin lock and inject the prepared heparin into the hub or cap to ensure patency of the device, withdraw the needle and cover the catheter end for protection from trauma and dislodgement.

RIGHT ATRIAL CATHETER (RAC) INTRAVENOUS MEDICATIONS

An indwelling catheter is inserted through an incision in the right upper chest and directed through a subcutaneous tunnel into a deep vessel near the heart and maintained for long-term continuous or frequent intermittent IV administration of fluids, nutrients, and medications. Growth of tissue to the cuff around the portion in the subcutaneous tissue provides anchoring of the catheter in place. Catheters commonly used include the Hickman, Broviac and Groshong.

Site assessment and protection:

1. Note redness, edema, pain, and drainage at the site through a transparent dressing daily or during dressing changes; assess for temperature elevation.

2. Cover the site with plastic when bathing to protect from wetness.
3. Cover site with a shirt or clothing; avoid handling the tube end.
4. Report any signs of infection, damage, or occlusion to the catheter and clamp if a Hickman, Broviac is in place.

Patency and care of RAC:

1. Prepare syringe with a specified amount of heparin solution (Broviac), 5 ml saline (Groshong) as outlined in IM and SC injections to flush catheter (prescribed frequency is daily and following all medication administrations for Broviac, weekly and following all medication administrations for Groshong).
2. Use gloves and sterile technique for care of an RAC.
3. Cleanse injection cap of catheter with antiseptic, insert needle of syringe with the flushing solution into the cap center, and inject the contents slowly.
4. Remove the needle from the cap (Groshong) and while the injection of the last 0.2 ml of the prepared heparin is injected (Broviac) to ensure patency of the device.
5. To replace an injection cap (frequency determined by policy), clamp the tube in the area between the end of the tube and the skin (Broviac), on the area prepared for clamping found on some catheters, or not at all on the Groshong, cleanse around the tip below the cap with an antiseptic swab, remove the old cap, attach the new cap, and remove the clamp if used.
6. To change a transparent dressing (frequency determined by policy or if soiled or insecure), gently peel off dressing, assess skin and site, cleanse around insertion site with a circular motion from center outward using hydrogen peroxide swabs, and then again using antiseptic, allow to air dry; loop the tube at the insertion site with the cap below the area to be covered by the dressing, place the window frame type of dressing on the skin, gently pressing from top to bottom while eliminating any air bubbles, secure cap area in place with tape for easy access but covered with clothing.
7. To change a gauze dressing, follow same procedure as for a transparent dressing through cleansing of the site, apply antiseptic ointment around the insertion site, position gauze dressing over the site, loop catheter over the gauze and

cover with another gauze dressing, secure the edges with tape and leave the cap area exposed for easy access but covered with clothing.

Medication preparation and administration:

1. Prepare medication in syringe as outlined in IM and SC injections.
2. Cleanse cap with antiseptic, insert needle of syringe with the medication into the cap center, and inject the contents slowly over 3 to 4 minutes.
3. Remove the needle of the empty syringe from the cap and insert the needle of the prepared heparin or saline into cap and inject to ensure patency of the catheter, withdraw the needle and cover the catheter end with clothing for protection from trauma and dislodgement.

*Nursing Diagnoses (NANDA)**

Activity intolerance
Activity intolerance, risk for
Adaptive capacity, decreased: intracranial
Adjustment, impaired
Airway clearance, ineffective
Anxiety
Aspiration, risk for
Body image disturbance
Body temperature, altered, risk for
Bowel incontinence
Breastfeeding, effective
Breastfeeding, ineffective
Breastfeeding, interrupted

*Derived from revised Eleventh Conference of Official Nursing Diagnoses presented by the North American Nursing Diagnosis Association (NANDA), 1994.

Breathing pattern, ineffective
Cardiac output, decreased
Caregiver role strain
Caregiver role strain, risk for
Communication, impaired verbal
Community coping, potential for enhanced
Community coping, ineffective
Confusion, acute
Confusion, chronic
Constipation
Constipation, colonic
Constipation, perceived
Coping, defensive
Coping, family: potential for growth
Coping, ineffective family: compromised
Coping, ineffective family: disabling
Coping, ineffective individual
Decisional conflict (specify)
Denial, ineffective
Diarrhea
Disuse syndrome, risk for
Diversional activity deficit
Dysreflexia
Energy field disturbance
Environmental interpretation syndrome: impaired
Family processes, altered
Family processes, altered: alcoholism
Fatigue
Fear
Fluid volume deficit
Fluid volume deficit, risk for
Fluid volume excess
Gas exchange, impaired
Grieving, anticipatory
Grieving, dysfunctional
Growth and development, altered
Health maintenance, altered
Health-seeking behaviors (specify)
Home maintenance management, impaired
Hopelessness
Hyperthermia

Hypothermia
Incontinence, functional
Incontinence, reflex
Incontinence, stress
Incontinence, total
Incontinence, urge
Infant behavior, disorganized
Infant behavior, disorganized: risk for
Infant behavior, organized: potential for enhanced
Infant feeding pattern, ineffective
Infection, risk for
Injury, perioperative positioning, risk for
Injury, risk for
Knowledge deficit (specify)
Loneliness, risk for
Management of therapeutic regimen, community: ineffective
Management of therapeutic regimen, families: ineffective
Management of therapeutic regimen, individuals: effective
Management of therapeutic regimen, individuals: ineffective
Memory, impaired
Mobility, impaired physical
Noncompliance (specify)
Nutrition, altered: less than body requirements
Nutrition, altered: more than body requirements
Nutrition, altered: risk for more than body requirements
Oral mucous membrane, altered
Pain
Pain, chronic
Parent/infant/child attachment altered, risk for
Parental role conflict
Parenting, altered
Parenting, altered, risk for
Peripheral neurovascular dysfunction, risk for
Personal identity disturbance
Poisoning, risk for
Post-trauma response
Powerlessness
Protection, altered
Rape-trauma syndrome
Rape-trauma syndrome: compound reaction
Rape-trauma syndrome: silent reaction

Relocation stress syndrome
Role performance, altered
Self-care deficit, bathing/hygiene
Self-care deficit, dressing/grooming
Self-care deficit, feeding
Self-care deficit, toileting
Self-esteem disturbance
Self-esteem, chronic low
Self-esteem, situational low
Self-mutilation, risk for
Sensory/perceptual alterations (specify) (visual, auditory, kinesthetic, gustatory, tactile, olfactory)
Sexual dysfunction
Sexuality patterns, altered
Skin integrity, impaired
Skin integrity, impaired, risk for
Sleep pattern disturbance
Social interaction, impaired
Social isolation
Spiritual distress (distress of the human spirit)
Spiritual well-being, potential for enhanced
Suffocation, risk for
Swallowing, impaired
Thermoregulation, ineffective
Thought processes, altered
Tissue integrity, impaired
Tissue perfusion, altered (specify type) (renal, cerebral, cardiopulmonary, gastrointestinal, peripheral)
Trauma, risk for
Unilateral neglect
Urinary elimination, altered
Urinary retention
Ventilation, inability to sustain spontaneous
Ventilatory weaning process, dysfunctional
Violence, risk for: self-directed or directed at others

Resources for Home Care and Selected National Agencies

American Federation of Home Health Agencies
1320 Fenwick Lane, Suite 500
Silver Springs, MD 20910

American Hospital Association
Division of Ambulatory and Home Care Services
840 North Lake Shore Drive
Chicago, IL 60611

Council of Community Health Services
National League for Nursing
10 Columbus Circle
New York, NY 10019

National Association of Home Care
519 C Street, NE
Washington, DC 20002

Administration on Aging
Department of Health and Human Services
330 Independence Avenue, SW
Washington, DC 20201

National Council on the Aging
600 Maryland Avenue, SW
West Wing 100
Washington, DC 20024

American Geriatrics Society
770 Lexington Avenue, Suite 400
New York, NY 10021

American Heart Association
7320 Greenville Avenue
Dallas, TX 75231

American Lung Association
1740 Broadway
New York, NY 10019

American Cancer Society
777 Third Avenue
New York, NY 10017

American Diabetic Association
149 Madison Avenue
New York, NY 10016

United Ostomy Association
2001 West Beverly Boulevard
Los Angeles, CA 90057

Arthritis Foundation
3400 Peachtree Road, Suite 1101
Atlanta, GA 30326

American Parkinson's Disease Association
116 John Street
New York, NY 10038

National Multiple Sclerosis Society
733 Third Avenue
New York, NY 10017

Asthma and Allergy Foundation of America
1125 15 Street, NW, Suite 502
Washington, DC 20005

Mental Health Association
1800 North Kent Street
Arlington, VA 22209

Alcoholics Anonymous
15 East 26 Street, Room 1817
New York, NY 10010

Association for Alzheimer's Disease and Related Disorders
919 North Michigan Avenue, Suite 1000
Chicago, IL 60611

National Hospice Organization
North Monroe Street, Suite 901
Arlington, VA 22209

American Council of the Blind
1156 15 Street, NW, Suite 720
Washington, DC 20005

National Association for the Deaf
814 Thayer Avenue
Silver Spring, MD 20910

American Association of Retired Persons
1909 K Street, NW
Washington, DC 20049

National Kidney Foundation
1 Park Avenue
New York, NY 10016

Veterans Administration
810 Vermont Avenue, NW
Washington, DC 20420

Medic-Alert
PO Box 1009
Turlock, CA 95381

United Way
Regional or local offices

American Red Cross
Local offices

Durable medical equipment and supplies
Local listings (yellow pages)

Self-Determination Guidelines (Advance Directives)*

The Patient Self-Determination Act requires Medicare- and Medicaid-certified hospitals, long-term facilities, hospice care, home care agencies, health maintenance organizations, and other health care providers and organizations to give clients information about their right to make their own health care decisions, including the right to accept or refuse medical treatment. It also includes the provision for providers to educate their staffs on issues related to advance directives. The advance directive is a written statement completed in advance of a serious illness about how one wants medical decisions made. The act was incorporated into the Omnibus Budget Reconciliation Act of 1990 (OBRA 1990) and took effect on December 1, 1991. This does not preclude the need for advance directives for those receiving care from any agency or institution not certified by Medicare and Medicaid.

PROVISIONS OF THE LAW

1. Provide all adult individuals with written information about their rights under state law to make health decisions, including the right to execute advance directives. State laws are developed, and the federal law does not override any law that would allow a health provider to object on the basis of conscience to implementing an advance directive.
2. Inform patients, residents, and clients about the facility or agency policy on implementing advance directives. Written information must be provided at the time of admission to an inpatient entering a hospital, a resident of a nursing facility, an outpatient of a home health provider, an enrollee of a prepaid health plan, and a recipient of hospice care.
3. Document in the medical record whether or not an advance directive has been executed.

*Modified from Health Care Financing Administration Fact Sheet, Department of Health and Human Services, November 1991.

4. Do not discriminate against an individual on the basis of the existence of an advance directive.
5. Provide staff and community education on advance directives.

DEFINITION OF ADVANCE DIRECTIVE

It is a written statement completed in advance of a serious illness, or in the presence of a chronic illness, about how one wants medical decisions made. It allows one to state choices for health care or to name someone to make those choices if unable to make decisions about medical treatment now or in the future. It allows one to control medical treatment decisions and to say ''yes'' to treatment wanted or ''no'' to treatment not wanted.

TYPES OF ADVANCE DIRECTIVES

1. Living Will: A written form approved by a state that specifies the kind of medical care wanted or not wanted if the client becomes unable to make the decisions. A living will can be initiated by using a form developed by the state, completing and signing a preprinted form available in the community, developing one's own form, or writing a statement of treatment preference. Advice can be solicited from an attorney or physician to ensure that one's wishes are understood and followed.
2. Durable Power of Attorney for Health Care: A signed, dated, and witnessed paper naming another person, such as a spouse, daughter, son, or close friend, as the client's agent or proxy to make medical decisions if a client should become unable to make them. It may include instructions about any treatment the client wishes to avoid. Some states have specific laws allowing for health care power of attorney and provide printed forms.

APPLICATION TO HEALTH CARE IN THE HOME

Probably the most important directive applicable to the client at home with a serious chronic illness is the decision to call 911 emergency services in cases of heart or respiratory arrest and if CPR should be administered. Unless a directive is available to the respondents, CPR would be administered regardless of the consequences of such an action. The client would be well advised to clearly indicate his or her directive in this regard.

Other home care should be provided totally or in part according to the client's directive if possible, or care can be provided by a hospice or a long-term care facility.

GENERAL REMARKS

Some state laws make it better to have one or the other type of directive, and it may be possible to have both or to combine the two types (in a document that describes treatment choices in specific situations and names someone to make decisions for the client when necessary). Either of these can be changed or canceled at any time. Some states allow a change by oral statement.

An advance directive should be signed and dated, with copies given to the physician and others as needed. A copy should be given to the client's attorney if a durable power of attorney exists, a copy given to the physician to become a part of the permanent record, a copy given to an agent or proxy, and a copy placed in a safe place with easy access if needed. A card should be placed in the client's purse or wallet that states the existence of an advance directive, where it is located, and the name of the agent or proxy if appropriate.

Universal Precautions and Guidelines for Control of Body Substances

Universal precautions is a method to prevent or minimize exposure to blood and potentially infectious materials. Blood of infected individuals can contain pathogenic microorganisms (human immunodeficiency virus, hepatitis B virus) called bloodborne pathogens that can be transmitted to others by the blood and other body fluids. Body fluids include feces, urine, sweat, saliva, tears, sputum, nasal secretions, wound drainage, and vomitus that contain blood; semen and vaginal secretions; and chest, joint, spinal, and abdominal fluids. The standards require that every health worker or caregiver must take protective measures when in contact with any client, whether known or suspected to be infected. The goal is to practice controls that decrease the possibility of exposure by changing the way a task or procedure is performed. These include hand protection, personal protective clothing, handling of equipment and supplies, and other techniques to prevent transmission to a home health nurse or caregiver. The selection of protective safeguards to use or teach to the caregiver depends on specific situations. The following guidelines are outlined for home implementation.

HAND PROTECTION

Wash hands with soap and water, rinse, and dry before and after client contact for care or treatments, wash hands even if gloves are worn, and wash bare hands immediately following exposure to blood or body secretions or excretions (count to 10 for thorough wash).

Wear gloves if possibility of touching blood, body fluids, secretions, or excretions on any item or article or specimen exposed to these fluids exists.

Change gloves if soiled or torn prior to client contact.

Wear gloves if rash, cuts, or open areas are present on hands, or avoid any contact with body fluids or contaminants.

Wear gloves if collecting blood, urine, feces, or other specimens for dipstick or laboratory examination.

Wear gloves to administer parenteral medications or fluids; take precautions to prevent accidental sticks to hands.

PROTECTIVE WEAR

Wear disposable plastic apron or gown during direct or close contact if soiling of clothing is likely or if spattering of body fluids is possible.

Anticipate splashing of blood or body fluids and protect face with shield or goggles.

EQUIPMENT AND SUPPLIES

Gloves should not be washed, disinfected, and reused. Discard used gloves, dressings, cleansing articles, and other disposable supplies in a waterproof, leakproof bag for proper disposal.

Dispose of used lancets, syringes with needle attached and not recapped, cut, or bent, and other sharp articles in a hard container (coffee can with lid) and label for future disposal of hazardous material.

Dispose of catheters and bags, IV tubing and bags, and medication vials in labeled biohazard container for disposal.

Dispose of suction canister fluid by tightly closing and discarding without emptying contents in a biohazard container

Wash soiled linens, clothing, bathing articles, dishes, and eating utensils in hot water and detergent, rinse, and dry well for reuse.

Label specimen of blood or body fluids for special precautions, place in a bag, and label again before transport to laboratory.

DISINFECTION

Wash article in warm, soapy water, rinse inside and outside with hot running water to prepare for further disinfection:

Moist heat: boil in water in a covered container for 10 minutes after water has boiled for 1 hour.

Dry heat: place cloth-wrapped article on a flat pan and bake in an oven at 350 degrees for 1 hour.

Prepare commercial solution according to instructions and submerge article for 10 minutes, rinse well, and air dry on paper towel.

Spilled liquids: Cleanse liquids such as vomitus, blood, or others containing blood by putting on gloves, wiping with paper towels, preparing and pouring a solution of bleach and water (1 : 10) onto the area, wiping clean with paper towels, and finally placing used towels in a waterproof, leakproof bag with gloves and other used articles for disposal.

Bibliography

American Heart Association Scientific Publishing: *Basic life support for the adult victim,* Dallas, 1993, The Association.

Burrell LO: *Adult nursing in hospital and community settings,* East Norwalk, Conn, 1992, Appleton & Lange.

Collopy B, Dubler N, Zuckerman C: *The ethics of home care: autonomy and accommodation,* 1990, The Hastings Center.

Dee-Kelly PA, Heller S, Sibley M: Managed care: an opportunity for home care agencies, *Nurs Clin North Am* 29(3), 1994.

Department of Health and Human Services: *Health care financing administration fact sheets,* 1991, The Department.

Dombi W: Home care coverage through HMOs, *Caring.* 12(6), 1993.

Eliopoulos C: *Manual of gerontologic nursing,* St. Louis, 1995, Mosby.

Ferri RS: *Care planning for the older adult,* Philadelphia, 1994, WB Saunders.

Gingerich BS, Ondeck DA: *Clinical pathways for the multidisciplinary home care team,* Gaithersburg, Md, 1995, Aspen.

Giuliano K, Poirier C: Nursing case management: critical pathways to desirable patient outcomes, *Nurs Management,* 22(3): 52-55, 1991.

Gorski L. *High-tech home care manual,* Gaithersburg, Md, 1994, Aspen.

Haddad AM, Kapp MB: *Ethical and legal issues in home health care,* East Norwalk, Conn, 1990, Appleton & Lange.

Henry JB: *Clinical diagnosis and management by laboratory methods,* ed 18, Philadelphia, 1991, WB Saunders.

Humphrey CJ, Milone-Nuzzo P: *Home care nursing: an orientation to practice,* East Norwalk, Conn, 1991, Appleton & Lange.

Ignatavicius DD, Hausman KA: *Clinical pathways for collaborative practice,* Philadelphia, 1995, WB Saunders.

Marrelli TM: *Handbook of home health standards and documentation guidelines for reinbursement,* ed 2, St. Louis, 1994, Mosby.

Mosher C and others: Critical pathways, *Am J Nurs* 92(1):41-44, 1992.

North American Nursing Diagnosis Association: *Official nursing diagnoses: proceedings of the eleventh conference,* St. Louis, 1994, Mosby.

Pokalo C: Understanding of the patient self-determination act, *J Gerontol Nurs* 18(3):47, 1992.

Rogers-Seidl FF, editor: *Geriatric nursing care plans,* St. Louis, 1991, Mosby.

Scherman SL: *Community health nursing care plans: a guide for home health care professionals,* ed 2, Albany, NY, 1990, Delmar.

Woodyard LW Sheetz JE: Critical pathway patient outcomes: the missing standard, *J Nurs Care Qual,* 8(1):51-57, 1993.

Index

B

D

L

M

O

P

T

U